Post-stroke Rehabilitation

Post-stroke Rehabilitation

Noureddin Nakhostin Ansari
Gholamreza Hassanzadeh
Ardalan Shariat

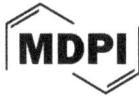

Basel • Beijing • Wuhan • Barcelona • Belgrade • Novi Sad • Cluj • Manchester

Noureddin Nakhostin Ansari
Department of Physiotherapy
Tehran University of
Medical Sciences
Tehran
Iran

Gholamreza Hassanzadeh
Department of Neuroscience
and Addiction Studies
School of Advanced
Technologies in Medicine
Tehran University of
Medical Sciences
Tehran
Iran

Ardalan Shariat
Department of Digital Health
Tehran University of
Medical Sciences
Tehran
Iran

Editorial Office
MDPI AG
Grosspeteranlage 5
4052 Basel, Switzerland

This is a reprint of articles from the Special Issue published online in the open access journal *Brain Sciences* (ISSN 2076-3425) (available at: www.mdpi.com/journal/brainsci/special_issues/89PRO96M4R).

For citation purposes, cite each article independently as indicated on the article page online and using the guide below:

Lastname, A.A.; Lastname, B.B. Article Title. *Journal Name* **Year**, *Volume Number*, Page Range.

ISBN 978-3-7258-2054-2 (Hbk)
ISBN 978-3-7258-2053-5 (PDF)
https://doi.org/10.3390/books978-3-7258-2053-5

© 2024 by the authors. Articles in this book are Open Access and distributed under the Creative Commons Attribution (CC BY) license. The book as a whole is distributed by MDPI under the terms and conditions of the Creative Commons Attribution-NonCommercial-NoDerivs (CC BY-NC-ND) license (https://creativecommons.org/licenses/by-nc-nd/4.0/).

Contents

About the Editors vii

Noureddin Nakhostin Ansari, Gholamreza Hassanzadeh and Ardalan Shariat
From Editorial Board of Special Issue Entitled "Post-Stroke Rehabilitation"
Reprinted from: *Brain Sci.* **2024**, *14*, 824, doi:10.3390/brainsci14080824 1

Noureddin Nakhostin Ansari, Fatemeh Bahramnezhad, Albert T. Anastasio, Gholamreza Hassanzadeh and Ardalan Shariat
Telestroke: A Novel Approach for Post-Stroke Rehabilitation
Reprinted from: *Brain Sci.* **2023**, *13*, 1186, doi:10.3390/brainsci13081186 4

Licong Chen, Lulu Zhang, Yidan Li, Quanquan Zhang, Qi Fang and Xiang Tang
Association of the Neutrophil-to-Lymphocyte Ratio with 90-Day Functional Outcomes in Patients with Acute Ischemic Stroke
Reprinted from: *Brain Sci.* **2024**, *14*, 250, doi:10.3390/brainsci14030250 7

Somaye Azarnia, Kamran Ezzati, Alia Saberi, Soofia Naghdi, Iraj Abdollahi and Shapour Jaberzadeh
The Effect of Uni-Hemispheric Dual-Site Anodal tDCS on Brain Metabolic Changes in Stroke Patients: A Randomized Clinical Trial
Reprinted from: *Brain Sci.* **2023**, *13*, 1100, doi:10.3390/brainsci13071100 18

Alex Martino Cinnera, Serena Marrano, Daniela De Bartolo, Marco Iosa, Alessio Bisirri and Enza Leone et al.
Convergent Validity of the Timed Walking Tests with Functional Ambulatory Category in Subacute Stroke
Reprinted from: *Brain Sci.* **2023**, *13*, 1089, doi:10.3390/brainsci13071089 28

Matthew J. Chilvers, Deepthi Rajashekar, Trevor A. Low, Stephen H. Scott and Sean P. Dukelow
Clinical, Neuroimaging and Robotic Measures Predict Long-Term Proprioceptive Impairments following Stroke
Reprinted from: *Brain Sci.* **2023**, *13*, 953, doi:10.3390/brainsci13060953 39

Victoria Tilton-Bolowsky, Melissa D. Stockbridge and Argye E. Hillis
Remapping and Reconnecting the Language Network after Stroke
Reprinted from: *Brain Sci.* **2024**, *14*, 419, doi:10.3390/brainsci14050419 56

Hao Meng, Michael Houston, Yingchun Zhang and Sheng Li
Exploring the Prospects of Transcranial Electrical Stimulation (tES) as a Therapeutic Intervention for Post-Stroke Motor Recovery: A Narrative Review
Reprinted from: *Brain Sci.* **2024**, *14*, 322, doi:10.3390/brainsci14040322 69

Ardalan Shariat, Mahboubeh Ghayour Najafabadi, Noureddin Nakhostin Ansari, Albert T. Anastasio, Kian Bagheri and Gholamreza Hassanzadeh et al.
Outcome Measures Utilized to Assess the Efficacy of Telerehabilitation for Post-Stroke Rehabilitation: A Scoping Review
Reprinted from: *Brain Sci.* **2023**, *13*, 1725, doi:10.3390/brainsci13121725 86

Ming-Jian Ko, Ya-Chi Chuang, Liang-Jun Ou-Yang, Yuan-Yang Cheng, Yu-Lin Tsai and Yu-Chun Lee
The Application of Soft Robotic Gloves in Stroke Patients: A Systematic Review and Meta-Analysis of Randomized Controlled Trials
Reprinted from: *Brain Sci.* **2023**, *13*, 900, doi:10.3390/brainsci13060900 103

Juan Carlos Chacon-Barba, Jose A. Moral-Munoz, Amaranta De Miguel-Rubio and David Lucena-Anton
Effects of Resistance Training on Spasticity in People with Stroke: A Systematic Review
Reprinted from: *Brain Sci.* **2024**, *14*, 57, doi:10.3390/brainsci14010057 117

Mansoureh Sadat Dadbakhsh, Afarin Haghparast, Noureddin Nakhostin Ansari, Amin Nakhostin-Ansari and Soofia Naghdi
Translation, Adaptation, and Determining the Intra-Rater Reliability of the Balance Evaluation Systems Test (BESTest) for Persian Patients with Chronic Stroke
Reprinted from: *Brain Sci.* **2023**, *13*, 1674, doi:10.3390/brainsci13121674 131

About the Editors

Noureddin Nakhostin Ansari

Dr. Nakhosin Ansari is interested in research investigating the effects of physiotherapy and electrophysical interventions in stroke. Over the past few years, he has examined the effects of dry needling in improving muscle spasticity in stroke and is keen to expand the application of dry needling in multiple sclerosis. His research is currently focused on the biomechanical and electrophysiological effects of dry needling on muscle flexibility. His other main area of research interest is the reliability and validity of clinical spasticity instruments. His other research interests include the adaptation and validation of tests/questionnaires.

Gholamreza Hassanzadeh

Dr. Hassanzadeh is a Professor of Anatomy at Tehran University of Medical Sciences. He teaches neuroanatomy and currently serves as the Head of the Department of Neuroscience and Addiction Studies and the Department of Digital Health at Tehran University of Medical Sciences. Additionally, he holds the position of Secretary of the Anatomy Board in the Ministry of Health and Medical Education. Dr. Hassanzadeh is also the Head of the Iranian Association of Medical Sciences Education. His research primarily focuses on neuroinflammation and neurodegenerative disorders.

Ardalan Shariat

Dr. Shariat is an Assistant Professor in the Department of Digital Health, and his research focus is on different aspects of telehealth for the prevention and treatment of patients, as well as healthy individuals, using non-pharmacological methods. His other main area of research interest includes the prevention and treatment of musculoskeletal issues among patients and healthy individuals with a focus on exercise.

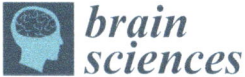

Editorial

From Editorial Board of Special Issue Entitled "Post-Stroke Rehabilitation"

Noureddin Nakhostin Ansari [1,2], Gholamreza Hassanzadeh [3,4,5] and Ardalan Shariat [3,*]

1. Department of Physiotherapy, School of Rehabilitation, Tehran University of Medical Sciences, Tehran P.O. Box 14155-6559, Iran; nakhostin@sina.tums.ac.ir
2. Research Center for War-Affected People, Tehran University of Medical Sciences, Tehran P.O. Box 14155-6559, Iran
3. Department of Digital Health, School of Medicine, Tehran University of Medical Sciences, Tehran P.O. Box 14618-84513, Iran; hassanzadeh@tums.ac.ir
4. Department of Anatomy, School of Medicine, Tehran University of Medical Sciences, Tehran P.O. Box 14176-13151, Iran
5. Department of Neuroscience and Addiction Studies, School of Advanced Technologies in Medicine, Tehran University of Medical Sciences, Tehran P.O. Box 55469-14177, Iran
* Correspondence: ardalansh2002@gmail.com

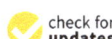

Citation: Nakhostin Ansari, N.; Hassanzadeh, G.; Shariat, A. From Editorial Board of Special Issue Entitled "Post-Stroke Rehabilitation". *Brain Sci.* **2024**, *14*, 824. https://doi.org/10.3390/brainsci14080824

Received: 19 July 2024
Accepted: 11 August 2024
Published: 16 August 2024

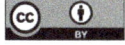

Copyright: © 2024 by the authors. Licensee MDPI, Basel, Switzerland. This article is an open access article distributed under the terms and conditions of the Creative Commons Attribution (CC BY) license (https://creativecommons.org/licenses/by/4.0/).

Diseases affecting the nervous system are diverse. A recent global burden of disease study found that nervous system diseases were the leading cause of disability-adjusted life-years (DALYs) in 2021 [1]. Among the ten conditions with the highest age-standardised DALYs in 2021, stroke was ranked first [1]. Furthermore, it is noteworthy that low- and middle-income countries bear the highest burden of stroke [2,3]. With increasing global DALYs, effective strategies for the prevention, medical treatment, and rehabilitation of nervous system diseases, particularly stroke, are imperative. It is subsequently crucial to swiftly identify and treat stroke patients, especially in remote or rural areas, to minimise subsequent complications. The time taken to intervene in cases of stroke is particularly critical in reducing the risk of long-term disability and mortality [4].

This Special Issue presents the latest achievements related to post-stroke rehabilitation though the publication of 11 papers, comprising several types of articles including original studies, reviews, and a brief report written by experts from Iran, the USA, China, Australia, Italy, Spain, Taiwan, the Netherlands, the UK, and Canada.

An editorial written by Nakhostin Ansari et al., entitled "Telestroke: a novel approach for post-stroke rehabilitation", highlights the importance of telemedicine in the current world of patient's rehabilitation post stroke (Contribution 1). In a retrospective cohort study entitled "Association of the neutrophil-to-lymphocyte ratio with 90-day functional outcomes in patients with acute ischemic stroke", Cheng et al. identify the potential factors associated with functional prognosis in acute ischemic stroke (Contribution 2).

In a paper by Azarnia et al., the authors designed a double-blind, randomised clinical trial with attention to the effectiveness of uni-hemispheric dual-site anodal tDCS on brain metabolic changes in stroke patients (Contribution 3). After this, Cinnera et al., in their paper entitled "Convergent validity of the timed walking tests with functional ambulatory category in subacute stroke", assess the convergent validity of three different walking tests for patients post stroke (Contribution 4). Then, Chilvers et al. published an interesting paper entitled "Clinical, neuroimaging and robotic measures predict long-term proprioceptive impairments following stroke" with a focus on robotic measures to predict proprioceptive impairments among patients post stroke (Contribution 5).

Authors from Johns Hopkins University, in their paper entitled "Remapping and reconnecting the language network after stroke", review the literature on neurotypical individuals and individuals with post-stroke aphasia (Contribution 6). Following this, a narrative review entitled "Exploring the prospects of transcranial electrical stimulation (tES) as a therapeutic intervention for post-stroke motor recovery: a narrative review", conducted by authors from the USA, explores the mechanisms underlying commonly employed tES techniques and evaluates their prospective advantages and challenges in applications in motor recovery after stroke (Contribution 7). Then, Shariat et al., in their scoping review paper entitled "Outcome measures utilized to assess the efficacy of telerehabilitation for post-stroke rehabilitation: a scoping review", determine the outcome measures used in TR studies and define which parts of the International Organization of Functioning are measured in trials (Contribution 8). Then, Ko et al., from Taiwan, present a systematic review and meta analyses entitled "The application of soft robotic gloves in stroke patients: a systematic review and meta-analysis of randomized controlled trials" and determine the effectiveness of soft robotic gloves (SRGs) in improving the motor recovery and functional abilities in patients with post-stroke hemiparesis (Contribution 9). Moreover, Chacon-Barba et al., from Spain, published their systematic review entitled "Effects of resistance training on spasticity in people with stroke: a systematic review" in which they analyse the effects of resistance training, compared with no treatment, conventional therapy, or other therapies, in people with stroke-related spasticity (Contribution 10).

Finally, Dadbakhsh et al. conclude this Special Issue with their brief review entitled "Translation, adaptation, and determining the intra-rater reliability of the balance evaluation systems test (BESTest) for Persian patients with chronic stroke" (Contribution 11).

Overall, this Special Issue highlights the need to focus on multiple variables related to the assessment and rehabilitation of post-stroke patients, utilising not only traditional methods, but also advanced technologies such as telehealth and robotics.

We believe that continuing research in this field is imperative for conducting more in-depth investigations, particularly concerning cost and feasibility, especially for those living in rural areas who lack access to specialists and hospitals in big cities. In this context, the development of novel protocols and approaches, such as telehealth, should be given significant consideration.

Author Contributions: Conceptualization, N.N.A., A.S. and G.H.; methodology, N.N.A., A.S. and G.H.; formal analysis, N.N.A., A.S. and G.H.; data curation, N.N.A., A.S. and G.H.; writing—original draft preparation, N.N.A., A.S. and G.H.; writing—review and editing, N.N.A., A.S. and G.H.; visualization, N.N.A.; supervision, A.S.; project administration, N.N.A. and A.S. and G.H. All authors have read and agreed to the published version of the manuscript.

Funding: This research received no external funding.

Conflicts of Interest: The authors declare no conflicts of interest.

List of Contributions:

1. Nakhostin Ansari, N.; Bahramnezhad, F.; Anastasio, A.T.; Hassanzadeh, G.; Shariat, A. Tele-stroke: A Novel Approach for Post-Stroke Rehabilitation. *Brain Sci.* **2023**, *13*, 1186.
2. Chen, L.; Zhang, L.; Li, Y.; Zhang, Q.; Fang, Q.; Tang, X. Association of the Neutrophil-to-Lymphocyte Ratio with 90-Day Functional Outcomes in Patients with Acute Ischemic Stroke. *Brain Sci.* **2024**, *14*, 250.
3. Azarnia, S.; Ezzati, K.; Saberi, A.; Naghdi, S.; Abdollahi, I.; Jaberzadeh, S. The Effect of Uni-Hemispheric Dual-Site Anodal tDCS on Brain Metabolic Changes in Stroke Patients: A Randomized Clinical Trial. *Brain Sci.* **2023**, *13*, 1100.
4. Cinnera, A.M.; Marrano, S.; De Bartolo, D.; Iosa, M.; Bisirri, A.; Leone, E.; Stefani, A.; Koch, G.; Ciancarelli, I.; Paolucci, S.; et al. Convergent validity of the timed walking tests with functional ambulatory category in subacute stroke. *Brain Sci.* **2023**, *13*, 1089.
5. Chilvers, M.J.; Rajashekar, D.; Low, T.A.; Scott, S.H.; Dukelow, S.P. Clinical, neuroimaging and robotic measures predict long-term proprioceptive impairments following stroke. *Brain Sci.* **2023**, *13*, 953.
6. Tilton-Bolowsky, V.; Stockbridge, M.D.; Hillis, A.E. Remapping and Reconnecting the Language Network after Stroke. *Brain Sci.* **2024**, *14*, 419.
7. Meng, H.; Houston, M.; Zhang, Y.; Li, S. Exploring the Prospects of Transcranial Electrical Stimulation (tES) as a Therapeutic Intervention for Post-Stroke Motor Recovery: A Narrative Review. *Brain Sci.* **2024**, *14*, 322.

8. Shariat, A.; Najafabadi, M.G.; Nakhostin Ansari, N.; Anastasio, A.T.; Bagheri, K.; Hassanzadeh, G.; Farghadan, M. Outcome Measures Utilized to Assess the Efficacy of Telerehabilitation for Post-Stroke Rehabilitation: A Scoping Review. *Brain Sci.* **2023**, *13*, 1725.
9. Ko, M.-J.; Chuang, Y.-C.; Ou-Yang, L.-J.; Cheng, Y.-Y.; Tsai, Y.-L.; Lee, Y.-C. The application of soft robotic gloves in stroke patients: A systematic review and meta-analysis of randomized controlled trials. *Brain Sci.* **2023**, *13*, 900.
10. Chacon-Barba, J.C.; Moral-Munoz, J.A.; De Miguel-Rubio, A.; Lucena-Anton, D. Effects of Resistance Training on Spasticity in People with Stroke: A Systematic Review. *Brain Sci.* **2024**, *14*, 57.
11. Dadbakhsh, M.S.; Haghparast, A.; Nakhostin Ansari, N.; Nakhostin-Ansari, A.; Naghdi, S. Translation, Adaptation, and Determining the Intra-Rater Reliability of the Balance Evaluation Systems Test (BESTest) for Persian Patients with Chronic Stroke. *Brain Sci.* **2023**, *13*, 1674.

References

1. Steinmetz, J.D.; Seeher, K.M.; Schiess, N.; Nichols, E.; Cao, B.; Servili, C.; Cavallera, V.; Cousin, E.; Hagins, H.; Moberg, M.E.; et al. Global, regional, and national burden of disorders affecting the nervous system, 1990–2021: A systematic analysis for the Global Burden of Disease Study 2021. *Lancet Neurol.* **2024**, *23*, 344–381. [CrossRef] [PubMed]
2. Tinker, R.J.; Smith, C.J.; Heal, C.; Bettencourt-Silva, J.H.; Metcalf, A.K.; Potter, J.F.; Myint, P.K. Predictors of mortality and disability in stroke-associated pneumonia. *Acta Neurol. Belg.* **2021**, *121*, 379–385. [CrossRef] [PubMed]
3. Phipps, M.S.; Cronin, C.A. Management of acute ischemic stroke. *BMJ* **2020**, *368*. [CrossRef] [PubMed]
4. Garcia-Esperon, C.; Chew, B.L.A.; Minett, F.; Cheah, J.; Rutherford, J.; Wilsmore, B.; Parsons, M.W.; Levi, C.R.; Spratt, N.J. Impact of an outpatient telestroke clinic on management of rural stroke patients. *Aust. J. Rural. Health* **2022**, *30*, 337–342. [CrossRef] [PubMed]

Disclaimer/Publisher's Note: The statements, opinions and data contained in all publications are solely those of the individual author(s) and contributor(s) and not of MDPI and/or the editor(s). MDPI and/or the editor(s) disclaim responsibility for any injury to people or property resulting from any ideas, methods, instructions or products referred to in the content.

Editorial

Telestroke: A Novel Approach for Post-Stroke Rehabilitation

Noureddin Nakhostin Ansari [1,2], Fatemeh Bahramnezhad [3], Albert T. Anastasio [4], Gholamreza Hassanzadeh [5,6,7] and Ardalan Shariat [5,*]

[1] Department of Physiotherapy, School of Rehabilitation, Tehran University of Medical Sciences, Tehran P.O. Box 14155-6559, Iran; nakhostin@tums.ac.ir
[2] Research Center for War-Affected People, Tehran University of Medical Sciences, Tehran P.O. Box 14155-6559, Iran
[3] Department of Critical Care Nursing, School of Nursing and Midwifery, Tehran University of Medical Sciences, Tehran P.O. Box 14197-3317, Iran; bahramnezhad.f@gmail.com
[4] Department of Orthopaedic Surgery, Duke University, Durham, NC 27710, USA; albert.anastasio@duke.edu
[5] Department of Digital Health, School of Medicine, Tehran University of Medical Sciences, Tehran P.O. Box 14618-84513, Iran; hassanzadeh@tums.ac.ir
[6] Department of Anatomy, School of Medicine, Tehran University of Medical Sciences, Tehran P.O. Box 14176-13151, Iran
[7] Department of Neuroscience and Addiction Studies, School of Advanced Technologies in Medicine, Tehran University of Medical Sciences, Tehran P.O. Box 55469-14877, Iran
* Correspondence: a-shariat@sina.tums.ac.ir

Despite the tremendous technologic advancements of recent years, the prevalence of stroke has increased significantly worldwide from 1990 to 2019 (a 70.0% increase in stroke and a 43.0% increase in stroke deaths). Moreover, the highest global burden of stroke is borne by low- and middle-income countries [1,2]. Rapid identification and treatment of these patients, especially in remote or rural areas, is imperative to reduce subsequent complications. The time-to-intervention for stroke is of particular importance in reducing the risk of long-term disability and mortality [3].

Virtual communication related to the distribution and provision of healthcare (referred to as "telehealth") has become an essential component to providing equitable care and treatment services to individuals who may be unable to access care in person more readily. The telehealth concept encompasses virtual healthcare provision, communications and collaborations, research and development, education, disaster readiness, administration, and management [4]. The health resource services administration (HRSA) has defined telehealth as "the use of electronic information and telecommunications technologies to support long-distance clinical health care, patient and professional health-related education, public health and health administration" [5]. Across the literature, the terms "telemedicine" and "telehealth" are sometimes used interchangeably [6], despite a slight difference between the two terms. While telemedicine is a more limited term, referring only to remote clinical services, telehealth is a broad term which encompasses both virtual non-clinical services and clinical services [4]. As described by Khandpur et al., non-clinical aspects of telehealth can include the provision of remote training sessions, administrative meetings, and continuing health education [7].

The World Health Organization (WHO) has also commented on the emergence of "eHealth", referring to "cost-effective and secure use of information and communications technologies in support of health and health-related fields, including health-care services, health surveillance, health literature, and health education, knowledge and research". By this definition, eHealth can incorporate various forms of information and communication technology (ICT). Thus, applications and health promotion websites in addition to screening, assessment, and video-chat tools can all be considered forms of eHealth [8].

During the COVID-19 Pandemic, the use of telehealth became commonplace, as patients sought to avoid the risk of exposure to the viral vector. Telehealth was used to provide primary care [9] and psychiatric [10] services throughout the course of the Pandemic. Moreover, telehealth was used extensively for the prevention and treatment of various types of musculoskeletal discomforts [11]. Within the field of rehabilitation after neurological insult, the development of telestroke in 1996 has brought about a revolution in the treatment of patients with stroke. Telestroke allows physicians and advanced practice providers to begin examining and treating patients with stroke remotely utilizing various forms of technology (e.g., video conferencing, digital cameras, smartphones, tablets, and other technologies) well before reaching the hospital [12,13].

Further emphasis on education for suspectable populations, screening and monitoring for signs and symptoms of neurological change, and management advancements and insights can all continue to improve the care of patients with stroke. Improvements within the domain of telestroke can also revolutionize stroke care. Training efforts for high-risk individuals in the use of modern technologies can result in improved prevention and treatment of this disease [14]. Researchers and healthcare practitioners must consider all three levels of prevention: primary, secondary, and tertiary prevention to improve the efficiency of telestroke capabilities. Broadly speaking, primary prevention through the use of telestroke involves the careful provision of primary care through virtual platforms, including discussion regarding risk mitigation through the use of diet and exercise interventions [15] as well as pharmacotherapy targeting hypertension [16] and hypercholesterolemia [16]. Secondary prevention can also be achieved through the use of telecommunications for screening and identification of patients at risk for impending neurological insult. Patients can then follow up in the clinical setting for advanced imaging or invasive diagnostic tests. Finally, tertiary prevention once patients have been diagnosed with stroke can be at least in part administered through the use of telestroke, as patients require close follow up and rehabilitative consultations [17].

In addition to efforts geared towards the level of physicians and rehabilitative practitioners, telenursing can be effective in reducing the global burden of disease from stroke [18]. Today, the capabilities of different aspects of telehealth, such as telenursing and teleconsultation have expanded markedly [19]. Therefore, linking these entities with telestroke, especially in the discussion of primary prevention, can bring great utility in preventing the occurrence and complications of stroke, especially in developing and low-income countries.

To these aims, for this special series for *Brain Sciences* on post-stroke rehabilitation, we invite experts in the field of neurorehabilitation to submit their valuable papers including original articles and reviews. The main purpose of this issue is to highlight the novel efforts for patients who are post-stroke using new technologies. In addition, the series will include contributions using traditional methods as well. We look forward to fostering the ongoing discussion regarding the provision of stroke-related care via virtual means.

Author Contributions: Conceptualization, G.H. and A.S.; Writing—Original Draft Preparation, F.B. and N.N.A.; Writing—Review & Editing, A.T.A. and A.S.; Supervision, G.H. and N.N.A. All authors have read and agreed to the published version of the manuscript.

Conflicts of Interest: The authors declare no conflict of interest.

References

1. Tinker, R.J.; Smith, C.J.; Heal, C.; Bettencourt-Silva, J.H.; Metcalf, A.K.; Potter, J.F.; Myint, P.K. Predictors of mortality and disability in stroke-associated pneumonia. *Acta Neurol. Belg.* **2021**, *121*, 379–385. [PubMed]
2. Phipps, M.S.; Cronin, C.A. Management of acute ischemic stroke. *BMJ* **2020**, *368*, l6983. [PubMed]
3. Garcia-Esperon, C.; Chew, B.L.A.; Minett, F.; Cheah, J.; Rutherford, J.; Wilsmore, B.; Parsons, M.W.; Levi, C.R.; Spratt, N.J. Impact of an outpatient telestroke clinic on management of rural stroke patients. *Aust. J. Rural. Health* **2022**, *30*, 337–342. [CrossRef] [PubMed]
4. Bitar, H.; Alismail, S. The role of eHealth, telehealth, and telemedicine for chronic disease patients during COVID-19 pandemic: A rapid systematic review. *Digit. Health* **2021**, *7*, 20552076211009396. [PubMed]
5. Fong, B.; Fong, A.C.M.; Li, C.K. *Telemedicine Technologies: Information Technologies in Medicine and Telehealth*; John Wiley & Sons: Hoboken, NJ, USA, 2011.

6. Fatehi, F.; Wootton, R. Telemedicine, telehealth or e-health? A bibliometric analysis of the trends in the use of these terms. *J. Telemed. Telecare* **2012**, *18*, 460–464. [CrossRef] [PubMed]
7. Khandpur, R.S. *Telemedicine Technology and Applications (mHealth, TeleHealth and eHealth)*; PHI Learning Pvt. Ltd.: New Delhi, Delhi, 2017.
8. Stevens, W.J.M.; van der Sande, R.; Beijer, L.J.; Gerritsen, M.G.M.; Assendelft, W.J.J. eHealth apps replacing or complementing health care contacts: Scoping review on adverse effects. *J. Med. Internet Res.* **2019**, *21*, e10736. [PubMed]
9. Huang, J.; Graetz, I.; Millman, A.; Gopalan, A.; Lee, C.; Muelly, E.; Reed, M.E. Primary care telemedicine during the COVID-19 pandemic: Patient's choice of video versus telephone visit. *JAMIA Open* **2022**, *19*, ooac002.
10. Reay, R.E.; Looi, J.C.L.; Keightley, P. Telehealth mental health services during COVID-19: Summary of evidence and clinical practice. *Australas. Psychiatry* **2020**, *28*, 514–516. [PubMed]
11. Shariat, A.; Hajialiasgari, F.; Alizadeh, A.; Anastasio, A.T. The role of telehealth in the care of musculoskeletal pain conditions after COVID-19. *Work* **2023**, *74*, 1261–1264. [PubMed]
12. Simmons, C.A.; Poupore, N.; Nathaniel, T.I. Age Stratification and Stroke Severity in the Telestroke Network. *J. Clin. Med.* **2023**, *12*, 1519. [CrossRef] [PubMed]
13. Brown, C.; Terrell, K.; Goodwin, R.; Nathaniel, T. Stroke Severity in Ischemic Stroke Patients with a History of Diastolic Blood Pressure Treated in a Telestroke Network. *J. Cardiovasc. Dev. Dis.* **2022**, *9*, 345. [CrossRef] [PubMed]
14. Richard, J.V.; Mehrotra, A.; Schwamm, L.H.; Wilcock, A.D.; Uscher-Pines, L.; Majersik, J.J.; Zachrison, K.S. Improving Population Access to Stroke Expertise Via Telestroke: Hospitals to Target and the Potential Clinical Benefit. *J. Am. Heart Assoc.* **2022**, *11*, e025559. [PubMed]
15. Nguyen, L.T.K.; Do, B.N.; Vu, D.N.; Pham, K.M.; Vu, M.-T.; Nguyen, H.C.; Nguyen, Q.M.; Tran, C.Q. Physical activity and diet quality modify the association between comorbidity and disability among stroke patients. *Nutrients* **2021**, *13*, 1641. [CrossRef] [PubMed]
16. Johansson, B.B. Hypertension mechanisms causing stroke. *Clin. Exp. Pharmacol. Physiol.* **1999**, *26*, 563–565. [PubMed]
17. Rubin, M.N.; Wellik, K.E.; Channer, D.D.; Demaerschalk, B.M. Systematic review of telestroke for post-stroke care and rehabilitation. *Curr. Atheroscler. Rep.* **2013**, *15*, 343. [CrossRef] [PubMed]
18. Jagolino-Cole, A.L.; Zha, A.M.; Sangha, N.; Song, S.S.; Majersik, J.J. Careers in Telestroke: Toward a Virtual and Tangible Purpose. *Stroke* **2023**, *54*, e220–e223. [PubMed]
19. Alizadeh, R.; Anastasio, A.T.; Shariat, A.; Bethell, M.; Hassanzadeh, G. Teleexercise for geriatric patients with failed back surgery syndrome. *Front. Public. Health* **2023**, *11*, 1140506. [CrossRef] [PubMed]

Disclaimer/Publisher's Note: The statements, opinions and data contained in all publications are solely those of the individual author(s) and contributor(s) and not of MDPI and/or the editor(s). MDPI and/or the editor(s) disclaim responsibility for any injury to people or property resulting from any ideas, methods, instructions or products referred to in the content.

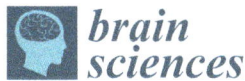

Article

Association of the Neutrophil-to-Lymphocyte Ratio with 90-Day Functional Outcomes in Patients with Acute Ischemic Stroke

Licong Chen [1,†], Lulu Zhang [1,†], Yidan Li [1], Quanquan Zhang [1], Qi Fang [1,2,*] and Xiang Tang [1,*]

1. Department of Neurology, The First Affiliated Hospital of Soochow University, Suzhou 215000, China; 20215232103@stu.suda.edu.cn (L.C.); zll@suda.edu.cn (L.Z.); 20215232104@stu.suda.edu.cn (Y.L.); zhangquanquan@suda.edu.cn (Q.Z.)
2. Department of Neurology, Dushu Lake Hospital Affiliated to Soochow University, Suzhou 215000, China
* Correspondence: fangqi_008@126.com (Q.F.); tangxiang163yx@163.com (X.T.); Tel.: +86-13606213892 (Q.F.); +86-15950553968 (X.T.)
† These authors contributed equally to this work.

Abstract: The neutrophil-to-lymphocyte ratio (NLR), an inflammatory marker, plays an important role in the inflammatory mechanisms of the pathophysiology and progression of acute ischemic stroke (AIS). The aim of this study was to identify the potential factors associated with functional prognosis in AIS. A total of 303 AIS patients were enrolled in this study; baseline information of each participant, including demographic characteristics, medical history, laboratory data, and 90-day functional outcome, was collected. Multivariate logistic regression analysis revealed that NLR, systolic blood pressure (SBP) and National Institutes of Health Stroke Scale (NIHSS) score were found to be independent factors for poor functional outcomes. Receiver operating characteristic (ROC) curve analysis was performed to estimate the predictive value of the NLR for 90-day functional outcome, with the best predictive cutoff value being 3.06. In the multivariate logistic regression analysis, three models were constructed: Model 1, adjusted for age, sex, SBP, and TOAST classification (AUC = 0.694); Model 2, further adjusted for the NIHSS score at admission (AUC = 0.826); and Model 3, additionally adjusted for the NLR (AUC = 0.829). The NLR at admission was an independent predictor of 90-day prognosis in patients with AIS. The risk factors related to poor 90-day functional outcomes were higher SBP, higher NLR, and a greater NIHSS score.

Keywords: acute ischemic stroke; inflammation; neutrophil-to-lymphocyte ratio; 90-day functional outcome

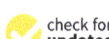

Citation: Chen, L.; Zhang, L.; Li, Y.; Zhang, Q.; Fang, Q.; Tang, X. Association of the Neutrophil-to-Lymphocyte Ratio with 90-Day Functional Outcomes in Patients with Acute Ischemic Stroke. *Brain Sci.* **2024**, *14*, 250. https://doi.org/10.3390/brainsci14030250

Academic Editors: Rocco Salvatore Calabrò, Ardalan Shariat, Noureddin Nakhostin Ansari and Gholamreza Hassanzadeh

Received: 1 February 2024
Revised: 18 February 2024
Accepted: 21 February 2024
Published: 4 March 2024

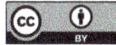

Copyright: © 2024 by the authors. Licensee MDPI, Basel, Switzerland. This article is an open access article distributed under the terms and conditions of the Creative Commons Attribution (CC BY) license (https://creativecommons.org/licenses/by/4.0/).

1. Introduction

Globally, stroke is the second leading cause of death and the third leading cause of death and disability [1]. Timely prediction and intervention can effectively reduce the disability rate among patients. The pathogenesis of acute ischemic stroke (AIS) involves multiple factors, including in situ thrombotic occlusion, artery-to-artery embolism, local branch occlusion, the inflammatory response, ischemia–reperfusion injury, and other contributing mechanisms [2]. Studies have shown that immune responses play an important role in the pathophysiology and progression of AIS, particularly with regard to brain injury and tissue repair [3–5]. In fact, inflammation and immune mechanisms can be involved throughout all stages of the disease [6].

In recent studies, novel inflammatory markers, including the neutrophil-to-lymphocyte ratio (NLR), C-reactive protein (CRP), the CRP-to-lymphocyte ratio (CLR), the platelet-to-lymphocyte ratio (PLR), and the systemic immune-inflammation index (SII), have been acknowledged as surrogate markers of systemic inflammation, and they have been valuable indicators for the diagnosis and prognosis of diverse infectious diseases, including cancer [7–9], heart disease [10,11], acute respiratory distress syndrome (ARDS) [12], and

COVID 2019 [13]. According to recent studies, these markers can also predict the complications of stroke. The NLR is significantly associated with the clinical prognosis of stroke patients, including both patient outcomes following endovascular therapy (EVT) [14] and the risk of hemorrhagic transformation (HT) [15]. In addition, increased systemic inflammation is associated with the risk of progressive stroke [16,17] and the severity of cerebral edema early after reperfusion therapy in stroke patients [18].

The aim of this study was to identify potential factors associated with 90-day functional outcomes and explore the relationships between these factors and functional prognosis in AIS. This study focused on common clinical inflammatory markers, including NLR, CLR, SII, CRP, FIB, PLR, HCY, and WBC and ultimately validated the utility of the NLR as a reliable prognostic indicator for AIS patients. Furthermore, our study integrated clinical factors, biomarkers, and imaging to construct a highly accurate prediction model, emphasizing that prompt and effective clinical intervention can significantly improve patient outcomes.

2. Materials and Methods

2.1. Study Design and Participants

This was a single-center retrospective cohort study of all consecutive AIS patients admitted to our stroke unit between July 2021 and October 2022. The inclusion criteria were established based on the confirmation of AIS diagnosis through diffusion-weighted imaging (DWI). The exclusion criteria were as follows: (1) had fever or an infectious disease on admission or a history of immune system disease, (2) lacked complete imaging, laboratory, or follow-up data, (3) had a life expectancy of less than 3 months or were unable to complete the study for other reasons, and (4) were unable to comprehend or adhere to study protocols or follow-up procedures due to mental, cognitive, or emotional impairments. Finally, a total of 303 AIS patients fulfilled the inclusion criteria and were included in the study (Figure 1).

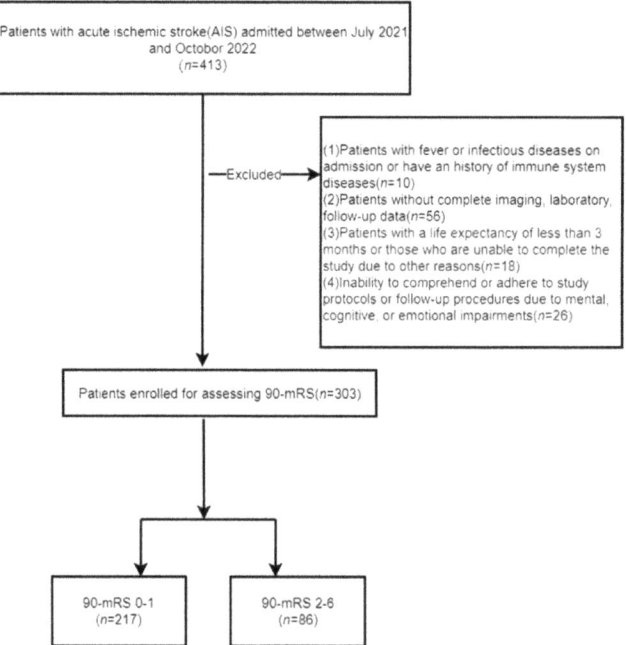

Figure 1. Details on study recruitment. AIS: acute ischemic stroke; mRS: modified Rankin scale.

This study was conducted according to the guidelines of the Declaration of Helsinki and approved by the Research Ethics Committee of the First Affiliated Hospital of Soochow University.

2.2. Data Collection

Basic information on each participant who met the inclusion and exclusion criteria was collected, including age, sex, systolic blood pressure (SBP), diastolic blood pressure (DBP), medical history (including hypertension, diabetes mellitus, smoking, alcoholic habit, history of stroke, atrial fibrillation, and other heart diseases), and clinical data on admission (including relevant laboratory indicators, stroke severity at admission as measured by the NIHSS score, stroke etiology established based on the TOAST classification, computed tomography perfusion imaging (CTP)-positive, HT, and thrombolytic treatment).

The laboratory data included triglyceride (TG), total cholesterol (TC), low-density lipoprotein cholesterol (LDL-C), albumin, blood platelet count, creatinine, uric acid, hemoglobin A1c, fasting blood glucose (FBG), fibrinogen (FIB), homocysteine (HCY), white blood cell (WBC), CRP, NLR, CLR, PLR and SII. The NLR was calculated as the neutrophil count/lymphocyte count. The CLR was calculated as the CRP/lymphocyte count. The PLR was calculated as the platelet count/lymphocyte count. The SII was calculated as the platelet count × neutrophil count/lymphocyte count. All blood samples were obtained within 24 h of admission.

The modified Rankin scale (mRS) scores ranged from 0 to 6, with a score of 0 indicating no symptoms, a score of 1 indicating no clinically significant disability, a score of 2 indicating slight disability, a score of 3 indicating moderate disability, a score of 4 indicating moderately severe disability, a score of 5 indicating severe disability, and a score of 6 indicating death. We defined mRS scores of 0–1 at 90 days after AIS onset as excellent functional outcomes and mRS scores of 2–6 as poor functional outcomes.

2.3. Statistical Tests

SPSS version 26.0 (SPSS, Inc., Chicago, IL, USA) was used for the statistical analysis. The patients were categorized into two groups based on their mRS score at 90 days: those with excellent functional outcomes (mRS: 0–1) and those with poor functional outcomes (mRS: 2–6). The normality of the distribution was assessed using the Shapiro–Wilk test. Continuous variables are presented as the mean ± standard deviation (SD), while nonnormally distributed variables are presented as medians and interquartile ranges. Categorical data were examined using the chi-squared test. The difference between two groups was analyzed using a *t*-test for normally distributed continuous variables or the Mann–Whitney *U* test for continuous variables that do not follow a normal distribution. Univariate logistic regression and multivariate logistic regression analyses were also conducted to evaluate the association between the NLR and 90-day clinical outcomes, and odds ratios (ORs) and 95% confidence intervals (95% CIs) were calculated. Receiver operating characteristic (ROC) curve analysis was performed to estimate the predictive value of the NLR for 90-day functional outcomes, and the optimal cutoff value was determined based on the maximum Youden index. In the multivariate logistic regression analysis, three models were constructed: Model 1, adjusted for age, sex, SBP, and TOAST classification; Model 2, further adjusted for the NIHSS score at admission; and Model 3, additionally adjusted for the NLR.

3. Results
3.1. Demographics and Baseline Characteristics of All Participants

As shown in Table 1, significant differences between the two groups were described by age, and patients with poor functional outcomes were older than patients with excellent functional outcomes (t = 2.10; $p < 0.05$). Patients with higher SBP (t = 2.97, $p < 0.05$) and higher TC (t = 2.15, $p < 0.05$) were more likely to suffer from poor functional outcomes. Poor functional outcome patients showed higher NIHSS scores (Z = 8.47, $p < 0.01$) and a higher NLR (Z = 5.43, $p < 0.01$). Another association was found between the two groups according to the TOAST classification ($\chi^2 = 17.46$, $p < 0.01$), and patients who were CTP negative ($\chi^2 = 10.36$, $p < 0.01$) seemed to have poor functional outcomes.

Table 1. Clinical baseline characteristic of AIS patients according to 90-day mRS.

Demographic and Clinical Data	Excellent Functional Outcome ($n = 217$)	Poor Functional Outcome ($n = 86$)	$t/Z/\chi^2$	p
Age (years)	63.91 ± 13.02	67.30 ± 11.89	$t = 2.10$	0.037 *
Sex male/female	149/68	56/30	$\chi^2 = 0.35$	0.552
SBP † (mmHg)	146.66 ± 19.88	154.51 ± 22.68	$t = 2.97$	0.003 *
DBP † (mmHg)	83.52 ± 11.86	84.64 ± 12.83	$t = 0.72$	0.470
History of hypertension yes/no	146/71	56/30	$\chi^2 = 0.13$	0.719
History of diabetes yes/no	63/154	23/63	$\chi^2 = 0.16$	0.690
Alcoholic habit yes/no	42/175	14/72	$\chi^2 = 0.39$	0.534
Smoking yes/no	55/162	19/67	$\chi^2 = 0.35$	0.552
History of AF † yes/no	20/197	8/78	$\chi^2 = 0.00$	0.981
Other heart diseases yes/no	12/205	4/82	$\chi^2 = 0.10$	0.758
Previous stroke yes/no	38/179	14/72	$\chi^2 = 0.07$	0.798
TG † (mmol/L)	[1.37 (1.03, 1.76)]	[1.36 (0.99, 2.04)]	$Z = 0.13$	0.900
TC † (mmol/L)	4.40 ± 1.05	4.69 ± 1.14	$t = 2.15$	0.032 *
LDL-C † (mmol/L)	2.73 ± 0.98	2.89 ± 1.09	$t = 1.27$	0.205
Albumin (g/L)	39.11 ± 3.44	39.68 ± 3.72	$t = 1.28$	0.202
Prealbumin (g/L)	238.31 ± 50.48	234.57 ± 63.79	$t = 0.49$	0.628
Blood platelet (10^9/L)	[208 (172, 249)]	[199 (165, 256)]	$Z = 0.65$	0.514
Creatinine (μmol/L)	[69.1 (58.8, 77.6)]	[71.6 (57.8, 83.9)]	$Z = 1.45$	0.149
Uric acid (μmol/L)	329.39 ± 96.65	347.08 ± 122.05	$t = 1.20$	0.231
FBG † (μmol/L)	[5.38 (4.77, 6.74)]	[5.75 (4.98, 7.44)]	$Z = 1.93$	0.054
CRP † (mg/L)	[2.46 (0.95, 8.05)]	[7.49 (2.58, 15.36)]	$Z = 4.518$	0.000 *
CLR †	[1.38 (0.58, 4.90)]	[5.11 (1.61, 10.64)]	$Z = 5.216$	0.000 *
HCY † (μmol/L)	[9.90 (8.20, 12.10)]	[11.75 (9.60, 13.75)]	$Z = 3.314$	0.001 *
WBC † (10^9/L)	[6.97 (5.61, 8.54)]	[8.18 (6.60, 10.00)]	$Z = 3.371$	0.001 *
NLR †	[2.62 (1.94, 3.99)]	[3.93 (2.83, 6.01)]	$Z = 5.43$	0.000 *
SII †	[529.74 (373.78, 841.03)]	[847.39 (531.30, 1375.46)]	$Z = 4.555$	0.000 *
PLR †	[124.64 (92.75, 171.93)]	[149.77 (113.44, 202.28)]	$Z = 3.140$	0.002 *
FIB † (g/L)	[2.80 (2.30, 3.32)]	[3.22 (2.69, 3.95)]	$Z = 3.940$	0.000 *
Hemoglobin A1c ‡ (%)	[6.1 (5.6, 7.3)]	[6.1 (5.7, 7.2)]	$Z = 0.38$	0.703
NIHSS † score	[2 (1, 5)]	[7 (4, 11)]	$Z = 8.47$	0.000 *
TOAST classification †	98/23/80/16/0	59/10/12/5/0	$\chi^2 = 17.46$	0.001 *
CTP † -positive yes/no #	102/64	55/11	$\chi^2 = 10.36$	0.006 *
Thrombolytic yes/no	53/164	28/58	$\chi^2 = 2.08$	0.149
HT † yes/no †	5/212	2/84	$\chi^2 = 0.88$	0.831

Continuous data are shown as the mean ± SD, minimum and maximum values in patients with statistical significance based on two sample t tests. Categorical data differences are represented with statistical significance based on the chi-square test (χ^2 and p) or Fisher's exact test (Z and p). * $p < 0.05$. † SBP: systolic blood pressure; DBP: diastolic blood pressure; AF: atrial fibrillation; TG: triglyceride; TC: total cholesterol; LDL-C: low-density lipoprotein cholesterol; FBG: fasting blood glucose; CRP: C-reactive protein; CLR: the CRP-to-lymphocyte ratio; HCY: homocysteine; WBC: white blood cell; NLR: the neutrophil-to-lymphocyte ratio; SII: the systemic immune-inflammation index; PLR: the platelet-to-lymphocyte ratio; FIB: fibrinogen; TOAST refers to five classifications: (1) large-artery atherosclerosis, (2) cardioembolism, (3) small-vessel occlusion, (4) stroke of other determined etiology, and (5) stroke of undetermined etiology. NIHSS: National Institutes of Health Stroke Scale; CTP: computed tomography perfusion imaging; HT: hemorrhagic transformation. ‡ We defined modified Rankin scale (mRS) scores of 0–1 at 90 days after AIS onset as excellent functional outcomes and mRS scores of 2–6 as poor functional outcomes. A total of 217 patients with excellent functional outcomes and 86 patients with poor functional outcomes underwent HCY tests, while 208 patients with excellent functional outcomes and 83 patients with poor functional outcomes underwent hemoglobin A1c tests. # A total of 166 patients with excellent functional outcomes and 66 patients with poor functional outcomes underwent CTP tests.

3.2. Comparison of Derived Blood Lymphocyte Parameters

As shown in Figure 2 and Table 2, ROC curve analysis revealed that the cutoff levels of NLR [AUC = 0.717 (0.648 to 0.786)], CLR [AUC = 0.697 (0.625 to 0.768)], SII [AUC = 0.694 (0.626 to 0.763)], CRP [AUC = 0.663 (0.587 to 0.738)], FIB [AUC = 0.661] (0.589 to 0.734)], PLR [AUC = 0.639 (0.567 to 0.710)], HCY [AUC = 0.624 (0.550 to 0.698)], and WBC [AUC = 0.622 (0.547 to 0.697)] were 3.06, 3.87, 769.83, 4.44, 3.03, 125.09, 11.15, 7.43. The NLR had a significantly greater AUC than did the CLR, SII, CRP, FIB, PLR, HCY and WBC in predicting 90-day functional outcomes in patients with AIS.

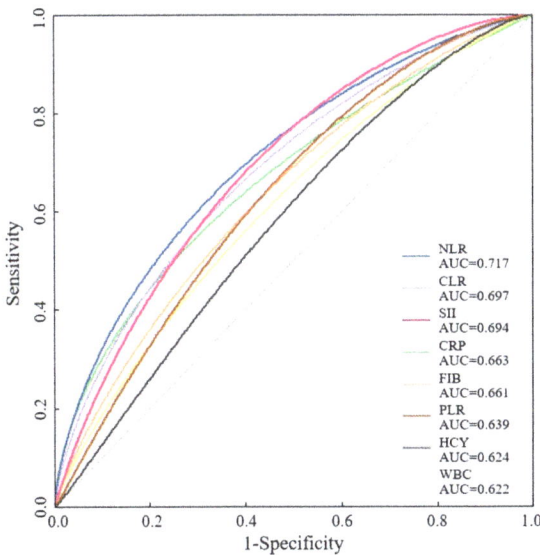

Figure 2. ROC curves of the derived blood inflammatory parameters to predict 90-day functional outcomes.

Table 2. ROC analysis results of the derived blood lymphocyte parameters.

	AUC-ROC	95% CI	Cut-Off Level	p Value
NLR	0.717	0.648, 0786	3.06	<0.001
CLR	0.697	0.625, 0.768	3.87	<0.001
SII	0.694	0.626, 0.763	769.83	<0.001
CRP	0.663	0.587, 0.738	4.4	<0.001
FIB	0.661	0.589, 0.734	3.03	<0.001
PLR	0.639	0.567, 0.710	125.09	<0.001
HCY	0.624	0.550, 0.698	11.15	0.002
WBC	0.622	0.547, 0.697	7.43	0.002

NLR: the neutrophil-to-lymphocyte ratio; CLR: the CRP-to-lymphocyte ratio; SII: the systemic immune-inflammation index; CRP: C-reactive protein; FIB: fibrinogen; PLR: the platelet-to-lymphocyte ratio; HCY: homocysteine; WBC: white blood cell.

3.3. Analysis of Risk Factors Associated with Unfavorable Prognosis in AIS Patients

To avoid the influence of multiple comparisons, we chose $p < 0.05$ in Table 1 when performing multivariate logistic regression analysis. We selected the NLR, which has the most influential prognostic value among inflammatory factors. The three variables (NIHSS score, TOAST classification and NLR) with the most significant associations, SBP, TC and CTP-positivity were combined with age and sex and used to construct a prediction scale using a multivariate logistic model. As shown in Table 3, the SBP (OR = 1.015, $p < 0.01$), NLR (OR = 1.145, $p < 0.01$) and NIHSS score (OR = 1.241, $p < 0.01$) showed the most significant associations with poor functional outcomes according to multivariate statistical analysis, and the other variables, including age, sex, and TOAST classification, showed no associations.

Table 3. Multivariable logistic regression model for predicting patients with 90-day mRS.

Variables	Odd Ratio	95% CI	p Value
Age	1.016	0.99, 1.05	0.313
Sex	0.903	0.46, 1.77	0.766
SBP (mmHg)	1.015	1.00, 1.03	0.043
NLR	1.148	1.04, 1.27	0.008
NIHSS score	1.255	1.16, 1.36	0.000
Large-artery atherosclerosis	1.458	0.36, 5.96	0.599
Cardio-embolism	0.524	0.10, 2.90	0.459
Small-vessel occlusion	0.467	0.10, 2.10	0.320
TC	1.260	0.95, 1.67	0.104
CTP-positive	0.550	0.31, 1.43	0.221
CTP-negative	0.775	0.35, 1.74	0.536

SBP: systolic blood pressure; NLR: the neutrophil-to-lymphocyte ratio; NIHSS: National Institutes of Health Stroke Scale; TC: total cholesterol; CTP: computed tomography perfusion imaging.

3.4. Comparison of Functional Outcomes of AIS Patients with High or Low NLR

A ROC curve was drawn to estimate the predictive value of the NLR for 90-day poor functional outcomes. We observed that the area under the curve was 0.7 (95% CI 0.636–0.765), and the best predictive cutoff value was 3.06, with a sensitivity of 70.3% and a specificity of 67.0%. As shown in Figure 3, we divided patients into two groups around the cutoff value, and the scores on mRS are shown for the patients in the two groups who had data for the primary outcome.

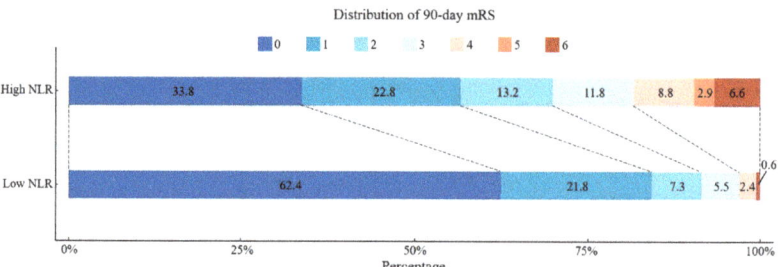

Figure 3. Distribution of functional outcomes at 90 days in patients with high NLR and low NLR. A high NLR is defined as an NRL greater than or equal to 3.06, and a low NLR is defined as an NLR less than 3.06. NLR: the neutrophil-to-lymphocyte ratio; mRS: modified Rankin scale.

3.5. Comparison of Various Models in Predicting 90-Day Functional Outcome with AIS

A ROC analysis was performed to examine the accuracy of the prediction scale of the 90-day mRS. As shown in Figure 4, SBP, TOAST classification, NIHSS score and NLR together showed a significantly high AUC (area under the ROC curve) of 0.829, which indicated the higher accuracy of the 90-day functional outcome prediction scale. The AUC of the predictions based on SBP and TOAST classification (green curve, AUC = 0.694) and on the SBP, TOAST classification and NIHSS score (orange curve, AUC = 0.826) are also presented. Age and sex effects were included in the multivariate logistic model to construct prediction scales.

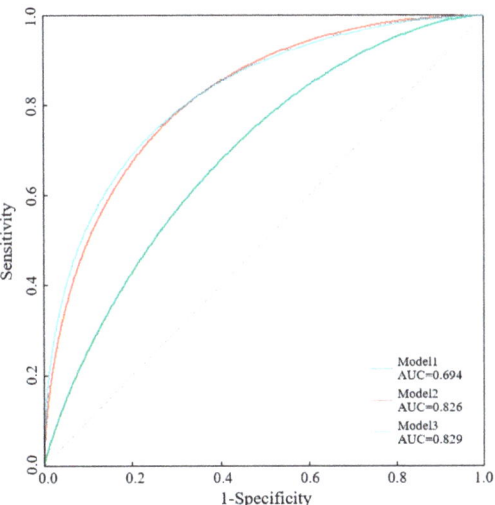

Figure 4. ROC curves generated for stroke with 90-day poor functional outcomes. ROC curve is generated for SBP, TOAST classification, NIHSS score and NLR (age and sex effects included) with 90-day poor functional outcomes (blue line, AUC = 0.829) based on multiple logistic regression. ROC curves are generated for SBP and TOAST classification (green, AUC = 0.694), SBP, TOAST classification and NIHSS score (orange, AUC = 0.826) with age and sex effects included.

4. Discussion

In this study, which included 303 patients with AIS, we found potential clinical risk factors for 90-day poor functional outcomes following AIS, including older age, higher SBP, higher TC, higher NIHSS score, TOAST classification, CTP-positive and a higher NLR. Among the various inflammatory markers examined, such as CLR, SII, CRP, FIB, SCY, WBC and PLR, the NLR exhibited a superior ability to predict the 90-day functional outcome, with an area under the curve of approximately 0.717 and an optimal cutoff value of 3.06. Furthermore, the NLR, age, sex, SBP, NIHSS score and TOAST classification substantially enhanced the accuracy of the prediction of functional outcome in patients with AIS at 90 days.

The majority of studies conducted both domestically and internationally have consistently proven that hypertension is the most important risk factor for cerebral infarction. Many studies have shown that elevated blood pressure is associated with adverse outcomes in patients with AIS who receive intravenous thrombolysis (IVT) or EVT [19–21]. Our study also indicates that SBP serves as an independent risk factor for poor functional outcomes in AIS patients, with a higher SBP correlating to a greater likelihood of experiencing unfavorable clinical outcomes.

A few studies have shown that elevated TC levels are associated with outcomes of ischemic stroke. A study involving 513 patients with AIS found that post-stroke mortality was negatively correlated with TC, with higher TC being a protective factor for post-stroke prognosis [22]. Our study also indicates an association between TC and stroke prognosis, although it does not act as an independent risk factor. The NIHSS score is the predominant clinical scale utilized for evaluating stroke severity. Generally, a higher NIHSS score is related to a more severe stroke. Multiple studies have shown a strong association between the NIHSS score upon admission and 90-day functional outcomes [23,24]. Our study confirms this finding. The TOAST classifies cerebral infarction into five distinct types based on the etiology of the condition [25]. The stratification of risk factors, treatment selection and prognostic assessment for various types of cerebral infarction can be facilitated according to the TOAST classification.

CTP is a medical imaging method, enabling the estimation of irreversible ischemic core damage as well as potentially salvageable ischemic penumbra [26]. CTP may aid in the selection of EVT and the prediction of the prognosis of stroke patients. The DAWN [27] and DEFUSE 3 [28] trials have demonstrated the efficacy of EVT in patients with stroke occurring more than 6 h prior, as these patients exhibit a favorable CTP penumbral pattern. However, our study revealed that CTP is associated with functional outcomes in AIS patients but is not an independent risk factor in the multivariate logistic regression analysis of AIS patients. One potential explanation is that the prognosis of AIS patients is influenced by numerous factors such as age, lesion extent, early treatments, and rehabilitation measures. Therefore, relying solely on CTP may not accurately predict prognosis. In addition, it may be related to different subjects. Our subjects received various treatments, including IVT, EVT or antiplatelet therapy alone.

The majority of strokes are caused by atherosclerosis, which leads to stenosis or occlusion of the cerebellum. This subsequently results in ischemia and hypoxia in brain tissue, leading to damage in corresponding functional areas. In recent years, growing evidence has suggested that inflammation plays a pivotal role in the initiation and progression of stroke [29,30]. After ischemia, the damaged brain tissue triggers a local inflammatory response, leading to the release of inflammatory mediators. Neutrophils, monocytes, and other immune cells accumulate and secrete metalloproteinases (MMPs), perforin, cytokines, and neutrophil extracellular traps (NETs), thereby causing damage to brain tissue. Simultaneously, thrombin is activated, disrupting endothelial barrier function and initiating complement system activation [4,31]. Blood analysis, the most commonly used clinical test, has significant value in determining the prognosis of stroke. By incorporating the ratio of various inflammatory indicators, such as the NLR, PLR, and CLR, this approach has been shown to provide greater predictive value than relying solely on individual inflammatory markers [32].

Previous studies have demonstrated the association between the NLR and stroke prognosis. The initial investigation of the relationship between the NLR and short-term mortality in stroke patients demonstrated that the NLR serves as an independent prognostic indicator of short-term mortality in AIS patients, with higher NLRs significantly associated with increased stroke-related mortality [33–36]. Min-Su Kim et al. discovered a similar finding, indicating an optimal NLR threshold value of 2.09 [37]. Our study also provided evidence that the NLR is an independent factor for 3-month clinical functional outcomes in patients with AIS. Furthermore, an increased NLR may also predict infarction size irrespective of its etiology [38]. Lattanzi et al. reported that patients with AIS and a higher NLR at admission exhibited a greater propensity for early neurological deterioration (END), with an optimal NLR threshold value of 6.4 [39]. Furthermore, multiple studies have substantiated the association between an increased NLR and HT in patients with AIS. Goyal et al. reported that the NLR was a significant independent predictor of symptomatic intracranial hemorrhage (sICH) and 3-month mortality in patients with large vessel occlusion who underwent EVT [40]. Similarly, Milena Switonska et al. also discovered that NLR at admission can accurately predict sHT in AIS patients undergoing revascularization [41]. Slaven Pikija et al. confirmed this conclusion and highlighted that the critical value of ICH is 3.89 [42]. Additionally, a high NLR is associated with an increased likelihood of stroke complications, including poststroke depression [43], stroke-associated pneumonia [44,45], delirium after stroke [46] and poststroke cognitive impairment [47,48].

The relationship between inflammation, including systemic and intravascular inflammation, and acute ischemic stroke is currently a focal point of attention. Our study focused on common clinical inflammatory markers such as NLR, CLR, SII, CRP, FIB, PLR, HCY and WBC, ultimately finding that the NLR exhibited the strongest correlation with a poor prognosis following stroke. Our study also encompassed clinical factors, laboratory indicators, including inflammation markers, and imaging in order to identify risk factors that impact the prognosis of AIS and establish a predictive model. The present model enhances the accuracy of predicting functional outcomes during the early stages of AIS, facilitating timely intervention and reducing disability rates later in disease progression. Combined with the findings of previous studies and our study, these findings further substantiated the role of immune inflammation in stroke.

This study has several limitations. First, our study was a single-center retrospective study, which resulted in the exclusion of a large number of patients and potential selection bias. Furthermore, our study did not differentiate between various reperfusion treatments, such as IVT or EVT, nor did it consider the potential impact of END on patients. Moreover, we did not include information regarding poststroke complications, which could have contributed to adverse clinical outcomes. Additionally, dynamic changes in the NLR were not monitored. Future research should further address the shortcomings mentioned above.

5. Conclusions

Our study demonstrated that the NLR was an independent predictor of 90-day prognosis in patients with AIS and identified potential factors associated with 90-day functional outcomes; these factors were utilized to construct highly accurate prediction models. The NLR may serve as a simple and low-cost marker for predicting functional outcomes in patients with AIS.

Author Contributions: Conceptualization, Q.F., Q.Z. and X.T.; data collection L.C., L.Z. and Y.L.; formal analysis, L.C. and L.Z.; investigation, L.C. and Y.L.; writing—original draft preparation, L.C. and L.Z.; writing—review and editing, Q.F., Q.Z. and X.T. All authors have read and agreed to the published version of the manuscript.

Funding: This research was funded by the National Natural Science Foundation of China (no. 82001125, Xiang Tang), Natural Science Foundation of Jiangsu Province (no. BK20180201, Xiang Tang), Xingwei Kejiao science and technology project of Suzhou (no. KJXW2023013, Lulu Zhang), Xingwei Kejiao Science and Technology project of Suzhou (no. KJXW2021005, Quanquan Zhang) and General Project of Basic Science (Natural Science) in the universities of Jiangsu province, (no. 23KJB320016, Quanquan Zhang).

Institutional Review Board Statement: This study was conducted according to the guidelines of the Declaration of Helsinki and approved by the Research Ethics Committee of First Affiliated Hospital of SooChow University (protocol code 20230458, approved on 14 November 2023).

Informed Consent Statement: Informed consent was obtained from all subjects in this study.

Data Availability Statement: The data presented in this study are available in article.

Acknowledgments: The authors thank all of the patients who participated in this study and their families.

Conflicts of Interest: The authors declare no conflicts of interest.

References

1. Feigin, V.L.; Stark, B.A.; Johnson, C.O.; Roth, G.A.; Bisignano, C.; Abady, G.G.; Abbasifard, M.; Abbasi-Kangevari, M.; Abd-Allah, F.; Abedi, V.; et al. Global, regional, and national burden of stroke and its risk factors, 1990–2019: A systematic analysis for the Global Burden of Disease Study 2019. *Lancet Neurol.* **2021**, *20*, 795–820. [CrossRef]
2. Kim, J.S.; Nah, H.W.; Park, S.M.; Kim, S.K.; Cho, K.H.; Lee, J.; Lee, Y.S.; Kim, J.; Ha, S.W.; Kim, E.G.; et al. Risk factors and stroke mechanisms in atherosclerotic stroke: Intracranial compared with extracranial and anterior compared with posterior circulation disease. *Stroke* **2012**, *43*, 3313–3318. [CrossRef]
3. Cui, J.; Li, H.; Chen, Z.; Dong, T.; He, X.; Wei, Y.; Li, Z.; Duan, J.; Cao, T.; Chen, Q.; et al. Thrombo-Inflammation and Immunological Response in Ischemic Stroke: Focusing on Platelet-Tregs Interaction. *Front. Cell. Neurosci.* **2022**, *16*, 955385. [CrossRef] [PubMed]
4. Iadecola, C.; Buckwalter, M.S.; Anrather, J. Immune responses to stroke: Mechanisms, modulation, and therapeutic potential. *J. Clin. Investig.* **2020**, *130*, 2777–2788. [CrossRef]
5. Qiu, Y.M.; Zhang, C.L.; Chen, A.Q.; Wang, H.L.; Zhou, Y.F.; Li, Y.N.; Hu, B. Immune Cells in the BBB Disruption After Acute Ischemic Stroke: Targets for Immune Therapy? *Front. Immunol.* **2021**, *12*, 678744. [CrossRef]
6. Endres, M.; Moro, M.A.; Nolte, C.H.; Dames, C.; Buckwalter, M.S.; Meisel, A. Immune Pathways in Etiology, Acute Phase, and Chronic Sequelae of Ischemic Stroke. *Circ. Res.* **2022**, *130*, 1167–1186. [CrossRef]
7. Schobert, I.T.; Savic, L.J.; Chapiro, J.; Bousabarah, K.; Chen, E.; Laage-Gaupp, F.; Tefera, J.; Nezami, N.; Lin, M.; Pollak, J.; et al. Neutrophil-to-lymphocyte and platelet-to-lymphocyte ratios as predictors of tumor response in hepatocellular carcinoma after DEB-TACE. *Eur. Radiol.* **2020**, *30*, 5663–5673. [CrossRef] [PubMed]

8. Guo, J.; Fang, J.; Huang, X.; Liu, Y.; Yuan, Y.; Zhang, X.; Zou, C.; Xiao, K.; Wang, J. Prognostic role of neutrophil to lymphocyte ratio and platelet to lymphocyte ratio in prostate cancer: A meta-analysis of results from multivariate analysis. *Int. J. Surg.* **2018**, *60*, 216–223. [CrossRef]
9. Wang, J.-H.; Chen, Y.-Y.; Kee, K.-M.; Wang, C.-C.; Tsai, M.-C.; Kuo, Y.-H.; Hung, C.-H.; Li, W.-F.; Lai, H.-L.; Chen, Y.-H. The Prognostic Value of Neutrophil-to-Lymphocyte Ratio and Platelet-to-Lymphocyte Ratio in Patients with Hepatocellular Carcinoma Receiving Atezolizumab Plus Bevacizumab. *Cancers* **2022**, *14*, 343. [CrossRef]
10. Tamaki, S.; Nagai, Y.; Shutta, R.; Masuda, D.; Yamashita, S.; Seo, M.; Yamada, T.; Nakagawa, A.; Yasumura, Y.; Nakagawa, Y.; et al. Combination of Neutrophil-to-Lymphocyte and Platelet-to-Lymphocyte Ratios as a Novel Predictor of Cardiac Death in Patients with Acute Decompensated Heart Failure with Preserved Left Ventricular Ejection Fraction: A Multicenter Study. *J. Am. Hear. Assoc.* **2023**, *12*, e026326. [CrossRef]
11. Mirna, M.; Schmutzler, L.; Topf, A.; Hoppe, U.C.; Lichtenauer, M. Neutrophil-to-lymphocyte ratio and monocyte-to-lymphocyte ratio predict length of hospital stay in myocarditis. *Sci. Rep.* **2021**, *11*, 18101. [CrossRef]
12. Zhang, W.; Wang, Y.; Li, W.; Wang, G. The Association between the Baseline and the Change in Neutrophil-to-Lymphocyte Ratio and Short-Term Mortality in Patients with Acute Respiratory Distress Syndrome. *Front. Med.* **2021**, *8*, 636869. [CrossRef]
13. Wang, S.; Fu, L.; Huang, K.; Han, J.; Zhang, R.; Fu, Z. Neutrophil-to-lymphocyte ratio on admission is an independent risk factor for the severity and mortality in patients with coronavirus disease 2019. *J. Infect.* **2020**, *82*, e16–e18. [CrossRef] [PubMed]
14. Pinčáková, K.; Krastev, G.; Haring, J.; Mako, M.; Mikulášková, V.; Bošák, V. Low Lymphocyte-to-Monocyte Ratio as a Possible Predictor of an Unfavourable Clinical Outcome in Patients with Acute Ischemic Stroke after Mechanical Thrombectomy. *Stroke Res. Treat.* **2022**, *2022*, 9243080. [CrossRef] [PubMed]
15. Song, Q.; Pan, R.; Jin, Y.; Wang, Y.; Cheng, Y.; Liu, J.; Wu, B.; Liu, M. Lymphocyte-to-monocyte ratio and risk of hemorrhagic transformation in patients with acute ischemic stroke. *Neurol. Sci.* **2020**, *41*, 2511–2520. [CrossRef]
16. Gong, P.; Liu, Y.; Gong, Y.; Chen, G.; Zhang, X.; Wang, S.; Zhou, F.; Duan, R.; Chen, W.; Huang, T.; et al. The association of neutrophil to lymphocyte ratio, platelet to lymphocyte ratio, and lymphocyte to monocyte ratio with post-thrombolysis early neurological outcomes in patients with acute ischemic stroke. *J. Neuroinflammation* **2021**, *18*, 51. [CrossRef] [PubMed]
17. Mao, X.; Yu, Q.; Liao, Y.; Huang, Q.; Luo, S.; Li, S.; Qiu, Y.; Wu, Y.; Zhang, J.; Chen, Q.; et al. Lymphocyte-to-Monocyte Ratio Is Independently Associated with Progressive Infarction in Patients with Acute Ischemic Stroke. *BioMed Res. Int.* **2022**, *2022*, 2290524. [CrossRef]
18. Ferro, D.; Matias, M.; Neto, J.; Dias, R.; Moreira, G.; Petersen, N.; Azevedo, E.; Castro, P. Neutrophil-to-Lymphocyte Ratio Predicts Cerebral Edema and Clinical Worsening Early After Reperfusion Therapy in Stroke. *Stroke* **2021**, *52*, 859–867. [CrossRef]
19. Malhotra, K.; Ahmed, N.; Filippatou, A.; Katsanos, A.H.; Goyal, N.; Tsioufis, K.; Manios, E.; Pikilidou, M.; Schellinger, P.D.; Alexandrov, A.W.; et al. Association of Elevated Blood Pressure Levels with Outcomes in Acute Ischemic Stroke Patients Treated with Intravenous Thrombolysis: A Systematic Review and Meta-Analysis. *J. Stroke* **2019**, *21*, 78–90. [CrossRef]
20. Samuels, N.; van de Graaf, R.A.; Mulder, M.J.H.L.; Brown, S.; Roozenbeek, B.; van Doormaal, P.J.; Goyal, M.; Campbell, B.C.V.; Muir, K.W.; Agrinier, N.; et al. Admission systolic blood pressure and effect of endovascular treatment in patients with ischaemic stroke: An individual patient data meta-analysis. *Lancet Neurol.* **2023**, *22*, 312–319. [CrossRef]
21. Malhotra, K.; Goyal, N.; Katsanos, A.H.; Filippatou, A.; Mistry, E.A.; Khatri, P.; Anadani, M.; Spiotta, A.M.; Sandset, E.C.; Sarraj, A.; et al. Association of Blood Pressure With Outcomes in Acute Stroke Thrombectomy. *Hypertension* **2020**, *75*, 730–739. [CrossRef]
22. Olsen, T.S.; Christensen, R.H.; Kammersgaard, L.P.; Andersen, K.K. Higher total serum cholesterol levels are associated with less severe strokes and lower all-cause mortality: Ten-year follow-up of ischemic strokes in the Copenhagen Stroke Study. *Stroke* **2007**, *38*, 2646–2651. [CrossRef]
23. Rangaraju, S.; Frankel, M.; Jovin, T.G. Prognostic Value of the 24-Hour Neurological Examination in Anterior Circulation Ischemic Stroke: A post hoc Analysis of Two Randomized Controlled Stroke Trials. *Interv. Neurol.* **2015**, *4*, 120–129. [CrossRef] [PubMed]
24. Heitsch, L.; Ibanez, L.; Carrera, C.; Binkley, M.M.; Strbian, D.; Tatlisumak, T.; Bustamante, A.; Ribó, M.; Molina, C.; Dávalos, A.; et al. Early Neurological Change After Ischemic Stroke Is Associated With 90-Day Outcome. *Stroke* **2021**, *52*, 132–141. [CrossRef]
25. Adams, H.P., Jr.; Bendixen, B.H.; Kappelle, L.J.; Biller, J.; Love, B.B.; Gordon, D.L.; Marsh, E.E., 3rd. Classification of subtype of acute ischemic stroke. Definitions for use in a multicenter clinical trial. TOAST. Trial of Org 10172 in Acute Stroke Treatment. *Stroke* **1993**, *24*, 35–41. [CrossRef] [PubMed]
26. Campbell, B.C.V.; Majoie, C.B.L.M.; Albers, G.W.; Menon, B.K.; Yassi, N.; Sharma, G.; van Zwam, W.H.; van Oostenbrugge, R.J.; Demchuk, A.M.; Guillemin, F.; et al. Penumbral imaging and functional outcome in patients with anterior circulation ischaemic stroke treated with endovascular thrombectomy versus medical therapy: A meta-analysis of individual patient-level data. *Lancet Neurol.* **2018**, *18*, 46–55. [CrossRef]
27. Nogueira, R.G.; Jadhav, A.P.; Haussen, D.C.; Bonafe, A.; Budzik, R.F.; Bhuva, P.; Yavagal, D.R.; Ribo, M.; Cognard, C.; Hanel, R.A.; et al. Thrombectomy 6 to 24 Hours after Stroke with a Mismatch between Deficit and Infarct. *N. Engl. J. Med.* **2018**, *378*, 11–21. [CrossRef]
28. Albers, G.W.; Marks, M.P.; Kemp, S.; Christensen, S.; Tsai, J.P.; Ortega-Gutierrez, S.; McTaggart, R.A.; Torbey, M.T.; Kim-Tenser, M.; Leslie-Mazwi, T.; et al. Thrombectomy for Stroke at 6 to 16 Hours with Selection by Perfusion Imaging. *N. Engl. J. Med.* **2018**, *378*, 708–718. [CrossRef] [PubMed]
29. Stoll, G.; Nieswandt, B. Thrombo-inflammation in acute ischaemic stroke—Implications for treatment. *Nat. Rev. Neurol.* **2019**, *15*, 473–481. [CrossRef]

30. Shi, K.; Tian, D.-C.; Li, Z.-G.; Ducruet, A.F.; Lawton, M.T.; Shi, F.-D. Global brain inflammation in stroke. *Lancet Neurol.* **2019**, *18*, 1058–1066. [CrossRef]
31. Westendorp, W.F.; Dames, C.; Nederkoorn, P.J.; Meisel, A. Immunodepression, Infections, and Functional Outcome in Ischemic Stroke. *Stroke* **2022**, *53*, 1438–1448. [CrossRef]
32. Curbelo, J.; Bueno, S.L.; Galván-Román, J.M.; Ortega-Gómez, M.; Rajas, O.; Fernández-Jiménez, G.; Vega-Piris, L.; Rodríguez-Salvanes, F.; Arnalich, B.; Díaz, A.; et al. Inflammation biomarkers in blood as mortality predictors in community-acquired pneumonia admitted patients: Importance of comparison with neutrophil count percentage or neutrophil-lymphocyte ratio. *PLoS ONE* **2017**, *12*, e0173947. [CrossRef]
33. Bolton, W.S.; Gharial, P.K.; Akhunbay-Fudge, C.; Chumas, P.; Mathew, R.K.; Anderson, I.A. Day 2 neutrophil-to-lymphocyte and platelet-to-lymphocyte ratios for prediction of delayed cerebral ischemia in subarachnoid hemorrhage. *Neurosurg. Focus* **2022**, *52*, E4. [CrossRef]
34. Chen, C.; Gu, L.; Chen, L.; Hu, W.; Feng, X.; Qiu, F.; Fan, Z.; Chen, Q.; Qiu, J.; Shao, B. Neutrophil-to-Lymphocyte Ratio and Platelet-to-Lymphocyte Ratio as Potential Predictors of Prognosis in Acute Ischemic Stroke. *Front. Neurol.* **2021**, *11*, 525621. [CrossRef]
35. Giede-Jeppe, A.; Madžar, D.; Sembill, J.A.; Sprügel, M.I.; Atay, S.; Hoelter, P.; Lücking, H.; Huttner, H.B.; Bobinger, T. Increased Neutrophil-to-Lymphocyte Ratio is Associated with Unfavorable Functional Outcome in Acute Ischemic Stroke. *Neurocritical Care* **2019**, *33*, 97–104. [CrossRef]
36. Tokgoz, S.; Kayrak, M.; Akpinar, Z.; Seyithanoğlu, A.; Güney, F.; Yürüten, B. Neutrophil Lymphocyte Ratio as a Predictor of Stroke. *J. Stroke Cerebrovasc. Dis.* **2013**, *22*, 1169–1174. [CrossRef] [PubMed]
37. Kim, M.-S.; Heo, M.Y.; Joo, H.J.; Shim, G.Y.; Chon, J.; Chung, S.J.; Soh, Y.; Yoo, M.C. Neutrophil-to-Lymphocyte Ratio as a Predictor of Short-Term Functional Outcomes in Acute Ischemic Stroke Patients. *Int. J. Environ. Res. Public Health* **2023**, *20*, 898. [CrossRef] [PubMed]
38. Tokgoz, S.; Keskin, S.; Kayrak, M.; Seyithanoglu, A.; Ogmegul, A. Is neutrophil/lymphocyte ratio predict to short-term mortality in acute cerebral infarct independently from infarct volume? *J. Stroke Cerebrovasc. Dis.* **2014**, *23*, 2163–2168. [CrossRef] [PubMed]
39. Lattanzi, S.; Norata, D.; Broggi, S.; Meletti, S.; Świtońska, M.; Słomka, A.; Silvestrini, M. Neutrophil-to-Lymphocyte Ratio Predicts Early Neurological Deterioration after Endovascular Treatment in Patients with Ischemic Stroke. *Life* **2022**, *12*, 1415. [CrossRef] [PubMed]
40. Goyal, N.; Tsivgoulis, G.; Chang, J.J.; Malhotra, K.; Pandhi, A.; Ishfaq, M.F.; Alsbrook, D.; Arthur, A.S.; Elijovich, L.; Alexandrov, A.V. Admission Neutrophil-to-Lymphocyte Ratio as a Prognostic Biomarker of Outcomes in Large Vessel Occlusion Strokes. *Stroke* **2018**, *49*, 1985–1987. [CrossRef] [PubMed]
41. Świtońska, M.; Piekuś-Słomka, N.; Słomka, A.; Sokal, P.; Żekanowska, E.; Lattanzi, S. Neutrophil-to-Lymphocyte Ratio and Symptomatic Hemorrhagic Transformation in Ischemic Stroke Patients Undergoing Revascularization. *Brain Sci.* **2020**, *10*, 771. [CrossRef]
42. Pikija, S.; Sztriha, L.K.; Killer-Oberpfalzer, M.; Weymayr, F.; Hecker, C.; Ramesmayer, C.; Hauer, L.; Sellner, J. Neutrophil to lymphocyte ratio predicts intracranial hemorrhage after endovascular thrombectomy in acute ischemic stroke. *J. Neuroinflammation* **2018**, *15*, 319. [CrossRef]
43. Chen, H.; Luan, X.; Zhao, K.; Qiu, H.; Liu, Y.; Tu, X.; Tang, W.; He, J. The association between neutrophil-to-lymphocyte ratio and post-stroke depression. *Clin. Chim. Acta* **2018**, *486*, 298–302. [CrossRef]
44. Chen, L.-Z.; Luan, X.-Q.; Wu, S.-Z.; Xia, H.-W.; Lin, Y.-S.; Zhan, L.-Q.; He, J.-C. Optimal time point for neutrophil-to-lymphocyte ratio to predict stroke-associated pneumonia. *Neurol. Sci.* **2023**, *44*, 2431–2442. [CrossRef]
45. Nam, K.-W.; Kim, T.J.; Lee, J.S.; Kwon, H.-M.; Lee, Y.-S.; Ko, S.-B.; Yoon, B.-W. High Neutrophil-to-Lymphocyte Ratio Predicts Stroke-Associated Pneumonia. *Stroke* **2018**, *49*, 1886–1892. [CrossRef] [PubMed]
46. Kotfis, K.; Bott-Olejnik, M.; Szylińska, A.; Rotter, I. Could Neutrophil-to-Lymphocyte Ratio (NLR) Serve as a Potential Marker for Delirium Prediction in Patients with Acute Ischemic Stroke? A Prospective Observational Study. *J. Clin. Med.* **2019**, *8*, 1075. [CrossRef] [PubMed]
47. Zha, F.; Zhao, J.; Chen, C.; Ji, X.; Li, M.; Wu, Y.; Yao, L. A High Neutrophil-to-Lymphocyte Ratio Predicts Higher Risk of Poststroke Cognitive Impairment: Development and Validation of a Clinical Prediction Model. *Front. Neurol.* **2022**, *12*, 755011. [CrossRef] [PubMed]
48. Lee, M.; Lim, J.-S.; Kim, C.-H.; Lee, S.-H.; Kim, Y.; Lee, J.H.; Jang, M.U.; Oh, M.S.; Lee, B.-C.; Yu, K.-H. High Neutrophil–Lymphocyte Ratio Predicts Post-stroke Cognitive Impairment in Acute Ischemic Stroke Patients. *Front. Neurol.* **2021**, *12*, 693318. [CrossRef] [PubMed]

Disclaimer/Publisher's Note: The statements, opinions and data contained in all publications are solely those of the individual author(s) and contributor(s) and not of MDPI and/or the editor(s). MDPI and/or the editor(s) disclaim responsibility for any injury to people or property resulting from any ideas, methods, instructions or products referred to in the content.

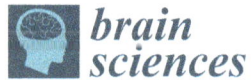

Article

The Effect of Uni-Hemispheric Dual-Site Anodal tDCS on Brain Metabolic Changes in Stroke Patients: A Randomized Clinical Trial

Somaye Azarnia [1], Kamran Ezzati [2], Alia Saberi [2], Soofia Naghdi [3], Iraj Abdollahi [4,*] and Shapour Jaberzadeh [5]

1 Department of Physiotherapy, Iranian Research Centre on Aging, University of Social Welfare and Rehabilitation Sciences, Tehran 19857-13834, Iran; azarnia.pt.82@gmail.com
2 Neuroscience Research Centre, Poorsina Hospital, Faculty of Medicine, Guilan University of Medical Sciences, Rasht 41937-13111, Iran
3 Department of Physiotherapy, Faculty of Rehabilitation, Tehran University of Medical Sciences, Tehran 65111-11489, Iran; naghdi@sina.tums.ac.ir
4 Department of Physiotherapy, Faculty of Rehabilitation, University of Social Welfare and Rehabilitation Sciences, Tehran 19857-13834, Iran
5 Department of Physiotherapy, Faculty of Medicine, Nursing and Health Sciences, Monash University, Melbourne, VIC 3800, Australia; shapour.jaberzadeh@monash.edu
* Correspondence: ir.abdollahi@uswr.ac.ir

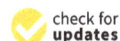

Citation: Azarnia, S.; Ezzati, K.; Saberi, A.; Naghdi, S.; Abdollahi, I.; Jaberzadeh, S. The Effect of Uni-Hemispheric Dual-Site Anodal tDCS on Brain Metabolic Changes in Stroke Patients: A Randomized Clinical Trial. *Brain Sci.* **2023**, *13*, 1100. https://doi.org/10.3390/brainsci13071100

Academic Editor: Farsin Hamzei

Received: 19 June 2023
Revised: 14 July 2023
Accepted: 18 July 2023
Published: 20 July 2023

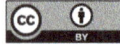

Copyright: © 2023 by the authors. Licensee MDPI, Basel, Switzerland. This article is an open access article distributed under the terms and conditions of the Creative Commons Attribution (CC BY) license (https://creativecommons.org/licenses/by/4.0/).

Abstract: Uni-hemispheric concurrent dual-site anodal transcranial direct current stimulation (UHCDS a-tDCS) of the primary motor cortex (M_1) and the dorsolateral prefrontal cortex (DLPFC) may enhance the efficacy of a-tDCS after stroke. However, the cellular and molecular mechanisms underlying its beneficial effects have not been defined. We aimed to investigate the effect of a-tDCS$_{M1\text{-}DLPFC}$ on brain metabolite concentrations (N-acetyl aspartate (NAA), choline (Cho)) in stroke patients using magnetic resonance spectroscopy (MRS). In this double-blind, sham-controlled, randomized clinical trial (RCT), 18 patients with a first chronic stroke in the territory of the middle cerebral artery trunk were recruited. Patients were allocated to one of the following two groups: (1) Experimental 1, who received five consecutive sessions of a-tDCS$_{M1\text{-}DLPFC}$ M_1 (active)-DLPFC (active). (2) Experimental 2, who received five consecutive sessions of a-tDCS$_{M1\text{-}DLPFC}$ M1 (active)-DLPFC (sham). MRS assessments were performed before and 24 h after the last intervention. Results showed that after five sessions of a-tDCS$_{M1\text{-}DLPFC}$, there were no significant changes in NAA and Cho levels between groups (Cohen's d = 1.4, Cohen's d = 0.93). Thus, dual site a-tDCS$_{M1\text{-}DLPFC}$ did not affect brain metabolites compared to single site a-tDCS M_1.

Keywords: transcranial direct current stimulation; metabolism; stroke; magnetic resonance spectroscopy

1. Introduction

Stroke is the second leading cause of death worldwide [1]. More than 50% of survivors suffer from chronic disability [2]. Motor impairment is the most common physical complication. However, improving motor function in stroke patients remains a challenge [3]. Recently, neurorehabilitation has progressed towards direct brain stimulation, and studies have suggested that brain modulation may have beneficial effects on motor training [4]. Non-invasive brain stimulation (NIBS) aims to transcranially modulate the excitability of specific brain areas [5]. Transcranial direct current stimulation (tDCS) is a form of NIBS that delivers low-intensity direct current through the scalp and facilitates cell plasticity by acting on the neuronal network [6–8]. A recent meta-analysis demonstrated the efficacy of tDCS for motor recovery in stroke patients [9].

Changing the parameters of tDCS to achieve the maximum effect is clinically important. One of the most important parameters is electrode placement. Studies have shown that stimulation of brain areas functionally connected to the primary motor cortex (M_1)

increases corticospinal excitability (CSE) [10]. A related method, called uni-hemispheric concurrent dual-site a-tDCS (UHCDS a-tDCS) stimulates two functionally connected brain regions simultaneously [11]. We chose M_1 and the dorsolateral prefrontal cortex (DLPFC). The DLPFC is largely responsible for attention, executive function, and working memory [12]. There is evidence of a strong link between executive function and the prefrontal cortex [13]. It is possible that DLPFC stimulation in addition to M_1 has an additive effect on motor recovery via functional connectivity to M_1, which is thought to be stronger than M_1 stimulation alone.

Neuroimaging evidence suggests that changes in neuronal and glial metabolism may play an important role in both functional decline and recovery of brain function. Proton magnetic resonance spectroscopy (H-MRS) can detect changes in the metabolic levels of neurotransmitters such as N-acetyl aspartate (NAA), choline (Cho), and creatine (Cr), and can provide a good picture of the metabolic state of damaged tissue [14].

N-acetyl aspartate (NAA) is used as a non-invasive marker of neurological health. Stroke survivors have shown decreased levels of brain NAA [15], suggesting a loss of neurons.

NAA deficiency is associated with reduced levels of ATP, acetyl CoA and other metabolites involved in energy metabolism [11]. The researchers found that the recovery of NAA levels was only observed in conjunction with the regeneration of ATP [15]. Cr, found in neurons and glial cells, plays an important role in maintaining the high levels of energy required to maintain membrane potentials [11]. Cho and its metabolites can affect functions such as maintaining the structural integrity of cell membranes and transmembrane signaling [12,13].

Hone-Blanchet et al. showed that anodal tDCS to the left DLPFC and cathodal tDCS to the right DLPFC in healthy subjects had rapid excitatory effects during stimulation and increased the amount of NAA in the left DLPFC [16]. Carlson et al. reported decreases in glutamate/glutamine and Cr after cathodal tDCS compared to sham tDCS [17].

The present study aims to extend the previous MRS research with metabolites in stroke patients. The aim of this study is to investigate whether the addition of DLPFC stimulation to M_1 (UHCDS a-tDCS$_{M1\text{-}DLPFC}$) can alter brain metabolite concentrations. We hypothesized that the levels of brain metabolites such as NAA, creatine, and choline would change significantly after UHCDS a-tDCS$_{M1\text{-}DLPFC}$ treatment compared to baseline levels.

2. Materials and Methods

2.1. Participants and Study Design

Eighteen patients with a first chronic stroke (>6 months post-stroke) in the MCA territory were enrolled in this double-blind, randomized clinical trial. The study sample was recruited from 533 patients who were admitted to Pars Hospital with a diagnosis of stroke between 20 June 2021 and 20 July 2022, diagnosed by a physiotherapist and a neurologist based on the admission criteria.

Ischemic stroke was confirmed clinically and by neuroimaging. Patients had no history of chronic neurological or cardiac disease and were not taking any medication that could alter their cognitive state. The severity of wrist flexor Spasticity was 1 or higher on the Modified Modified Ashworth Scale (MMAS). They were able to communicate verbally with the therapist. They did not have severe cognitive and memory impairment according to the Persian version of the Mini-Mental State Examination (MMSE) (MMAS $\geq$ 23). Figure 1 shows the study procedure.

Patients were assured that they could withdraw from the study at any time. All patients gave written informed consent to participate in the study. The study was approved by the Ethics Committee of the University of Social Welfare and Rehabilitation (IR: USWR.REC.1400.185).

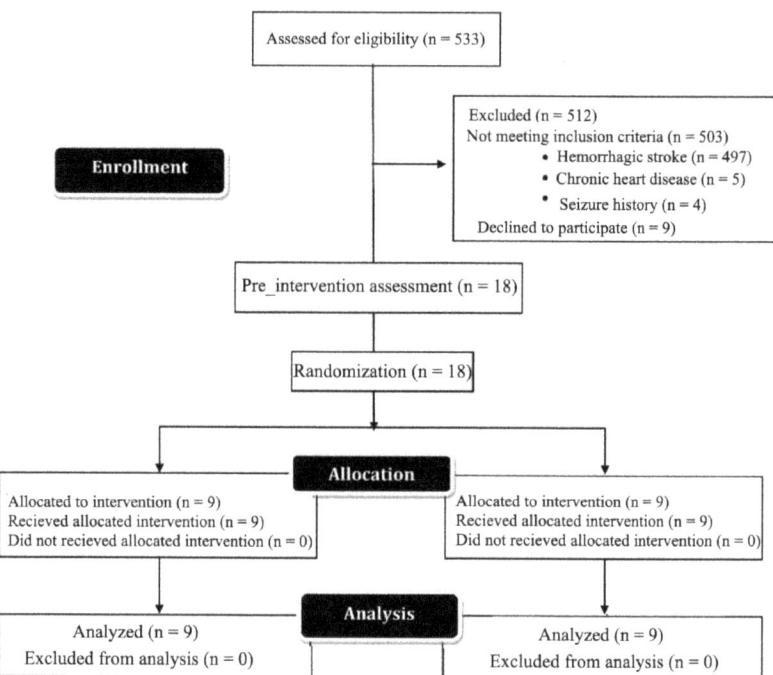

Figure 1. Consort diagram of patients.

Randomization

The assessor and the participants were kept blinded to the group allocation. Randomization was carried out using the Randomization.com website (accessed on 20 March 2023). The patients were randomized into two groups: Experimental 1 and Experimental 2, using a computer-generated randomization block. (1) Experimental 1 received five consecutive sessions of a-tDCS M_1-DLPFC M_1 (active)-DLPFC (active). (2) Experimental 2 received five consecutive sessions of a-tDCS M_1-DLPFC M_1 (active)-DLPFC (sham). All patients were assessed by MRS before and 24 h after five consecutive sessions of tDCS intervention. All patients completed the intervention period and there were no dropouts. Figure 1 demonstrates the CONSORT flow diagram depicting the phases of enrollment, intervention allocation, follow-up, and data analysis in this two-group parallel randomized trial (Figure 1).

2.2. H-MRS Protocol

MRS data were acquired using a Siemens 1.5 T scanner (Erlangen, Germany) with an eight-channel receive-only head coil. A conventional 3-dimensional brain image (sagittal T1 MPRAGE, TR/TE = 1800/3.5, field of view (FOV) = 256 × 256 × 160 mm^3, resolution = 1 × 1 × 1 mm^3) was acquired for all patients before the MRS sequence as a reference image for volume of interest (VOI) positioning. For single-voxel spectroscopy (SVS), MRS was acquired using a point-resolved spectroscopy (PRESS) sequence. Two 2 × 2 × 2 cm^3 voxels were located in the primary motor cortex (M_1), dorsolateral prefrontal cortex (DLPFC). Voxels were carefully placed to avoid contact with subcutaneous fat, skull, vasculature, arachnoid space, and cerebrospinal fluid. Manual shimming was performed on all acquisitions. Parameters were set to TR/TE = 1500/135 and NEX = 128. Six saturation bands were placed around the VOI to suppress external volume signals. The average duration of each H-MRS acquisition was 10 ± 2 min (5 min for each region) with no complications.

MRS Data Processing

Data were pre-processed by applying a water removal algorithm to the reference offset of 4.65 ppm to remove residual water signals. SVS raw data were fitted using TARQUIN (Gerg Reynolds and Martin Wilson, version 4.3.10). The predefined data set of NAA, Cho, and Cr target metabolites was selected for peak fitting and metabolite concentration. The metabolite ratios of NAA/Cr and Cho/Cr were calculated by dividing the metabolite values in the same spectrum for the M_1 region.

2.3. Transcranial Direct Current Stimulation

Two single-channel tDCS devices delivered direct current stimulation through two saline-soaked electrodes. Electrode placement was determined using the international 10–20 system of electroencephalography. In both groups, the active electrodes were placed on M_1 (C3/C4) and DLPFC (F3/F4) according to the involved hemisphere, and the reference electrodes were placed on the supraorbital area of the uninvolved side (Figure 2) [10]. According to the previous research [18], a constant current of 1 mA was applied for 20 min. In the sham group "experimental 2", the stimulation was switched off after 30 s only in the DLPFC region. The standard 5×7 cm^2 electrode was used as the reference electrode. To localize the excitability of the motor cortex and increase the excitability of the corticospinal tract, an active electrode of 4×4 cm^2 was applied to the M_1 and DLPFC regions [10,19].

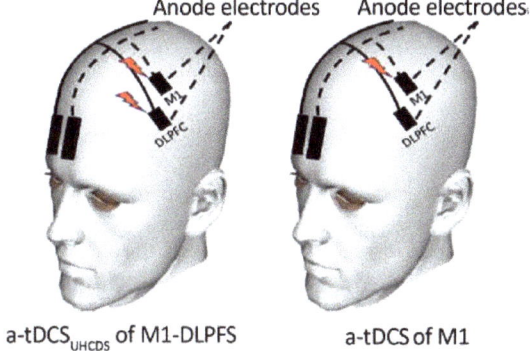

Figure 2. This figure is adapted from (The effects of anodal-tDCS on corticospinal excitability enhancement and its after-effects: Conventional vs. uni-hemispheric concurrent dual-site stimulation, Vaseghi et al., 2015 [10]).

Ref. [20] Schematic illustration of electrode montage in experimental 1: UHCDS a-tDCS$_{M1\text{-DLPFC}}$ and experimental 2: UHCDS a-tDCS$_{M1\text{-DLPFC}}$ ($M_{1active}$-DLPFC $_{sham}$); The reference electrodes were placed over the contralateral supraorbital area in two conditions. In both groups, the active electrodes were positioned over M_1 and dorsolateral prefrontal cortex (DLPFC).

2.4. Measurement of Metabolites

MRS is an objective, non-invasive technique to detect and quantify changes in certain biochemical compounds such as NAA, Cr, and Cho in brain tissue. MRS data were collected from M_1 for all patients.

2.5. Experimental Procedures

The study procedures consisted of three steps: baseline assessment, intervention period, and post-intervention period. In the first step, MRS data were collected from patients in both groups at baseline. In the next step, all patients received five sessions of tDCS according to the group allocation.

The stimulation dose was selected based on a previously published study. In the [10,18] post-intervention period, patients underwent MRS 24 h after the last tDCS session (Figure 3).

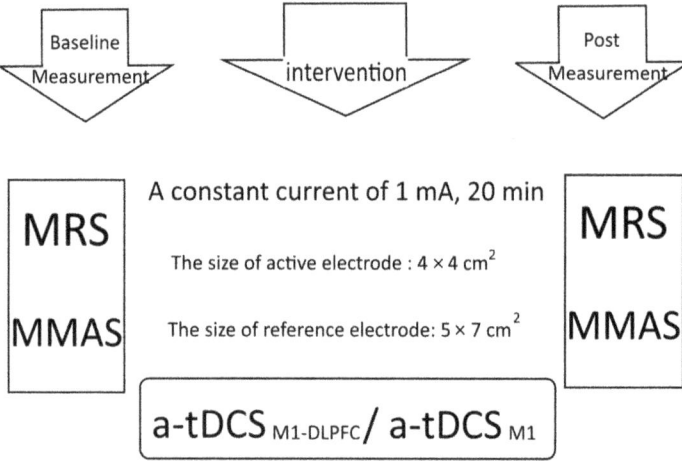

Figure 3. Experimental design for the comparison of conventional a-tDCS and UHCDS a-tDCS M_1-DLPFC. MMAS: Modified Modified Ashworth Scale, MRS: Magnetic resonance spectroscopy.

2.6. Outcome Measures and Data Analysis

The primary outcome was the concentration of brain metabolites (NAA, Cr, Cho) and the metabolite ratio (NAA/Cr, Cho/Cr) in M_1 tested by H-MRS. Metabolite levels on local brain H-MRS are often reported as ratios rather than absolute concentrations. The most common denominator is the Cr level, which is thought to be stable under normal conditions as well as under some pathological conditions [21]. Therefore, we examined NAA/Cr and Cho/Cr.

Data analysis was performed using SPSS software version 26 (IBM SPSS Statistics for Windows, version 26, IBM Corp, Armonk, NY, USA). Continuous variables were summarized as mean ± standard deviation. The Shapiro-Wilk test was used to determine the normal distribution of quantitative data. The test results indicated that the MRS data were not normally distributed. Non-parametric Mann-Whitney U test and Wilcoxon signed rank test were used to compare MRS data between/within groups.

Group differences were examined by ANCOVA controlling for baseline metabolite. $p < 0.05$ was considered statistically significant. The sample size was calculated using G*Power software (version 3:1, Heinrich-Heine-University) based on the effect size (d = 2.0) derived from the Rayen study (power of 0.90 and α = 0.05). We compensated for 20% of the dropouts.

3. Results

Eighteen stroke patients (10 female, 8 male) with a mean age of 60.94 ± 6.92 years were enrolled. The mean time since stroke onset was 34.28 ± 8.91 weeks. Table 1 shows that there were no statistical differences between the two study groups in terms of demographic characteristics, comorbidities, and spasticity level. This study assessed the mean NAA, Cr, Cho, NAA/Cr, and NAA/Cho between/within the two groups at baseline and after intervention in M_1.

Table 1. Summary of the Clinical Data.

		Study Group			p-Value
		Experimental 1 (n = 9)	Experimental 2 (n = 9)	Total (n = 18)	
		N(%)	N(%)	N(%)	
Gender	Female	3(33.3)	7(77.8)	10(55.6)	0.15 *
	Male	6(66.7)	2(22.2)	8(44.4)	
Age	Mean(SD)	61.8(6.25)	60.0(7.79)	60.9(6.92)	0.57 †
Weeks since stroke	Mean(SD)	32.4(4.88)	36.1(11.72)	34.2(8.91)	0.39 †
MMSE	Med (range)	30(29,30)	30(29,30)	30(29,30)	0.99 ‡
MMAS	Med (range)	2(1,4)	1(1,2)	2(1,4)	0.06 ‡
		Comorbidity diseases			
Hypertension	Yes	4(44.4)	3(33.3)	7(38.9)	0.99 *
Diabetes mellitus	Yes	2(22.2)	4(44.4)	6(33.3)	0.62 *
Dyslipidemia	Yes	3(33.3)	2(22.2)	5(27.8)	0.99 *

* Fisher's Exact Test; † Independent T-Test; ‡ Mann-Whitney U.

3.1. Between-Group Comparison

The results showed significantly higher NAA and Cho concentrations in M_1 after the intervention ($p = 0.040$, $p = 0.050$ respectively), with large effect sizes for NAA and Cho, 1.41 and 0.93 respectively. Metabolite ratio results showed a non-significant difference in NAA/Cr and Cho/Cr after intervention ($p = 0.113$, $p = 0.387$).

3.2. Comparison within Groups

The result showed significant changes in NAA, Cr, and Cho in group Experimental 2 ($p = 0.008$), and the concentration of metabolites was increased. In group Experimental 1 there were significant differences in Cr. Cr concentration was decreased (Table 2). For changes in metabolite ratios, there was a significant difference in NAA/Cr in both groups. However, changes in Cho/Cr ($p = 0.004$) were only observed in group Experimental 2 (Figure 4).

Table 2. Differences between baseline and post-intervention of brain metabolites in the M_1 between two groups.

Brain Metabolites	Time	Mean(SD)		p-Value	
		Experimental 1	Experimental 2	p-value †	p-value *
NAA	Baseline	158.4(59.6)	194.1(12.4)	0.43	0.04
	Post-intervention	190.9(35.3)	229.2(14.5)	0.04	
	p-Value	0.08	0.008		
Cr	Baseline	166.73(25.21)	135.23(14.60)	0.004	0.04
	Post-intervention	146.95(12.15)	152.58(15.15)	0.43	
	p-Value	0.02	0.008		
Cho	Baseline	142.98(23.58)	126.09(23.98)	0.22	0.008
	Post-intervention	137.62(20.07)	159.39(26.27)	0.05	
	p-Value	0.59	0.008		

* ANCOVA; † Mann-Whitney U.

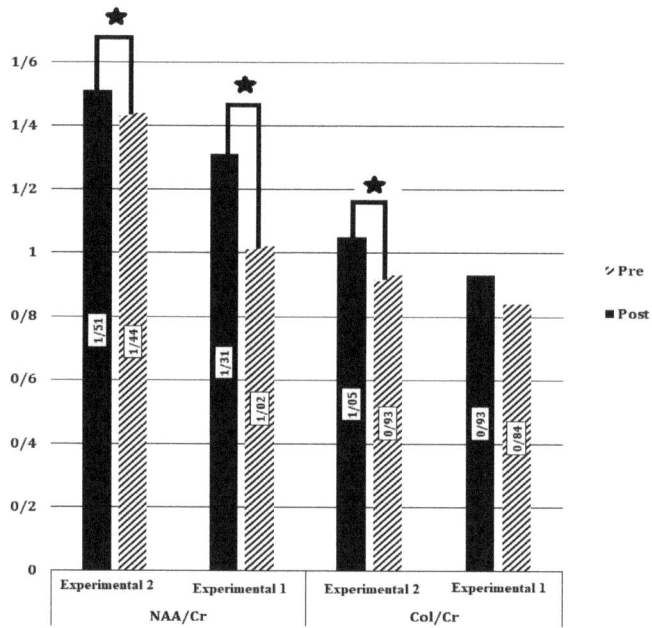

Figure 4. Metabolite ratio (NAA/Cr, Col/Cr) changes in M_1. Data are presented as the mean of brain metabolites compared between baseline and post-tDCS intervention. ★: Significant difference.

4. Discussion

To our knowledge, this is the first study investigating changes in brain metabolites after uni-hemispheric concurrent dual-site a-tDCS in chronic stroke patients.

The main findings of the results were significantly higher NAA, Cr, and Cho concentration in the M_1, in the group single-site a-tDCS$_{M1}$ compared to a-tDCS$_{M1\text{-DLPFC}}$, as measured by 1.5 T MR spectroscopy.

Previous literature has investigated bi-hemispheric single-site tDCS in healthy subjects [16,21,22] and children with spastic cerebral palsy (CP) [23,24]. Studies have shown that a-tDCS increases the levels of NAA and Cho [16,24]. Our study was also consistent with the previous study, and the group Experimental 2 that received the single-site stimulation had a significant increase in metabolites after the intervention. Hone-Blanchet et al. [16] showed that the online effect of a single session of a-tDCS on the DLPFC increased the amount of NAA. Auvichayapat et al. [24] reported an increase in Cr, Cho, and NAA after tDCS in the basal ganglia of CP patients. N-acetyl aspartate is usually considered a neuronal marker because it is only found in mature neurons.

Researchers have found an association between low levels of brain NAA concentration and poor motor function in patients after stroke, and increased levels of NAA were also predictive of recovery [25]. Glodzik-Sobanska et al. showed that an increase in NAA in stroke patients was associated with neurological improvement [24]. Perhaps an increase in NAA after a-tDCS is due to an increase in neuronal excitability leading to long-term potentiation, such as plasticity. However, the study of metabolites in dual-site stimulation has not been investigated. Previous fMRI studies have shown that dual-site stimulation increases corticospinal excitability up to twofold [26,27].

Our results also showed an increase in Cho concentration in both groups, particularly significant in Experimental group 2. This finding is consistent with Auvichayapat et al. [24] Cho is a membrane marker and its metabolites play an important role in a variety of mechanisms, such as maintaining the structural integrity of the cell membrane, methyl metabolism, and transmembrane signaling. In this case, choline repletion may affect neuronal connections and facilitate neuroplasticity in the adult CNS.

The lesser increase of NAA and Cho in the group receiving dual-site a-tDCS of both the DLPFC and M_1 region could be explained by the concept of homeostasis—that is, the ability of the human brain to regulate changes in synaptic plasticity to avoid drastic changes in its function. Homeostasis maintains stable function against changes in the activity of the number and strength of synapses. Homeostatic plasticity is increasingly recognized as a regulator of neural change within physiological limits [24]. In this context, researchers emphasize homeostatic plasticity as a tool to prevent the instability of the neural network that occurs in neurorehabilitation. Thus, dual-site stimulation could not induce further changes by overshooting the physiological range.

5. Limitations

The limitations of this study should also be noted. Firstly, changes in brain metabolites were measured only 24 h after the last stimulation session, and at longer follow-up times or immediately after the intervention. Therefore, we were not able to investigate immediate and long-term effects. Secondly, a single voxel MRS was used with a 1.5 T MRI, which may have limited the collection of data from multiple brain regions simultaneously. It could be suggested that further studies use a multi-voxel 3 or 7 T MRI system to measure stimulation effects in multiple brain regions, and to investigate other metabolites. Thirdly, the tDCS intervention consisted of five consecutive days of 20 min tDCS applications, may not be sufficient to alter brain metabolites. Finally, chronic stroke patients were included in the current study, so it is suggested that future studies investigate the changes in metabolites in subacute patients and examine the levels of metabolites in both hemispheres.

6. Conclusions

This study aimed to investigate the effect of adding transcranial direct stimulation of the DLPFC to M_1 stimulation on changes in brain metabolites in the M_1 region. The results showed that there are no significant changes in the amount of brain metabolites after UHCDS a-tDCS$_{M1-DLPFC}$ compared to a-tDCS M_1.

Author Contributions: Conceptualization, I.A. and S.A.; methodology, S.N., S.J., A.S. and S.A.; formal analysis, K.E. and I.A.; data curation, K.E.; Resources, A.S.; writing—original draft preparation, S.A.; writing—review and editing, S.N., K.E. and S.J.; supervision, S.J. All authors have read and agreed to the published version of the manuscript.

Funding: This research received no external funding.

Institutional Review Board Statement: The study was approved by the ethics committee of the University of Social Welfare and Rehabilitation (IR: USWR.REC.1400.185).

Informed Consent Statement: Informed consent was obtained from all subjects involved in the study.

Data Availability Statement: Data available on request from the authors.

Acknowledgments: I would like to thank the following people without whom I could not have completed this research: Patients who cooperated in the implementation of the study, and the imaging department of Rasht Pars Hospital, especially Pejman Kiani, who is the manager of the department.

Conflicts of Interest: The authors report no competing financial interests that could have appeared to influence the work reported in this paper.

References

1. Feigin, V.L.; Lawes, C.M.; Bennett, D.A.; Barker-Collo, S.L.; Parag, V. Worldwide stroke incidence and early case fatality reported in 56 population-based studies: A systematic review. *Lancet Neurol.* **2009**, *8*, 355–369. [CrossRef] [PubMed]
2. Donkor, E.S. Stroke in the century: A snapshot of the burden, epidemiology, and quality of life. *Stroke Res. Treat.* **2018**, *2018*, 3238165.

3. Hatem, S.M.; Saussez, G.; Della Faille, M.; Prist, V.; Zhang, X.; Dispa, D.; Bleyenheuft, Y. Rehabilitation of motor function after stroke: A multiple systematic review focused on techniques to stimulate upper extremity recovery. *Front. Hum. Neurosci.* **2016**, *10*, 442. [CrossRef]
4. Liebetanz, D.; Nitsche, M.A.; Tergau, F.; Paulus, W. Pharmacological approach to the mechanisms of transcranial DC-stimulation-induced after-effects of human motor cortex excitability. *Brain* **2002**, *125*, 2238–2247. [CrossRef]
5. Miniussi, C.; Harris, J.A.; Ruzzoli, M. Modelling non-invasive brain stimulation in cognitive neuroscience. *Neurosci. Biobehav. Rev.* **2013**, *37*, 1702–1712. [CrossRef]
6. Lee, S.J.; Chun, M.H. Combination transcranial direct current stimulation and virtual reality therapy for upper extremity training in patients with subacute stroke. *Arch. Phys. Med. Rehabil.* **2014**, *95*, 431–438. [CrossRef] [PubMed]
7. Fusco, A.; Iosa, M.; Venturiero, V.; De Angelis, D.; Morone, G.; Maglione, L.; Bragoni, M.; Coiro, P.; Pratesi, L.; Paolucci, S. After vs. priming effects of anodal transcranial direct current stimulation on upper extremity motor recovery in patients with subacute stroke. *Restor. Neurol. Neurosci.* **2014**, *32*, 301–312. [CrossRef]
8. Rabadi, M.; Aston, C. Effect of Transcranial Direct Current Stimulation on Severely Affected Arm-Hand Motor Function in Patients After an Acute ischemic Stroke (667). *Neurology* **2020**, *94*. [CrossRef] [PubMed]
9. Bai, X.; Guo, Z.; He, L.; Ren, L.; McClure, M.A.; Mu, Q. Different therapeutic effects of transcranial direct current stimulation on upper and lower limb recovery of stroke patients with motor dysfunction: A meta-analysis. *Neural Plast.* **2019**, *2019*, 1372138. [CrossRef]
10. Vaseghi, B.; Zoghi, M.; Jaberzadeh, S. The effects of anodal-tDCS on corticospinal excitability enhancement and its after-effects: Conventional vs. unihemispheric concurrent dual-site stimulation. *Front. Hum. Neurosci.* **2015**, *9*, 533. [CrossRef]
11. Magistretti, P.J.; Allaman, I. A cellular perspective on brain energy metabolism and functional imaging. *Neuron* **2015**, *86*, 883–901. [CrossRef] [PubMed]
12. Chen, Y.; Lee, E.; Ungvari, G.; Lu, J.; Shi, L.; Wang, D.; Chu, W.; Mok, V.; Wong, K.; Tang, W. Atrophy of left dorsolateral prefrontal cortex is associated with poor performance in verbal fluency in elderly poststroke women. *Eur. Psychiatry* **2011**, *26*, 1180. [CrossRef]
13. Yuan, P.; Raz, N. Prefrontal cortex and executive functions in healthy adults: A meta-analysis of structural neuroimaging studies. *Neurosci. Biobehav. Rev.* **2014**, *42*, 180–192. [CrossRef]
14. Granata, F.; Pandolfo, G.; Vinci, S.; Alafaci, C.; Settineri, N.; Morabito, R.; Pitrone, A.; Longo, M. Proton magnetic resonance spectroscopy (H-MRS) in chronic schizophrenia. A single-voxel study in three regions involved in a pathogenetic theory. *Neuroradiol. J.* **2013**, *26*, 277–283. [CrossRef] [PubMed]
15. Vagnozzi, R.; Signoretti, S.; Cristofori, L.; Alessandrini, F.; Floris, R.; Isgro, E.; Ria, A.; Marziale, S.; Zoccatelli, G.; Tavazzi, B. Assessment of metabolic brain damage and recovery following mild traumatic brain injury: A multicentre, proton magnetic resonance spectroscopic study in concussed patients. *Brain* **2010**, *133*, 3232–3242. [CrossRef]
16. Hone-Blanchet, A.; Edden, R.A.; Fecteau, S. Online effects of transcranial direct current stimulation in real time on human prefrontal and striatal metabolites. *Biol. Psychiatry* **2016**, *80*, 432–438. [CrossRef]
17. Carlson, H.L.; Ciechanski, P.; Harris, A.D.; MacMaster, F.P.; Kirton, A. Changes in spectroscopic biomarkers after transcranial direct current stimulation in children with perinatal stroke. *Brain Stimul.* **2018**, *11*, 94–103. [CrossRef] [PubMed]
18. Hassanzahraee, M.; Nitsche, M.A.; Zoghi, M.; Jaberzadeh, S. Determination of anodal tDCS duration threshold for reversal of corticospinal excitability: An investigation for induction of counter-regulatory mechanisms. *Brain Stimul.* **2020**, *13*, 832–839. [CrossRef]
19. Bastani, A.; Jaberzadeh, S. Does anodal transcranial direct current stimulation enhance excitability of the motor cortex and motor function in healthy individuals and subjects with stroke: A systematic review and meta-analysis. *Clin. Neurophysiol.* **2012**, *123*, 644–657. [CrossRef]
20. Talimkhani, A.; Abdollahi, I.; Zoghi, M.; Ghane, E.T.; Jaberzadeh, S. The Effects of Unihemispheric Concurrent Dual-Site Transcranial Direct Current Stimulation on Motor Sequence Learning in Healthy Individuals: A Randomized, Clinical Trial. *Iran. Red Crescent Med. J.* **2018**, *20*, e64147. [CrossRef]
21. Choi, C.H.; Iordanishvili, E.; Shah, N.J.; Binkofski, F. Magnetic resonance spectroscopy with transcranial direct current stimulation to explore the underlying biochemical and physiological mechanism of the human brain: A systematic review. *Hum. Brain Mapp.* **2021**, *42*, 2642–2671. [CrossRef] [PubMed]
22. Koolschijn, R.S.; Emir, U.E.; Pantelides, A.C.; Nili, H.; Behrens, T.E.; Barron, H.C. The hippocampus and neocortical inhibitory engrams protect against memory interference. *Neuron* **2019**, *101*, 528–541. [CrossRef]
23. Rango, M.; Cogiamanian, F.; Marceglia, S.; Barberis, B.; Arighi, A.; Biondetti, P.; Priori, A. Myoinositol content in the human brain is modified by transcranial direct current stimulation in a matter of minutes: A ^{1}H-MRS study. *Magn. Reson. Med.* **2008**, *60*, 782–789. [CrossRef] [PubMed]
24. Auvichayapat, P.; Aree-Uea, B.; Auvichayapat, N.; Phuttharak, W.; Janyacharoen, T.; Tunkamnerdthai, O.; Boonphongsathian, W.; Ngernyam, N.; Keeratitanont, K. Transient changes in brain metabolites after transcranial direct current stimulation in spastic cerebral palsy: A pilot study. *Front. Neurol.* **2017**, *8*, 366. [CrossRef]
25. Austin, T.; Bani-Ahmed, A.; Cirstea, M.C. N-acetylaspartate biomarker of stroke recovery: A case series study. *Front. Neurol. Neurosci. Res.* **2021**, *2*, 100007. [PubMed]

26. Lang, N.; Siebner, H.R.; Ward, N.S.; Lee, L.; Nitsche, M.A.; Paulus, W.; Rothwell, J.C.; Lemon, R.N.; Frackowiak, R.S. How does transcranial DC stimulation of the primary motor cortex alter regional neuronal activity in the human brain? *Eur. J. Neurosci.* **2005**, *22*, 495–504. [CrossRef]
27. Meyerson, B.; Lindblom, U.; Linderoth, B.; Lind, G.; Herregodts, P. Motor cortex stimulation as treatment of trigeminal neuropathic pain. In *Advances in Stereotactic and Functional Neurosurgery 10: Proceedings of the 10th Meeting of the European Society for Stereotactic and Functional Neurosurgery Stockholm 1992*; Springer: Vienna, Austria, 1993; pp. 150–153.

Disclaimer/Publisher's Note: The statements, opinions and data contained in all publications are solely those of the individual author(s) and contributor(s) and not of MDPI and/or the editor(s). MDPI and/or the editor(s) disclaim responsibility for any injury to people or property resulting from any ideas, methods, instructions or products referred to in the content.

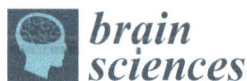

Article

Convergent Validity of the Timed Walking Tests with Functional Ambulatory Category in Subacute Stroke

Alex Martino Cinnera [1], Serena Marrano [1], Daniela De Bartolo [1,2,*], Marco Iosa [1,3], Alessio Bisirri [4], Enza Leone [5,6], Alessandro Stefani [7], Giacomo Koch [1,8], Irene Ciancarelli [9], Stefano Paolucci [1] and Giovanni Morone [9,10]

1. Santa Lucia Foundation, Scientific Institute for Research, Hospitalization and Health Care (IRCCS), 00179 Rome, Italy; a.martino@hsantalucia.it (A.M.C.); sere.marrano@gmail.com (S.M.); marco.iosa@uniroma1.it (M.I.); giacomo.koch@unife.it (G.K.); s.paolucci@hsantalucia.it (S.P.)
2. Department of Human Movement Sciences, Faculty of Behavioural and Movement Sciences, Amsterdam Movement Sciences & Institute for Brain and Behaviour Amsterdam, Vrije Universiteit Amsterdam, 1081 HV Amsterdam, The Netherlands
3. Department of Psychology, Sapienza University of Rome, 00185 Rome, Italy
4. Villa Sandra Institute, Via Portuense, 798, 00148 Rome, Italy; alessiobisirri@gmail.com
5. School of Allied Health Professions, Faculty of Medicine and Health Sciences, Keele University, Staffordshire ST5 5BG, UK; e.leone@keele.ac.uk
6. Centre for Biomechanics and Rehabilitation Technologies, Staffordshire University, Stoke-on-Trent ST4 2DF, UK
7. Department of System Medicine, Faculty of Medicine and Surgery, University of Rome Tor Vergata, 00133 Rome, Italy; stefani@uniroma2.it
8. Department of Neuroscience and Rehabilitation, University of Ferrara and Center for Translational Neurophysiology of Speech and Communication (CTNSC), Italian Institute of Technology (IIT), 44121 Ferrara, Italy
9. Department of Life, Health and Environmental Sciences, University of L'Aquila, 67100 L'Aquila, Italy; irene.ciancarelli@univaq.it (I.C.); giovanni.morone@univaq.it (G.M.)
10. San Raffaele Institute of Sulmona, Viale dell'Agricoltura, 67039 Sulmona, Italy
* Correspondence: d.debartolo@hsantalucia.it or d.de.bartolo@vu.nl; Tel.: +39-0651501181

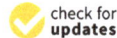

Citation: Cinnera, A.M.; Marrano, S.; De Bartolo, D.; Iosa, M.; Bisirri, A.; Leone, E.; Stefani, A.; Koch, G.; Ciancarelli, I.; Paolucci, S.; et al. Convergent Validity of the Timed Walking Tests with Functional Ambulatory Category in Subacute Stroke. Brain Sci. 2023, 13, 1089. https://doi.org/10.3390/brainsci13071089

Academic Editor: Noureddin Nakhostin Ansari

Received: 22 June 2023
Revised: 14 July 2023
Accepted: 16 July 2023
Published: 18 July 2023

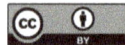

Copyright: © 2023 by the authors. Licensee MDPI, Basel, Switzerland. This article is an open access article distributed under the terms and conditions of the Creative Commons Attribution (CC BY) license (https://creativecommons.org/licenses/by/4.0/).

Abstract: Determining the walking ability of post-stroke patients is crucial for the design of rehabilitation programs and the correct functional information to give to patients and their caregivers at their return home after a neurorehabilitation program. We aimed to assess the convergent validity of three different walking tests: the Functional Ambulation Category (FAC) test, the 10-m walking test (10MeWT) and the 6-minute walking test (6MWT). Eighty walking participants with stroke (34 F, age 64.54 ± 13.02 years) were classified according to the FAC score. Gait speed evaluation was performed with 10MeWT and 6MWT. The cut-off values for FAC and walking tests were calculated using a receiver-operating characteristic (ROC) curve. Area under the curve (AUC) and Youden's index were used to find the cut-off value. Statistical differences were found in all FAC subgroups with respect to walking speed on short and long distances, and in the Rivermead Mobility Index and Barthel Index. Mid-level precision (AUC > 0.7; $p < 0.05$) was detected in the walking speed with respect to FAC score (III vs. IV and IV vs. V). The confusion matrix and the accuracy analysis showed that the most sensitive test was the 10MeWT, with cut-off values of 0.59 m/s and 1.02 m/s. Walking speed cut-offs of 0.59 and 1.02 m/s were assessed with the 10MeWT and can be used in FAC classification in patients with subacute stroke between the subgroups able to walk with supervision and independently on uniform and non-uniform surfaces. Moreover, the overlapping walking speed registered with the two tests, the 10MeWT showed a better accuracy to drive FAC classification.

Keywords: stroke; gait; walking speed; outcome measures; gait disorders; neurologic; correlation of data

1. Introduction

Stroke is a cerebrovascular disorder characterized by the sudden onset of clinical signs and symptoms [1] and represents the second leading cause of death and a major contributor to disability worldwide [2]. Intracerebral or subarachnoid hemorrhage represent 1/3 of strokes, whereas cerebral ischemia represents the remaining 2/3. Among ischemic strokes there are cardioembolic strokes and atherothrombotic strokes, both requiring hospitalization in the acute phase and associated with a high mortality risk [3]. Furthermore, the short-term prognosis of these two types of ischemic stroke is poor compared to that of other ischemic strokes. About half of stroke survivors experience severe and significant long-term daily life disability, such as difficulties with eating, bathing, and working, as well as participating in social activities [4–6]. Motor impairment of the lower limb is common after stroke and represents the most disabling aspect affecting the autonomy of these patients [7,8]. Indeed, walking dysfunction occurs in more than 80% of stroke survivors [9], resulting in long-term gait impairment which impacts the stroke survivor's quality of life [9,10]. To minimize this, recovery of functional mobility and walking function is a priority of the rehabilitation programs offered to people after stroke [11]. Given the clinical importance of walking, a standardized assessment is required [12]. To assess the patient's abilities, clinicians use disability assessment scales [13] and residual motor function scales [14]. However, the clinical motor assessment scales available today for post-stroke patients fail to assess their actual walking ability, and the walking parameters they do assess may not be truly representative of the patient's disability status [15]. To assess walking ability, many different scales, tests and clinical instruments have been proposed. The gold standard for the investigation of gait impairment is the stereophotogrammetric gait analysis combined with electromyography; the use of force platforms and wearable inertial devices have also recently become frequently used [15–17]. Despite the possible disadvantages of using clinical scales or timed tests, they are still measures of first choice among healthcare professionals. Therefore, while most clinical assessments are still based on these scales, it is important that they are adequate to quantify the post-stroke patient's deficit in a simple but accurate way. Among the clinical scales used, the Functional Ambulation Category (FAC) is one of the most common and simple tools to be used for people with locomotor deficit. The FAC scale distinguishes six levels of walking ability based on the amount of physical support required, with scores ranging from 0 (non-functional ambulation) to 5 (independent ambulation on any surface) [18,19]. This easily allows categorization of a patient's level of ambulation and is a familiar scale for many clinicians of different training. Among the most commonly used timed walking tests, there are the 10-m walking test (10MeWT) [20] and the 6-minute walking test (6MWT) [21]. In our previous study, congruency was found between walking speed (measured during 10-m walking test) and walking capacity (measured by 6-minute walking test), and together, these may be useful to assess the safety of patients with respect to the risk of repeated falls in the community, at the point of hospital discharge from a subacute rehabilitation unit [22].

The Functional Ambulation Category and walking tests based on comfortable walking speed are each valid measures of functional mobility in adults with stroke. Characterized by a limited number of items and ease of use, FAC results are strongly correlated to walking speed and endurance, with excellent test-retest reliability and intra-rater reliability among peer assessors [23]. Despite this, there are some aspects of this scale that deserve a deeper analysis, especially for patients not requiring physical assistance. In fact, the differences may be unclear among scores 3 (no need of physical assistance but requiring supervision of a guarding person for safety and verbal cueing), 4 (independent walking on level surface, requiring supervision for negotiating stairs and non-level surfaces) and 5 (independent walking also on stairs and non-level surfaces). Furthermore, the use of these scores could be prone to subjective interpretation and can be influenced by the level of caution needed by the therapist and the self-confidence of the patient. Currently, a deep analysis of the convergent validity between FAC-score and walking tests in subacute stroke is lacking [23]. Convergent validity refers to how closely a score (in our case, the FAC score) is related to the results of other tests that measure the same or similar construct (in our case walking speed measured by 10MeWT and 6MWT). The aim of this study was to evaluate the convergent validity between the FAC test and the 10MeWT and 6MWT, by assessing the stratification of the three levels of the FAC scores related to walking ability. We tested the correlation between the FAC score and gait speed of the two walking tests, finding a cut-off value helpful to pilot the clinical evaluation of the FAC score in patients able to walk independently (with or without supervision). This may meet the need of identifying objective parameters to classify similar patients with the same FAC-score independently by their walking confidence or by the physiotherapist's caution. Specific cut-off points determined by instrumented estimation of walking speed to optimize the convergent validity of the FAC test with walking tests, could also provide objective criteria to improve the reliability of clinical assessments of patients. Furthermore, clinicians may wish to combine the results of these timed tests (10MeWT and 6MWT with the score of the FAC) to obtain a more objective, combined, multidimensional evaluation tool.

2. Materials and Methods

All individuals admitted with stroke to our hospital between September 2018 and December 2020 were invited to participate in the study. Inclusion criteria included (1) first-ever stroke in the sub-acute stage (<180 days from stroke), confirmed with brain imaging test (Computerized Tomography (CT) or Magnetic Resonance Image (MRI)); (2) age between 18 to 85 years and (3) ability to walk. Exclusion criteria were: (1) concomitant lower peripheral motor neuron lesion or orthopedic disease in the lower limbs and (2) presence of moderate to severe cognitive impairment (assessed through the neuropsychological evaluation with the Mini-Mental State Examination < 24 [24]). A cross-sectional evaluation of walking ability was performed using the following tests: FAC, 10MeWT and 6MWT. Demographic characteristics (i.e., age) and clinical characterization via Barthel Index (BI) and Rivermead Mobility Index (RMI) were collected. All scales and tests were administered by an expert clinician with more than ten years of experience in the field of neurorehabilitation. All participants were stratified into three functional groups with respect to the FAC score obtained (FAC III, IV or V), in which FAC III includes ambulators, dependent on supervision, FAC IV includes independent ambulators on level surface only and FAC V includes independent ambulators. After stratification, each patient underwent the 10MeWT and 6MWT with a pause of ten minutes between two evaluations, with random first test assignment [25].

The 10MeWT was conducted at a comfortable gait speed, following a verbal start command when the patient is instructed to walk at a self-selected speed, using whatever walking aids might be needed, such as a walker or cane. Timing was recorded between 2 and 12 m on a total linear distance of 14 m [20,26,27]. The velocity was calculated as distance divided by time. For the 6MWT, participants walked unassisted in a hallway for six minutes. Instructions were scripted as "Walk as fast as comfortable for a period of six minutes. You are allowed to rest as much as you need, but time will not be stopped". Distance was measured at the end of 6 minutes [21,28,29]. Following the participant along the entire duration of the test, the assessor does not use other words of encouragement to influence the patients' walking speed. The protocol was approved by the local independent ethics committee, and all participants provided written informed consent prior to enrolment.

Statistical Analysis

The statistical analysis was performed using SPSS software (version 25, IBM, Armonk, CA, USA). All continuous data are summarized here as mean ± standard deviation (SD) and dichotomous data are reported as percentage. The normal distribution of data for each parameter was verified using the Kolmogorov–Smirnov test applying the Lilliefors correction for continuous data distribution [30] and considering as significant level the highest critical value $p = 0.20$. All normally distributed data ($p > 0.20$) were analyzed using a one-way analysis of variance (one-way ANOVA), while non-normally distributed data were analyzed using the Kruskal–Wallis test. The Kruskal–Wallis test for non-parametric statistics was used to compare the three subgroups (FAC III; IV; V) in terms of their clinical scores. All results with p value < 0.05 were considered significant and investigated with a post-hoc analysis. For the post-hoc analysis has been choosing the Bonferroni correction for multiple comparisons, (with a level of significance of $p < 0.0166$) and the Dwass–Steel–Critchlow–Fligner (DSCF) test for parametric and non-parametric data respectively. Pearson and Spearman correlation analyses were performed on walking speed tests and FAC scores for parametric and non-parametric data respectively. The value of correlation coefficient was categorized as: negligible, from 0 to 0.3; low, from 0.3 to 0.5; moderate, from 0.5 to 0.7; high, from 0.7 to 0.9 and very high from 0.9 to 1, according to Cohen (1988) [31]. Following the correlations, a receiver-operating characteristic (ROC) analysis was conducted on gait speed and FAC. We reported the area under the curve (AUC) and its p value. We classified the AUC as follows: $0.5 < AUC \leq 0.7$ indicates lower precision, $0.7 < AUC \leq 0.9$ indicates mid-level precision, $0.9 < AUC < 1$ indicates high precision, and $AUC = 1$ indicates complete test [32]. The cut-off values for walking features with respect to the FAC score were calculated using a receiver-operating characteristic (ROC). The Youden's index (J) was used to identify the best discriminatory cut-off value in the curve' coordinates via the following formula:

$$J = \text{Sensitivity} + \text{Specificity} - 1 \quad (1)$$

After the cut-off definition, all data were analyzed with a contingency table. The accuracy (ACC) was calculated to reflect predictiveness. The Matthew's correlation coefficient (MCC) was used to obtain both (negative and positive) prediction values. ACC and MCC were respectively calculated as follows:

$$ACC = (Tp + Tn)/(Tp + Tn + Fp + Fn) \quad (2)$$

$$MMC = [(Tp \times Tn) - (Fp*Fn)]/\sqrt{[(Tp + Fp)(Tp + Fn)(Tn + Fp)(Tn + Fn)]}, \quad (3)$$

where Tp are the true positive results; Tn are the true negative results; Fp are the false positive results and Fn are the false negative results.

3. Results

Eighty sub-acute stroke patients were recruited (age: 64.54 ± 13.02 years; 42.5% women; 80.06 ± 35.97 days from stroke [ranged from 19 to 180 days]; 50 with ischemic stroke [70% PACS; 14% TACS; 10% POCS; 6% LACS]) (complete demographic characteristics of the sample and the subgroups are available in Table 1). The Kolmogorov–Smirnov test showed a non-normal distribution for all variables except for age [0.07; $df = 79$; $p > 0.20$]. Following the distribution analysis result, the Kruskal–Wallis test was used to investigate the differences between the FAC subgroups (III vs. IV; IV vs. V; and III vs. V). Statistical analysis showed significant differences existed between each of the administered clinical tests across these three subgroups. These differences underline that the FAC score is related to other clinical scores as well as walking speed. In contrast, no statistical differences between FAC subgroups were observed in the demographic and baseline clinical characteristics, age, gender, lesion side, and stroke type (hemorrhagic or ischemic), which confirms overlapping in these characteristics among the three subgroups of study. Consequently, homogeneity across FAC subgroups indicates that these variables did not have an impact on FAC grouping. In contrast, the post-hoc analysis via DSCF test revealed a significant difference between each subgroup of FAC with respect to Barthel Index and RMI, but not in terms of stroke onset. With the latter, only the FAC III subgroup statistically differed with respect to the other subgroups of FAC IV and V.

Table 1. Demographic characteristics.

	Total Sample	FAC III	FAC IV	FAC V
Sample (n)	80	24	35	21
Male/Female (n)	46/34	11/13	21/14	14/7
Age (years) [a]	64.54 ± 13.02	66.13 ± 13.36	65.03 ± 12.85	61.95 ± 13.2
Isch./hemor. (n)	50/30	18/6	19/16	13/8
Side: Right/Left (n) [b]	43/37	14/10	15/20	14/7
Onset [a]	80.06 ± 35.97	108.05 ± 45.05 **	71.32 ± 23.96 *	62.55 ± 19.92 *
Barthel Index [a]	86.7 ± 18.19	70.29 ± 19.82 **	91.51 ± 14.43 **	97.95 ± 3.73 **
RMI [a]	10.57 ± 3.7	6.74 + 3.16 **	11.57 ± 2.58 **	13.19 ± 1.57 **
FAC [a]	3.96 ± 0.75	3	4	5
10MeWT (s) [a]	/	35.46 ± 27.85 **	15.94 ± 10.43 **	9.87 ± 2.82 **
10MeWT speed (m/s) [a]	/	0.45 ± 0.28 **	0.79 ± 0.31 **	1.08 ± 0.27 **
6MWT (m) [a]	/	160.71 ± 101.81 **	284.35 ± 110.57 **	367.24 ± 83.41 **
6MWT speed (m/s) [a]	/	0.45 ± 0.28 **	0.79 ± 0.31 **	1.02 ± 0.23 **

Abbreviations: n, number; SD, standard deviation; FAC, Functional Ambulation Category; RMI, Rivermead Mobility Index. * Statistically significant with only one subgroup (IV vs. III and V vs. III specifically); ** Statistically significant respect to the other two subgroups; [a] result expressed as mean ± standard deviation; [b] affected hemisphere.

3.1. Correlation Analysis

Non-parametric Spearman (rs) correlation analysis was used to investigate the nature of the relationship between two variables. The correlation analysis showed a significant moderately positive correlation between the FAC score and the walking speed assessed with the administration of the 10MeWT and the 6MWT ($rs = 0.67$, $p < 0.001$; $rs = 0.59$, $p < 0.001$ respectively). Furthermore, a high correlation was shown between the walking speed and the two tests ($rs = 0.927$, $p < 0.001$) (Figure 1). No other statistically significant correlations were found between walking speed and FAC score with respect to the demographic characteristics, confirming the trend observed in the statistical comparison of averages.

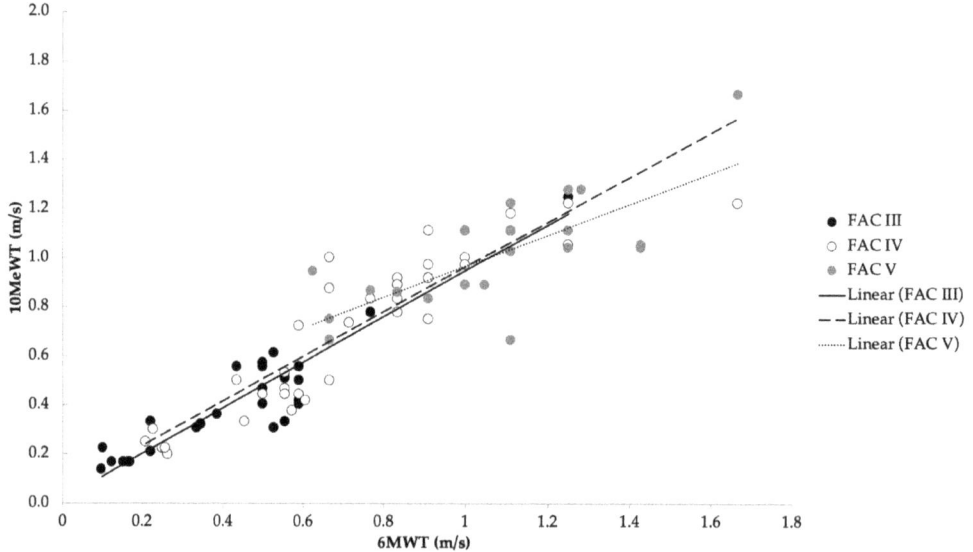

Figure 1. Correlation between average speed in the 10MeWT and 6MWT with respect to the three functional levels of FAC ($rs = 0.97$).

3.2. Receiving Operating Curve and Cut-Off Value

ROC analysis showed a mid-level precision (AUC > 0.70) with statistical significance ($p < 0.05$) in all comparisons of the FAC scores with respect to the walking speed (Figure 2A–D and Table 2).

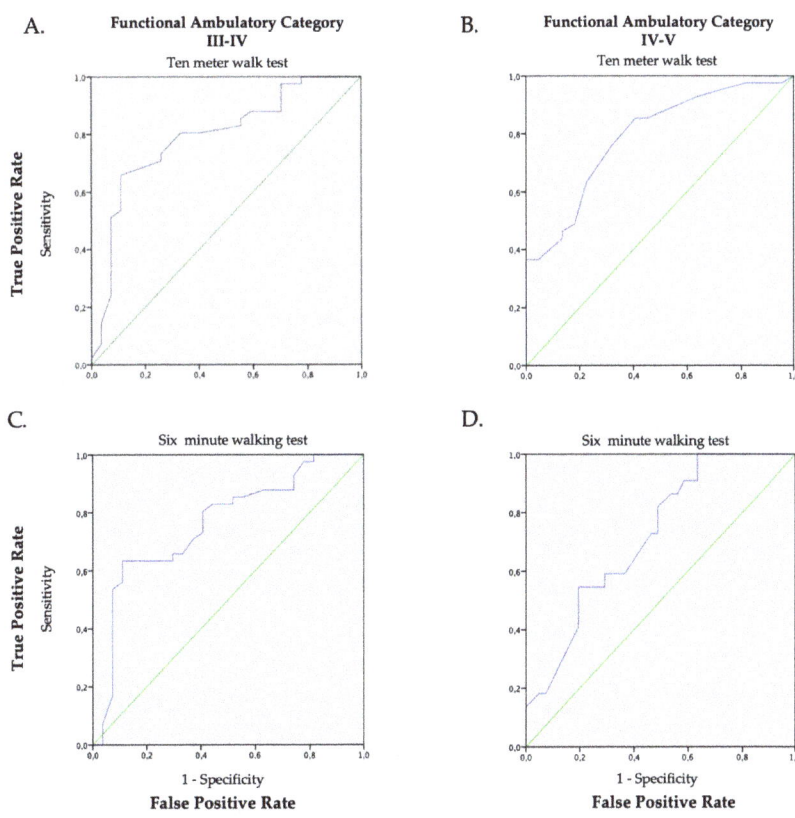

Figure 2. ROC graphs of the walking speed (average), the 10MeWT (Panel (**A**,**B**); AUC 0.79 $p < 0.001$ and AUC 0.79 $p < 0.001$) and the 6MWT (Panel (**C**,**D**); AUC 0.76 $p < 0.001$; AUC 0.72 $p = 0.004$) in relation to the FAC classification (Panel (**A**,**C**): FAC III vs. FAC IV; Panel (**B**,**D**): FAC IV vs. FAC V). The green line is the random classificatory, while the violet one is the prediction of the trade-offs between the true and false positive based on our data.

Table 2. Results of convergent validity analysis of walking speed tests with respect to functional walking levels of FAC.

	Cut-Off	AUC	*p*-Value	Sensitivity	Specificity	ACC	MCC
			FAC III vs. FAC IV				
10MeWT (m/s)	0.59	0.79	<0.001	0.89	0.34	0.75	0.54
6MWT (m/s)	0.66	0.76	<0.001	0.63	0.11	0.74	0.52
			FAC IV vs. FAC V				
10MeWT (s); ws (m/s)	9.76; 1.02	0.79	<0.001	0.85	0.41	0.76	0.46
6MWT (m); ws (m/s)	216; 0.6	0.72	0.004	1	0.63	0.58	0.40

Abbreviations: 10MeWT, 10-m walking test; 6MWT, six minutes walking test; FAC, Functional Ambulation Category; ACC, Accuracy; MCC, Matthew's correlation coefficient; m/s, meters per second.

Despite the mid-level precision in the capacity of both walking speed tests to detect a change in the FAC level, the accuracy was smaller for the 6MWT than for the 10MeWT. Furthermore, the accuracy of the 6MWT is greater between FAC III and FAC IV, than it is between FAC IV and FAC V (0.58); however, the accuracy for the 6MWT is lower than the 10MeWT in both comparisons. This finding was confirmed both in positive direction, and in bidirectional prediction (positive-negative) as indicated by a lowest value of the Matthew's correlation coefficient (MCC) (0.40). All results and the cut-off values identified via Youden's index are reported in Table 2.

3.3. Ischemic vs. Hemorrhagic

Investigating clinical data, comparing the hemorrhagic and clinical subgroups, we did not find any statistical difference. However, the walking speed analysis shows a different trend between the two subgroups and has been investigated with Wilcoxon rank-sum test for unpaired samples. Post-hoc analysis revealed a statistical difference in walking speed in both tests (10MeWT and 6MWT), exclusively in the subgroup of patients in the FAC V subgroup. Specifically, among patients able to walk independently, those who suffered a hemorrhagic stroke had a higher speed for both short and long distances compared to patients with ischemic stroke (all data are available in Table 3).

Table 3. Clinical difference between ischemic and hemorrhagic subgroups. We report statistical significant values as marked with an asterisk (*) for $p \leq 0.05$.

	Ischemic (50)	Hemorrhagic (30)	p-Value
Male/Female (n)	31/19	15/15	
Age (years) [a]	65.98 ± 12.58	62.13 ± 13.60	0.20
Onset (days) [a]	81.12 ± 40.28	78.42 ± 28.80	0.76
Barthel Index [a]	84.5 ± 20.61	90.37 ± 12.72	0.16
RMI [a]	10.24 ± 3.9	11.1 ± 2.78	0.30
FAC [a]	3.9 ± 0.78	4.06 ± 0.69	0.34
10MeWT ws [a]	0.72 ± 0.38	0.87 ± 0.36	0.07
6MWT ws [a]	0.69 ± 0.35	0.85 ± 0.34	0.06
Post-hoc analysis			
FAC III 10MeWT ws [a]	0.43 ± 0.31	0.51 ± 0.17	0.55
FAC III 6MWT ws [a]	0.42 ± 0.30	0.51 ± 0.19	0.51
FAC IV 10MeWT ws [a]	0.78 ± 0.33	0.81 ± 0.30	0.77
FAC IV 6MWT ws [a]	0.77 ± 0.31	0.80 ± 0.30	0.78
FAC V 10MeWT ws [a]	1.00 ± 0.25	1.24 ± 0.21	0.04 *
FAC V 6MWT ws [a]	0.93 ± 0.18	1.17 ± 0.20	0.01 *

Abbreviations: 10MeWT, 10-m walking test; 6MWT, six minutes walking test; RMI, Rivermead Mobility Index; FAC, Functional Ambulation Category; ws, walking speed; [a] result expressed as mean ± standard deviation.

4. Discussion

The present study aimed to investigate the convergent validity of two walking speed tests with FAC evaluation. The two-timed walking tests were highly correlated with each other, and moderately correlated with FAC scores. Despite these highly significant correlations, and the fact that the three FAC levels divides patients into three groups, each group walking with significantly different average walking speeds, there was an overlap among FAC scores in terms of walking speeds. The objective of our analysis was to identify the best cut-off values, by optimizing the clustering of subjects by their FAC scores. In fact, when the participants were grouped based on their FAC score, we found very similar values of walking speed between the two tests, except for subjects classified in the FAC V group. In fact, despite substantially overlapping AUC values, the accuracy and the positive-negative prediction revealed that the walking speed over a short distance (ten meters) is more sensitive to detect bidirectional classification in the FAC IV and V subgroup compared to the walking speed over a longer distance. These subjects, being the most independent, can maintain their speed for six minutes as confirmed by mean speed;

therefore, the incongruence in the cut-off value revealed an unsatisfactory bidirectional accuracy. Moreover, these two subgroups (FAC IV and V) can walk independently in a relatively short time after their stroke, especially compared to the FAC III subgroup. This information can be useful because it unmasks information that is not apparent from only comparing walking speeds over long distances. One possible explanation for the reduced accuracy level of the long-distance walking speed is that the results depend on the subject functional characteristics. The 6MWT was originally used to evaluate cardiopulmonary capacity [33], and later used in neurorehabilitation to assess walking capacity. As demonstrated in a previous work, subjects affected by subacute stroke may manage long-distance walking using various methods [34]. In fact, walking after stroke is demanding in terms of energy expenditure, even for less-affected subjects [34,35]. Some patients decrease velocity, especially in the second half of the test, to manage the latero-lateral oscillations of their trunk, while others maintain a stable velocity, accepting an increment of the trunk oscillation [36,37]. However, the latter motor behavior, while it leads to a higher walking capacity, is more correlated with the risk of falls. In a previous study, this incongruence in long-distance walking and the higher risk of fall was noted [22]. Notwithstanding, gait speed is fundamental in the prognosis of community ambulation outcomes among inpatients discharged from stroke rehabilitation care [38]. Our results suggest that these are not the only parameters that impact walking ability when assessed over long distances.

In summary, in the 10MeWT we found useful cut-off values (0.59 m/s and 1.02 m/s) with a good bidirectional predictive value with respect to all FAC subgroups considered. This positive convergent validity can support the gait evaluation of subacute patients, especially in the differentiation between the higher level of walking performance. In line with this observation, both FAC score and speed on the short distance are predictors of fall risk [39,40].

However, it should be reported that the patients able to walk everywhere independently (allocated in the FAC V subgroup) were highly heterogeneous and there was a statistical difference in walking speed between the etiopathogenesis of stroke (ischemic vs. hemorrhagic). Patients with hemorrhagic stroke with the maximum score of FAC showed a high average speed in both tests compared to subjects with ischemic stroke in the same FAC subgroup, notwithstanding an overlap in other clinical and demographics variables. This observation is reported previously in the literature, where hemorrhagic stroke showed a greater improvement in gait skills, and specifically in walking speed [41].

In the literature, walking measurements (functional walk distances and self-paced speed) were correlated with balance function, stroke specifics and global impairment score [42]. Our results are important because they add knowledge to the use of the short distance walking velocity tests in a specific pathological population, and because they are the most simple, inexpensive, and commonly used tests. A large body of literature agrees with the fact that a reduced walking speed is generally correlated to a major risk for disability, cognitive impairment, institutionalization, falls and mortality [43].

In summary, walking ability is fundamental for the patient's social participation when returning home after hospital and its assessment with simple scales and tests is important. Our data support the use of the FAC test and the 10MeWT especially in high level walking patients in the subacute phase of stroke, before social reintegration to potentially reduce their risk of falls.

4.1. Limitations

Our results are not generalizable to all stroke populations; in fact, the subacute phase of stroke differs from the chronic phase and is characterized as those without a stable functional status, with basic motor intentions and actual motor actions that are slightly misaligned. This complex relationship calls into question the locomotor body schema and its potential and necessary neuroplasticity modification during the recovery after stroke [44]. Present conclusions are based on collapsed data of hemorrhagic and ischemic stroke, albeit reproducing the distribution of pathogenesis of stroke [45] as in the general population. However, the recovery patterns are somewhat different (i.e., in walking speed). In the present study, the limited number of patients included in the subgroups (ischemic and hemorrhagic) did not allow for separated ROC analysis based on FAC scores and walking speed. Moreover, all scales and tests were assessed by only one clinician; thus, inter-rater reliability of the FAC test could not be calculated. However, there are reports in the literature that the FAC scale has good inter-rater reliability ($\kappa = 0.72$) [46]. This could have mitigated possible errors resulting from lack of agreement between multiple raters. Despite this, to confirm the current deductions, future studies should consider the above-mentioned limitations.

4.2. Future Perspective

Instrumental evaluation of walking speed would be useful to investigate the convergent validity with FAC test in future research. Specifically, the use of cutting-edge technologies would support investigators in a more accurate quantification of cut-off values which can be used in clinical practice [47–49]. Moreover, the correlation between instrumented walking speed cut-offs and other clinical scales (i.e., Fugl–Meyer Assessment scale, Berg Balance scale, National Institute of Health Stroke scale) will provide additional information about the involvement of motor, sensory, and joint functions and gait balance skills. Additionally, inter-rater reliability could be provided to evaluate the potential for bias in administration. Finally, stratification on a larger sample could reveal different characteristics about gait performance and more precise cut-off values. In particular, the differentiation between ischemic and haemorrhagic stroke and between lacunar and non-lacunar ischemic stroke can provide new insight about the correlation of pathophysiology and clinical gait features in these populations. This differentiation is important given the different clinical features reported for lacunar and non-lacunar stroke [50,51].

5. Conclusions

The evaluation of walking velocity is crucial in the routine assessment of functional status of patients following subacute stroke, and in designing personalized neurorehabilitation programs to improve post-discharge outcomes. From this investigation we found a good convergent validity between 10MeWT and FAC test scores, with a clear cut-off in terms of walking speed (0.59 and 1.02 m/s). The assessment on this short distance can be used to drive the attribution of the highest level of FAC score. In contrast, the convergent validity was lower between FAC score and the walking speed assessed over a long distance than in the 6MWT for FAC IV and V subgroups. This information suggests that it is necessary to carefully investigate patients with high functional levels over long distances, especially in the hemorrhagic stroke subgroup, who show a higher average speed compared to ischemic patients. Moreover, FAC IV and V subgroups start to walk independently about at the same time following stroke, making it more difficult to use the onset variable to drive their allocation. The assessment of walking autonomy using the FAC test is fundamental to describe the independency of patient; however, when there are some doubts about the FAC score, clinicians could evaluate the timed assessment of walking speed on a short linear distance (such as by the 10MeWT) to differentiate the gait level of the patient.

Author Contributions: Conceptualization, A.M.C. and G.M.; methodology, A.M.C. and M.I.; investigation, G.M.; data curation, S.M.; data analysis, A.M.C.; writing—original draft preparation, A.M.C., D.D.B. and E.L.; writing—review and editing, all authors; supervision, G.M.; project administration, G.M. All authors have read and agreed to the published version of the manuscript.

Funding: This research received no external funding.

Institutional Review Board Statement: The study was approved by the Local Independent Ethics Committee of IRCCS Santa Lucia Foundation (Rome, Italy) (protocol number: CE/PROG.819).

Informed Consent Statement: Written informed consent was obtained from all subjects involved in the study.

Data Availability Statement: The data that support the findings of this study are available on request to the corresponding author.

Acknowledgments: The authors would like to thank all patients and their family and caregivers.

Conflicts of Interest: The authors declare no conflict of interest.

References

1. Bushnell, C.; Bettger, J.P.; Cockroft, K.M.; Cramer, S.C.; Edelen, M.O.; Hanley, D.; Yenokyan, G. Chronic stroke outcome measures for motor function intervention trials: Expert panel recommendations. *Circ. Cardiovasc. Qual. Outcomes* **2015**, *8* (Suppl. S3), S163–S169. [CrossRef] [PubMed]
2. Kuriakose, D.; Xiao, Z. Pathophysiology and treatment of stroke: Present status and future perspectives. *Int. J. Mol. Sci.* **2020**, *21*, 7609. [CrossRef] [PubMed]
3. Mendis, S. Stroke disability and rehabilitation of stroke: World Health Organization perspective. *Int. J. Stroke* **2013**, *8*, 3–4. [CrossRef]
4. Pollock, A.; Baer, G.; Campbell, P.; Choo, P.L.; Forster, A.; Morris, J.; Pomeroy, V.M.; Langhorne, P. Physical rehabilitation approaches for the recovery of function and mobility following stroke. *Cochrane Database Syst. Rev.* **2014**, *4*, CD001920.
5. De Bartolo, D.; Morone, G.; Lupo, A.; Aloise, F.; Baricich, A.; Di Francesco, D.; Iosa, M. From paper to informatics: The Post Soft Care-App, an easy-to-use and fast tool to help therapists identify unmet needs in stroke patients. *Funct. Neurol.* **2018**, *33*, 200–205. [PubMed]
6. Kollen, B.; Van De Port, I.; Lindeman, E.; Twisk, J.; Kwakkel, G. Predicting improvement in gait after stroke: A longitudinal prospective study. *Stroke* **2005**, *36*, 2676–2680. [CrossRef]
7. Mohan, D.M.; Khandoker, A.H.; Wasti, S.A.; Ismail Ibrahim Ismail Alali, S.; Jelinek, H.F.; Khalaf, K. Assessment Methods of Post-stroke Gait: A Scoping Review of Technology-Driven Approaches to Gait Characterization and Analysis. *Front. Neurol.* **2021**, *12*, 650024. [CrossRef]
8. Duncan, P.W.; Zorowitz, R.; Bates, B.; Choi, J.Y.; Glasberg, J.J.; Graham, G.D.; Katz, R.C.; Lamberty, K.; Reker, D. Management of Adult Stroke Rehabilitation Care: A clinical practice guideline. *Stroke* **2005**, *36*, e100–e143. [CrossRef]
9. Dimyan, M.A.; Cohen, L.G. Neuroplasticity in the context of motor rehabilitation after stroke. *Nat. Rev. Neurol.* **2011**, *7*, 76–85. [CrossRef]
10. Martino Cinnera, A.; Bonnì, S.; Pellicciari, M.C.; Giorgi, F.; Caltagirone, C.; Koch, G. Health-related quality of life (HRQoL) after stroke: Positive relationship between lower extremity and balance recovery. *Top. Stroke Rehabil.* **2020**, *27*, 534–540. [CrossRef]
11. Schindl, M.R.; Forstner, C.; Kern, H.; Zipko, H.T.; Rupp, M.; Zifko, U.A. Evaluation of a German version of the Rivermead Mobility Index (RMI) in acute and chronic stroke patients. *Eur. J. Neurol.* **2000**, *7*, 523–528. [CrossRef]
12. Van Bloemendaal, M.; Bout, W.; Bus, S.A.; Nollet, F.; Geurts, A.C.; Beelen, A. Validity and reproducibility of the Functional Gait Assessment in persons after stroke. *Clin. Rehabil.* **2019**, *33*, 94–103. [CrossRef]
13. Ohura, T.; Hase, K.; Nakajima, Y.; Nakayama, T. Validity and reliability of a performance evaluation tool based on the modified Barthel Index for stroke patients. *BMC Med. Res. Methodol.* **2017**, *17*, 131. [CrossRef]
14. Lim, J.Y.; An, S.H.; Park, D.S. Walking velocity and modified rivermead mobility index as discriminatory measures for functional ambulation classification of chronic stroke patients. *Hong Kong Physiother. J.* **2019**, *39*, 125–132. [CrossRef]
15. De Bartolo, D.; Belluscio, V.; Vannozzi, G.; Morone, G.; Antonucci, G.; Giordani, G.; Santucci, S.; Resta, F.; Marinozzi, F.; Bini, F.; et al. Sensorized Assessment of Dynamic Locomotor Imagery in People with Stroke and Healthy Subjects. *Sensors* **2020**, *20*, 4545. [CrossRef]
16. Caldas, R.; Mundt, M.; Potthast, W.; de Lima Neto, F.B.; Markert, B. A systematic review of gait analysis methods based on inertial sensors and adaptive algorithms. *Gait Posture* **2017**, *57*, 204–210. [CrossRef]
17. Picerno, P.; Iosa, M.; D'Souza, C.; Benedetti, M.G.; Paolucci, S.; Morone, G. Wearable inertial sensors for human movement analysis: A five-year update. *Expert Rev. Med. Devices* **2021**, *18* (Suppl. S1), 79–94. [CrossRef]
18. Wade, D.T. Measurement in neurological rehabilitation. *Curr. Opin. Neurol. Neurosurg.* **1992**, *5*, 682–686.
19. Price, R.; Choy, N.L. Investigating the relationship of the functional gait assessment to spatiotemporal parameters of gait and quality of life in individuals with stroke. *J. Geriatr. Phys. Ther.* **2019**, *42*, 256–264. [CrossRef]
20. Collen, F.M.; Wade, D.T.; Bradshaw, C.M. Mobility after stroke: Reliability of measures of impairment and disability. *Int. Disabil. Stud.* **1990**, *12*, 6–9. [CrossRef]
21. Butland, R.J.; Pang, J.; Gross, E.R.; Woodcock, A.A.; Geddes, D.M. Two-, six-, and 12-minute walking tests in respiratory disease. *Br. Med. J. (Clin. Res. Ed.)* **1982**, *284*, 1607. [CrossRef] [PubMed]
22. Morone, G.; Iosa, M.; Pratesi, L.; Paolucci, S. Can overestimation of walking ability increase the risk of falls in people in the subacute stage after stroke on their return home? *Gait Posture* **2014**, *39*, 965–970. [CrossRef] [PubMed]
23. Mehrholz, J.; Wagner, K.; Rutte, K.; Meißner, D.; Pohl, M. Predictive validity and responsiveness of the functional ambulation category in hemiparetic patients after stroke. *Arch. Phys. Med. Rehabil.* **2007**, *88*, 1314–1319. [CrossRef] [PubMed]
24. Tombaugh, T.N.; McIntyre, N.J. The mini-mental state examination: A comprehensive review. *J. Am. Geriatr. Soc.* **1992**, *40*, 922–935. [CrossRef] [PubMed]

25. Matos Casano, H.A.; Anjum, F. Six-Minute Walk Test. 2023 April 27. In *StatPearls*; StatPearls Publishing: Treasure Island, FL, USA, 2023; PMID: 35015445.
26. Middleton, A.; Fritz, S.L.; Lusardi, M. Walking speed: The functional vital sign. *J. Aging Phys. Act.* **2015**, *23*, 314–322. [CrossRef]
27. Lindholm, B.; Nilsson, M.H.; Hansson, O.; Hagell, P. The clinical significance of 10-m walk test standardizations in Parkinson's disease. *J. Neurol.* **2018**, *265*, 1829–1835. [CrossRef]
28. Regan, E.; Middleton, A.; Stewart, J.C.; Wilcox, S.; Pearson, J.L.; Fritz, S. The six-minute walk test as a fall risk screening tool in community programs for persons with stroke: A cross-sectional analysis. *Top. Stroke Rehabil.* **2020**, *27*, 118–126. [CrossRef]
29. Dunn, A.; Marsden, D.L.; Nugent, E.; Van Vliet, P.; Spratt, N.J.; Attia, J.; Callister, R. Protocol variations and six-minute walk test performance in stroke survivors: A systematic review with meta-analysis. *Stroke Res. Treat.* **2015**, *2015*, 484813. [CrossRef]
30. Lilliefors, H.W. On the Kolmogorov-Smirnov test for normality with mean and variance unknown. *J. Am. Stat. Assoc.* **1967**, *62*, 399–402. [CrossRef]
31. Cohen, J. Set correlation and contingency tables. *Appl. Psychol. Meas.* **1988**, *12*, 425–434. [CrossRef]
32. Greiner, M.; Pfeiffer, D.; Smith, R.D. Principles and practical application of the receiver-operating characteristic analysis for diagnostic tests. *Prev. Vet. Med.* **2000**, *45*, 23–41. [CrossRef]
33. Hamilton, D.M.; Haennel, R.G. Validity and reliability of the 6-minute walk test in a cardiac rehabilitation population. *J. Cardiopulm. Rehabil. Prev.* **2000**, *20*, 156–164. [CrossRef]
34. Lefeber, N.; De Buyzer, S.; Dassen, N.; De Keersmaecker, E.; Kerckhofs, E.; Swinnen, E. Energy consumption and cost during walking with different modalities of assistance after stroke: A systematic review and meta-analysis. *Disabil. Rehabil.* **2020**, *42*, 1650–1666. [CrossRef]
35. Delussu, A.S.; Morone, G.; Iosa, M.; Bragoni, M.; Traballesi, M.; Paolucci, S. Physiological responses and energy cost of walking on the Gait Trainer with and without body weight support in subacute stroke patients. *J. Neuroeng. Rehabil.* **2014**, *11*, 54. [CrossRef]
36. Kołcz, A.; Urbacka-Josek, J.; Kowal, M.; Dymarek, R.; Paprocka-Borowicz, M. Evaluation of postural stability and transverse abdominal muscle activity in overweight post-stroke patients: A prospective, observational study. *Diabetes Metab. Syndr. Obes. Targets Ther.* **2020**, *13*, 451. [CrossRef]
37. Iosa, M.; Morone, G.; Fusco, A.; Pratesi, L.; Bragoni, M.; Coiro, P.; Multari, M.; Venturiero, V.; De Angelis, D.; Paolucci, S. Effects of walking endurance reduction on gait stability in patients with stroke. *Stroke Res. Treat.* **2012**, *2012*, 810415. [CrossRef]
38. Mulder, M.; Nijland, R.H.; van de Port, I.G.; van Wegen, E.E.; Kwakkel, G. Prospectively classifying community walkers after stroke: Who are they? *Arch. Phys. Med. Rehabil.* **2019**, *100*, 2113–2118. [CrossRef]
39. Morone, G.; Martino Cinnera, A.; Paolucci, T.; Beatriz, H.D.R.; Paolucci, S.; Iosa, M. Clinical features of fallers among inpatient subacute stroke: An observational cohort study. *Neurol. Sci.* **2020**, *41*, 2599–2604. [CrossRef]
40. Persson, C.U.; Hansson, P.O.; Sunnerhagen, K.S. Clinical tests performed in acute stroke identify the risk of falling during the first year: Postural stroke study in Gothenburg (POSTGOT). *J. Rehabil. Med.* **2011**, *43*, 348–353. [CrossRef]
41. Obembe, A.O.; Olaogun, M.O.B.; Adedoyin, R.A. Differences in gait between haemorrhagic and ischaemic stroke survivors. *J. Med. Med. Sci.* **2012**, *3*, 556–561.
42. Eng, J.J.; Chu, K.S.; Dawson, A.S.; Kim, C.M.; Hepburn, K.E. Functional walk tests in individuals with stroke: Relation to perceived exertion and myocardial exertion. *Stroke* **2002**, *33*, 756–761. [CrossRef] [PubMed]
43. Liu, B.; Hu, X.; Zhang, Q.; Fan, Y.; Li, J.; Zou, R.; Zhang, M.; Wang, X.; Wang, J. Usual walking speed and all-cause mortality risk in older people: A systematic review and meta-analysis. *Gait Posture* **2016**, *44*, 172–177. [CrossRef] [PubMed]
44. Cramer, S.C.; Sur, M.; Dobkin, B.H.; O'Brien, C.; Sanger, T.D.; Trojanowski, J.Q.; Vinogradov, S. Harnessing neuroplasticity for clinical applications. *Brain* **2011**, *134*, 1591–1609. [CrossRef] [PubMed]
45. Cassel, C.K.; Ek, K. Demography and epidemiology of age-associated neuronal impairment. In *Functional Neurobiology of Aging*; Academic Press: Cambridge, MA, USA, 2001; pp. 31–50.
46. Holden, M.K.; Gill, K.M.; Magliozzi, M.R.; Nathan, J.; Piehl-Baker, L. Clinical gait assessment in the neurologically impaired Reliability and meaningfulness. *Phys Ther.* **1984**, *64*, 35–40. [CrossRef]
47. Walsh, K.B. Non-invasive sensor technology for prehospital stroke diagnosis: Current status and future directions. *Int. J. Stroke* **2019**, *14*, 592–602. [CrossRef]
48. Verna, V.; De Bartolo, D.; Iosa, M.; Fadda, L.; Pinto, G.; Caltagirone, C.; De Angelis, S.; Tramontano, M. Te.M.P.O., an app for using temporal musical mismatch in post-stroke neurorehabilitation: A preliminary randomized con-trolled study. *NeuroRehabilitation* **2020**, *47*, 201–208. [CrossRef]
49. De Bartolo, D.; D'amico, I.; Iosa, M.; Aloise, F.; Morone, G.; Marinozzi, F.; Bini, F.; Paolucci, S.; Spadini, E. Validation of SuPerSense, a Sensorized Surface for the Evaluation of Posture Perception in Supine Position. *Sensors* **2023**, *23*, 424. [CrossRef]
50. Jiang, S.; Wu, S.; Zhang, S.; Wu, B. Advances in understanding the pathogenesis of lacunar stroke: From pathology and pathophysiology to neuroimaging. *Cerebrovasc. Dis.* **2021**, *50*, 588–596. [CrossRef]
51. Rudilosso, S.; Rodríguez-Vázquez, A.; Urra, X.; Arboix, A. The potential impact of neuroimaging and translational research on the clinical management of lacunar stroke. *Int. J. Mol. Sci.* **2022**, *23*, 1497. [CrossRef]

Disclaimer/Publisher's Note: The statements, opinions and data contained in all publications are solely those of the individual author(s) and contributor(s) and not of MDPI and/or the editor(s). MDPI and/or the editor(s) disclaim responsibility for any injury to people or property resulting from any ideas, methods, instructions or products referred to in the content.

Article

Clinical, Neuroimaging and Robotic Measures Predict Long-Term Proprioceptive Impairments following Stroke

Matthew J. Chilvers [1,2], Deepthi Rajashekar [1,2], Trevor A. Low [1,2], Stephen H. Scott [3,4,5] and Sean P. Dukelow [1,2,*]

1. Department of Clinical Neurosciences, Cumming School of Medicine, University of Calgary, 3330 Hospital Drive NW, Calgary, AB T2N 4N1, Canada; matthew.chilvers@ucalgary.ca (M.J.C.); deepthi.rajasheka1@ucalgary.ca (D.R.); talow@ucalgary.ca (T.A.L.)
2. Hotchkiss Brain Institute, University of Calgary, 3330 Hospital Drive NW, Calgary, AB T2N 4N1, Canada
3. Department of Biomedical and Molecular Sciences, Queens University, Kingston, ON K7L 3N6, Canada; steve.scott@queensu.ca
4. Centre for Neuroscience Studies, Queens University, Kingston, ON K7L 3N6, Canada
5. Providence Care Hospital, Kingston, ON K7L 3N6, Canada
* Correspondence: spdukelo@ucalgary.ca; Tel.: +1-403-944-5930

Abstract: Proprioceptive impairments occur in ~50% of stroke survivors, with 20–40% still impaired six months post-stroke. Early identification of those likely to have persistent impairments is key to personalizing rehabilitation strategies and reducing long-term proprioceptive impairments. In this study, clinical, neuroimaging and robotic measures were used to predict proprioceptive impairments at six months post-stroke on a robotic assessment of proprioception. Clinical assessments, neuroimaging, and a robotic arm position matching (APM) task were performed for 133 stroke participants two weeks post-stroke (12.4 ± 8.4 days). The APM task was also performed six months post-stroke (191.2 ± 18.0 days). Robotics allow more precise measurements of proprioception than clinical assessments. Consequently, an overall APM Task Score was used as ground truth to classify proprioceptive impairments at six months post-stroke. Other APM performance parameters from the two-week assessment were used as predictive features. Clinical assessments included the Thumb Localisation Test (TLT), Behavioural Inattention Test (BIT), Functional Independence Measure (FIM) and demographic information (age, sex and affected arm). Logistic regression classifiers were trained to predict proprioceptive impairments at six months post-stroke using data collected two weeks post-stroke. Models containing robotic features, either alone or in conjunction with clinical and neuroimaging features, had a greater area under the curve (AUC) and lower Akaike Information Criterion (AIC) than models which only contained clinical or neuroimaging features. All models performed similarly with regard to accuracy and F1-score (>70% accuracy). Robotic features were also among the most important when all features were combined into a single model. Predicting long-term proprioceptive impairments, using data collected as early as two weeks post-stroke, is feasible. Identifying those at risk of long-term impairments is an important step towards improving proprioceptive rehabilitation after a stroke.

Keywords: proprioception; stroke; prediction; robotics; modeling; stroke recovery; stroke outcomes

1. Introduction

1.1. Proprioception and Its Importance after Stroke

Proprioception, described by Sir Charles Sherrington [1], refers to the sense of limb position and movement, originating from receptors within the muscles and joints themselves [2]. The proprioceptive sense is important in allowing us to move our limbs freely in space and interact with our surroundings. Following stroke, proprioceptive impairments are common, typically observed in approximately 50% of stroke survivors [3,4]. Proprioceptive impairments have been associated with a reduced ability to perform activities of daily living (ADLs) post-stroke, independent of motor deficits [5–8]. Mitigating these impairments can be important for restoring independent quality of life. Recent studies assessing proprioception using robotic technology have, however, demonstrated that impairments are still apparent in 20–40% of stroke survivors six-months after stroke [9,10]. This is not necessarily surprising considering that evidence-based interventions for treating proprioception post-stroke are lacking (for an in-depth review, see [11,12]). Unfortunately, little is often done clinically to target proprioceptive recovery, and more than half of therapists believe that current treatments for somatosensory impairment are ineffective, lacking confidence in their ability to treat somatosensory deficits [13]. Early identification of individuals at high-risk of suffering chronic proprioceptive impairments is an important step towards personalized approaches to rehabilitation. Doing so would highlight those who would benefit from rehabilitation with some focus on restoring proprioception.

1.2. Predictors of Proprioceptive Impairment

Within stroke centres, clinical assessments and neuroimaging are a standard component of patient care, and thus are readily available for use in predicting patient outcomes. Previous literature has assessed the relationship of many clinical and neuroimaging measures with assessments of proprioception in the subacute stage post-stroke [7,14–18]. In particular, clinical measures of attention and activities of daily living, such as the Behavioural Inattention Test (BIT) and Functional Independence Measure (FIM), have been closely associated with measures of proprioception [7,14–18]. Furthermore, studies have investigated the relationship between neuroimaging measures, such as lesion volume and region-specific damage, and robotic assessments of proprioception [10,16,19–22]. Greater lesion volume has been linked with a worse proprioceptive performance post-stroke [16,19–21], while additional studies have used voxel-based lesion-symptom mapping (VLSM) to assess the statistical relationships between lesioned brain regions and proprioceptive performance after stroke [10,20–22]. In comparison to motor recovery, where many studies have tried to identify early predictors of recovery [23–28], few have focused on predicting long-term proprioceptive recovery [10,19,29].

1.3. Aims and Hypothesis

The utility of clinical, neuroimaging and robotic measures in predicting and classifying long-term proprioceptive outcomes has been under-explored. The purpose of this study, therefore, was to evaluate the ability of clinical, neuroimaging and robotic measures, collected within the first two weeks post-stroke, to predict proprioceptive impairments six-months post-stroke both independently of and in combination with each other. Considering the previously established associations between clinical measures, neuroimaging and proprioceptive measures, it was hypothesized that models containing just clinical or just neuroimaging features would reasonably predict six-month proprioceptive impairments. Furthermore, it was hypothesized that robotic features, alone and in conjunction with clinical and neuroimaging features, would lead to superior predictions in terms of accuracy and area under the receiver-operator characteristic (ROC) curve (AUC).

2. Materials and Methods

2.1. Participant Recruitment

Participants for the current study were recruited from a pool of participants taking part in a larger, ongoing prospective cohort study called RESTART, which documents stroke recovery using robotics and neuroimaging over the first six-month post-stroke.

2.1.1. Study Inclusion Criteria

Participant inclusion criteria for the current study was: (1) 18+ years of age, (2) first time ischemic or hemorrhagic unilateral stroke, (3) could follow task instructions, (4) completed a robotic arm position matching (APM) task at both two weeks and six months post-stroke, (5) had a clinical assessment collected at approximately two weeks post-stroke and (6) had clinical neuroimaging collected (Magnetic Resonance Imaging (MRI) or Computed Tomography (CT)).

2.1.2. Study Exclusion Criteria

Participant exclusion criteria were: (1) apraxia [30], (2) contraindications to neuroimaging, (3) other diagnosed neurological disorders (multiple sclerosis, Parkinson's disease, etc.), or (4) upper extremity orthopedic injury/pain that impacted their ability to perform the robotic assessments.

2.2. Robotic Assessment of Proprioception

Proprioception was assessed in the current study, using a robotic APM task [3,7], at two time points post-stroke, approximately two weeks (12.4 ± 8.4 days) and six months (191.2 ± 18.0 days) post-stroke. The APM task was performed in a Kinarm Exoskeleton robotic device (Kinarm., Kingston, ON, Canada). Participants sat in the wheelchair base of the robotic device with their arms supported in the horizontal plane by custom-fitted arm-troughs (Figure 1A). The linkages on the robot were then adjusted to fit each participant, such that the length of the robotic arms matched those of the participant and the robotic joints lined up with the participant's shoulders and elbows. Once each participant was set up, they were wheeled into the virtual reality environment, and vision of the arms was occluded by an opaque shutter and bib.

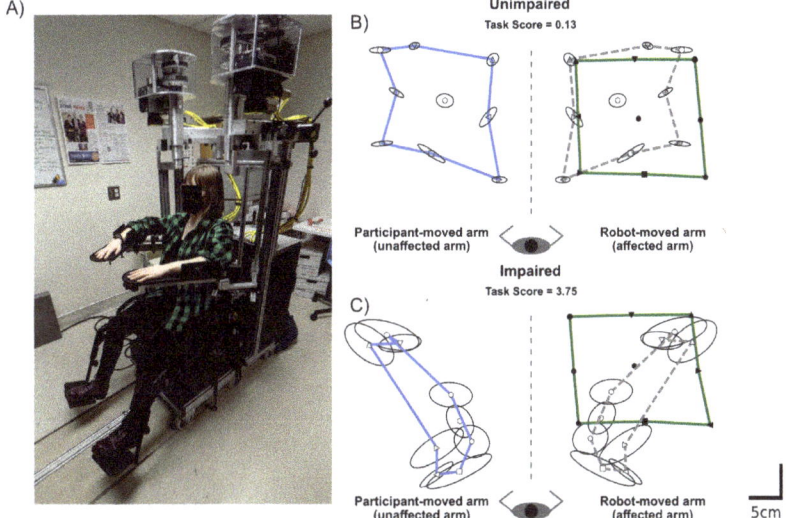

Figure 1. Robotic Assessment of Proprioception—(**A**) Kinarm Exoskeleton Lab (Kingston, ON, Canada) used to perform the robotic assessment of proprioception (Arm Position Matching task). (**B**) Exemplar Arm Position Matching task performance of an unimpaired stroke participant. The robot moved the affected right arm. Closed symbols indicate the mean nine target positions where the robot moved the participant's hand. For illustrative purposes, the green line connects the mean hand position of the eight outer targets. The participant matched with their unaffected left arm. Open symbols indicate the mean, matched hand position of the unaffected arm. Again, for illustrative purposes, the blue line connects the eight outer targets. Ellipsoids represent the variability (one standard deviation) in matched position around each target. For illustrative purposes, the participant's matched positions have been reflected across the midline onto the robot moved arm. The dashed grey line connects the reflected outer 8 targets. (**C**) Same format as B, except an exemplar from a stroke participant with an impairment on the Arm Position Matching task is provided.

The APM task began with the robot moving the participant's affected arm to one of nine-spatial targets. These targets were oriented in a 20 cm × 20 cm square, with eight outer targets surrounding a central target. Once the robot had finished moving the participant's affected arm to the first target, they were instructed to attempt to mirror match the position of the robot-moved (affected) arm, with their unaffected arm. Participants then verbalized that they felt that they were in a matched position, and the robot operator cued the robot to move the arm to the next target. The robot moved the participant's arm between the nine targets with a bell-shaped velocity profile and a maximum speed of 0.3–0.5 m/s. Each target was assessed in a pseudorandomized order, once per block. Six blocks were performed, so that there were 54 trials in the APM task. Exemplars of the APM task, from participants with and without an APM task impairment, are shown in Figure 1B,C, respectively.

Robotic assessments allow for objective measures of sensorimotor function, compared to standard clinical assessments [31]. As such, performance on the APM task was used as the primary measure of proprioception, to classify participants to those with and without impairments at six months post-stroke. Performance parameters from the APM task are described in Section 2.3. The APM task parameters used as features in the predictive models are described in Section 2.6.

2.3. Quantifying Proprioceptive Performance and Impairments

Performance on the APM task was quantified by a global measure called an APM Task Score, which was used to infer the presence of proprioceptive impairments. The APM Task Score is a composite measure, based on a number of parameters, each reflective of a different component of APM task performance. These parameters include: (1) Absolute Error, which quantifies the absolute distance in the mirror-matched position between the robot-moved arm and the participant-moved arm, (2) Variability, which measures the trial-to-trial variance in the participant's ability to match limb position, (3) Contraction Expansion, which describes the perception of the workspace in which the robot moved their affected arm as either shrunken or enlarged, and (4) Shift, which captures a perceived systematic shift of the robot moved arm. Each parameter was calculated in the x and y directions. Further details on these parameters and how they are calculated have been previously published [3,7,32].

Each parameter was first converted into a z-score based on a large normative data set, composed of 2229 previously collected APM task assessments from 799 control participants with no history of neurological disorders. For each parameter, data from the control set was first converted to a normal distribution by Box-Cox transformation and outliers were removed from the data that were outside ±3.29 SDs from the mean. Weighted linear regression models were used to remove the influence of age, sex and handedness [32–34]. Parameter z-scores were then calculated, with a z-score of zero equal to the mean performance of controls.

The next step was to convert these parameter z-scores into the APM Task Score. Parameter z-scores were first transformed such that for any given parameter, the best score was indicated by a score of zero and larger values indicative of worse performance [32–34]. Next, the root sum square (RSS) distance was calculated for each of these transformed scores and converted into a z-score by the same transformations used to convert parameter scores to z-scores. The final step in calculating the APM Task Score was to convert the z-score of the RSS distance into a zeta-score using the zeta-transformation [32]. Robotic analysis was performed using Dexterit-E version 3.9 (Kinarm, Kingston, ON, Canada).

The APM Task Score allows for comparisons in performance between stroke and control participants to be made, accounting for each participant's age, sex and handedness [32]. Since the APM Task Score is a normative score, based on a large control dataset (n = 799), it adopts the same features as a normal distribution. As such, 95% of healthy control participants, of the same age, sex and handedness as any given participant, have an APM Task Score less than 1.96 [32]. APM Task Scores greater than 1.96 indicated abnormal performance on the APM task and was used to infer if a participant had a proprioceptive impairment at six months. While the APM Task Score was used to quantify the binary proprioceptive outcome at six months, each of the parameter scores collected at two weeks were used as predictive features in the models trained. Further details on the APM Task Score, and each of these processes and calculations, have been extensively published and are best described in [34]. Additional documentation outlining these details can be freely downloaded at (https://kinarm.com/download/kst-summary-analysis-version-3-9/; accessed on 4 June 2022).

2.4. Clinical Assessment

Participants also completed a battery of clinical assessments two weeks post-stroke, collected along with the initial robotic assessment. Clinical assessments included the: Thumb Localization Test (TLT) [35], BIT [36] and FIM [37]. Scores from these clinical assessments were also used as features to predict proprioceptive impairments on the APM task at six months post-stroke, as described in Section 2.6.

The TLT was collected as a clinical measure of proprioception. In the TLT, with the participant's eyes closed, the clinician moves the affected arm to a fixed position and asks the participant to try to pinch the thumb of that limb with the opposing limb. The clinician gives a score ranging from zero to three (0 = quickly and accurately locates thumb, 1 = locates thumb with a minor corrective movement, 2 = locates thumb by chance or uses hand or other fingers as a guide, and 3 = unable to locate thumb at all, or uses arm as a guide). The BIT was collected due to the close association between hemispatial neglect and proprioceptive impairment [15–18]. The conventional sub-tests of the BIT were used, which included the following pencil and paper tasks: line bisection, line cancellation, letter cancellation, star cancellation, shape copying, and figure drawing. Lower scores indicate worse attentional deficits, with scores less than 130 indicative of hemispatial neglect. It has been previously established that proprioceptive impairments are linked with reduced participation in ADLs [5–7]. As such, the FIM was collected as a measure of ADLs and indicative of overall stroke severity. The FIM measures the performance of ADLs across 18 items, including measures of self-care, locomotion, communication, and social cognition.

2.5. Neuroimaging

For all participants, clinical MRI or CT imaging was collected in accordance with the acute stroke imaging procedure at the Foothill Medical Centre, Calgary, Alberta, Canada. The mean time from stroke to image acquisition was 2.9 ± 4.3 days. MRI images were collected on a 1.5 T or 3 T General Electric scanner. Acquisition sequences included fluid-attenuated inversion recovery (FLAIR) and diffusion-weighted imaging (DWI). CT images were collected on either a Siemens system or General Electric system.

Participants' lesions were marked on the original FLAIR or CT image, and the marking was verified by a stroke neurologist. The marked lesions were then normalized into Montreal Neurological Institute (MNI) space using the clinical toolbox (https://www.nitrc.org/projects/clinicaltbx; accessed on 13 January 2022) [38] in SPM12 (https://www.fil.ion.ucl.ac.uk/spm/software/spm12/; accessed on 13 January 2022). The normalized lesions were checked for accuracy by ensuring the alignment of the ventricles, anterior and posterior commissures and overall brain outline. Normalized lesions were then used to generate two neuroimaging measures, pertaining to each specific lesion, that were subsequently used as features in the prediction models.

Neuroimaging Measures

The first neuroimaging measure used was a simple calculation of lesion volume for each participant's lesion. A second neuroimaging measure was derived from Voxel-Based Lesion Symptom Mapping (VLSM) methodology [39]. Participants lesions and APM Task Scores, at two weeks post-stroke, were subject to an initial VLSM analysis. The VLSM analysis was performed using the NiiStat Toolbox (https://www.nitrc.org/projects/niistat; accessed 13 January 2019) in Matlab 2020a (Mathworks, Natick, MA, USA). At each voxel, participants were separated into those with and without lesions at that voxel. The voxel-wise significance was then determined for the difference in APM Task Scores between those with and without lesions to that voxel. To ensure statistical power, only voxels with minimum overlap of 5% (seven participants) were tested, which is an accepted threshold in the VLSM literature [20,40,41]. The result is a map where each voxel was assigned to a z-score from the corresponding statistical test. Next, to determine the structure-function relationship with respect to the APM Task Score, the mean z-score associated with all the voxels of each participant's lesion was calculated (VLSM mean Z). Therefore, for each participant, the VLSM mean Z score is a scalar metric, weighted to the relative importance of all the lesioned voxels to the APM Task Score.

2.6. Statistical Analysis

The purpose of this study was to assess the utility of clinical, neuroimaging and robotic measures, collected two weeks post-stroke, in predicting proprioceptive impairment on a robotic APM task six months post-stroke.

To first validate the linear relationships between each clinical, neuroimaging and robotic measure collected at two weeks and six-month APM Task Scores, simple linear regressions were conducted. For the TLT, Spearman's rank correlation coefficient was performed. Additionally, the relationship between demographic information (age, sex, affected side) was also assessed. For age, linear regression was also performed, whereas two sample t-tests were adopted for sex and affected side, assessing for differences in six-month APM Task Scores between males and females and left and right affected participants.

Next, participants were split into two groups, those impaired on the APM Task at six months (APM Task Score < 1.96) and those unimpaired on the APM task (APM Task Score > 1.96). For each clinical, robotic and neuroimaging measure, separate Mann–Whitney-U tests were conducted to test if group-level differences existed for each measure, between the impaired and unimpaired groups. To correct for multiple comparisons, a Bonferroni adjusted critical alpha of 0.00357 (14 comparisons) was used to infer significance.

Finally, to assess the utility of clinical, neuroimaging and robotic measures for predicting six-month proprioceptive outcomes (impaired vs. unimpaired), logistic regression classifiers were trained. Firstly, a *Basic model* containing demographic information was trained, which formed the basis for each subsequent model. Then, to assess the predictive utility of each individual modality, models containing only clinical, neuroimaging or robotic features were trained (*Clinical model*, *Imaging model*, *Robotic model*). All the features were also combined into an *Augmented model*, to assess whether the addition of specialized robotic measures would improve the prediction of impairments over current clinically available information such as clinical assessments and neuroimaging. Within the *Augmented model*, coefficients from the logistic regression were used to determine the relative importance of each feature towards aiding the prediction. The features included in each model are presented in Table 1. Classification models were trained using the Scikit toolbox (version 1.1.3) in Python (version 3.9.13) and were cross validated using stratified 10-fold cross validation.

The performance of each classification model was evaluated by calculating the classification accuracy, F1-score (to account for imbalances between the number of participants with and without impairments), area under the receiver-operator characteristic (ROC) curve (AUC), sensitivity, and specificity. It was anticipated that the *Augmented model* would yield more accurate predictions and reduce prediction error. To evaluate whether the potential benefits in prediction accuracy outweighed the cost of including additional features, Akaike information criterion (AIC) was also used to compare models, penalizing models with more features.

Table 1. Model variables—Features entered into each predictive model. TLT = Thumb Localisation Task, BIT = Behavioural Inattention Test, FIM = Functional Independence Measure, VLSM = Voxel-based Lesion Symptom Mapping.

Model	Measures Included
Basic model	Age, Sex, Affected Arm
Clinical model	Age, Sex, Affected Arm, TLT, BIT, FIM
Imaging model	Age, Sex, Affected Arm, VLSM mean Z, Lesion Volume
Robotic model	Age, Sex, Affected Arm, Absolute Error X, Absolute Error Y, Variability X, Variability Y, Contraction Expansion X, Contraction Expansion Y, Shift X, Shift Y
Augmented model	Age, Sex, Affected Arm, TLT, BIT, FIM, VLSM mean Z, Lesion Volume, Absolute Error X, Absolute Error Y, Variability X, Variability Y, Contraction Expansion X, Contraction Expansion Y, Shift X, Shift Y

3. Results

3.1. Participant Demographics and Other Predictors

A total of 133 participants were included in the current study (females = 42; Left affected arm = 78). Participant demographics are presented in Table 2. Participants were 60.2 ± 13.0 years of age. By six months post-stroke, 48 participants still had impairments on the APM task (36.1%). As such, a classification model that predicted every participant as impaired or unimpaired at six months (i.e., a single class/chance model), would have been 36.1% or 63.9% accurate, respectively. Lesion overlaps for participants impaired and unimpaired at six months are presented in Figure 2. At two weeks post-stroke, 26 participants had neglect (BIT scores < 130); however, only four participants still had neglect by six months, alleviating concerns that impairments on the APM task at six months could be due to participants still having neglect (Supplemental Figure S1).

Table 2. Demographics—Participant demographics. For Age, Lesion Volume, VLSM mean Z, Absolute Error, Variability, Contraction Expansion, Shift and six-month APM Task Score, values are presented as the mean ± standard deviation. For the BIT and FIM, values presented are the median with the range presented in parentheses. BIT = Behavioural Inattention Test, FIM = Functional Independence Measure, TLT = Thumb Localisation Task, APM = Arm Position Matching, VLSM = Voxel-based Lesion Symptom Mapping.

Age	60.2 ± 13.0
Sex	Males = 91, Females = 42
Affected Arm	Right = 55, Left = 78
TLT	0 = 50, 1 = 36, 2 = 33, 3 = 14
BIT	141 (58–146)
FIM	102 (35–126)
Lesion Volume (cc)	35.1 ± 53.5
VLSM Mean Z	1.652 ± 1.223
Absolute Error X (z-score)	1.42 ± 1.30
Absolute Error Y (z-score)	1.49 ± 1.28
Variability X (z-score)	2.15 ± 1.93
Variability Y (z-score)	2.67 ± 2.12
Contraction Expansion X	−1.71 ± 2.20
Contraction Expansion Y	−2.27 ± 3.77
Shift X	−0.40 ± 1.78
Shift Y	−0.64 ± 1.98
APM Task Score (six months)	1.90 ± 1.55

3.2. Examining the Linear Relationships between Clinical, Neuroimaging and Robotic Features and Six-Month APM Task Scores

First, the linear relationships between each feature collected at two weeks post-stroke and six-month APM Task Scores were independently validated (Supplemental Figures S2–S4). All clinical features collected two weeks post-stroke were significantly associated with six-month APM Task Scores (Supplemental Figure S2). For the TLT (rho = 0.499,

$p = 9.92 \times 10^{-10}$), higher scores (worse performance) were associated with higher APM Task Scores (worse performance). For the BIT ($R^2 = 0.253$, $p = 4.12 \times 10^{-10}$) and FIM ($R^2 = 0.239$, $p = 1.39 \times 10^{-9}$), lower clinical scores (worse performance) were associated with higher APM Task Scores (worse performance). Additionally, both neuroimaging features were significantly associated with six-month APM Task Scores (Supplemental Figure S2). Greater lesion volumes ($R^2 = 0.169$, $p = 5.29 \times 10^{-7}$) and VLSM mean Z scores ($R^2 = 0.205$, $p = 2.78 \times 10^{-8}$) were also all significantly associated with higher APM Task Scores (worse performance). Of the robotic features collected two weeks post-stroke, significant associations with six-month APM Task Scores were observed for Absolute Error X ($R^2 = 0.300$, $p = 5.46 \times 10^{-12}$), Absolute Error Y ($R^2 = 0.447$, $p = 9.21 \times 10^{-19}$), Variability X ($R^2 = 0.325$, $p = 4.64 \times 10^{-13}$), Variability Y ($R^2 = 0.423$, $p = 1.49 \times 10^{-17}$), Contraction Expansion X ($R^2 = 0.313$, $p = 1.58 \times 10^{-12}$) and Contraction Expansion Y ($R^2 = 0.382$, $p = 1.44 \times 10^{-15}$) (Supplemental Figure S3). There were no significant associations between two-week Shift X and Shift Y scores and six-month APM Task Scores.

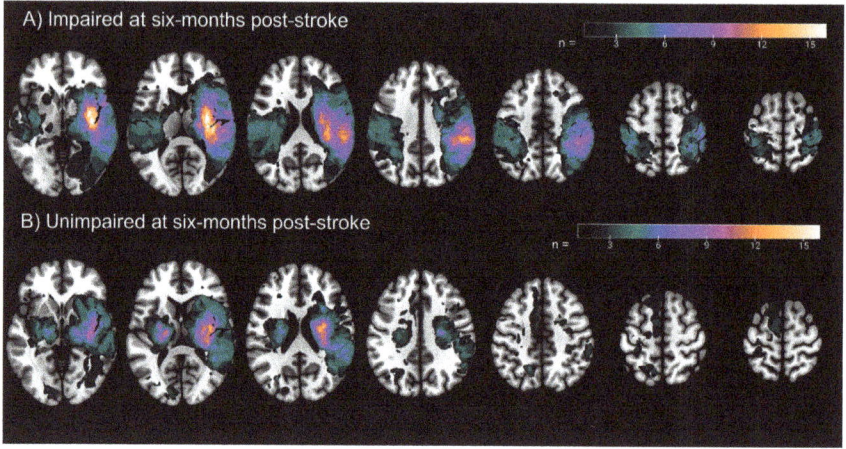

Figure 2. Lesion Overlaps—Lesion overlaps for (**A**) Participants impaired on the APM Task at six months post-stroke, and (**B**) Participants unimpaired on the APM Task at six months post-stroke. All lesions are normalised to Montreal Neurological Institute space and are presented in neurological convention (right hemisphere presented on the right). Color bar indicates the number of participants with lesions at each voxel. Axial slices (from left to right), z = −2, 10, 22, 34, 46, 58, 64.

For the demographic features, six-month APM Task Scores were significantly greater in left affected individuals than right affected individuals (t = 3.284, $p = 0.0013$) (Supplemental Figure S4). There were no differences between males and females (t = 1.815, $p = 0.0718$), nor a significant relationship with age ($R^2 = -0.00596$, $p = 0.641$) (Supplemental Figure S4).

3.3. Examining Differences in Clinical, Robotic and Neuroimaging Features between Those Impaired and Unimpaired on the APM Task Score

The second analysis assessed whether there were differences in clinical, neuroimaging and robotic features, collected two weeks post-stroke, between participants with and without APM task impairments (APM Task Scores > 1.96) at six months post-stroke. With the exception of age ($p = 0.974$), Shift X ($p = 0.294$) and Shift Y ($p = 0.944$), significant differences were observed for all measures (all p-values < 0.0005) between those with and without impairments on the APM task (Figure 3). For those with impairments, all measures were significantly higher (worse performance), except for BIT, FIM and Contraction Expansion X and Y, which were significantly lower (worse performance—in the case of Contraction Expansion, lower values indicate more contraction).

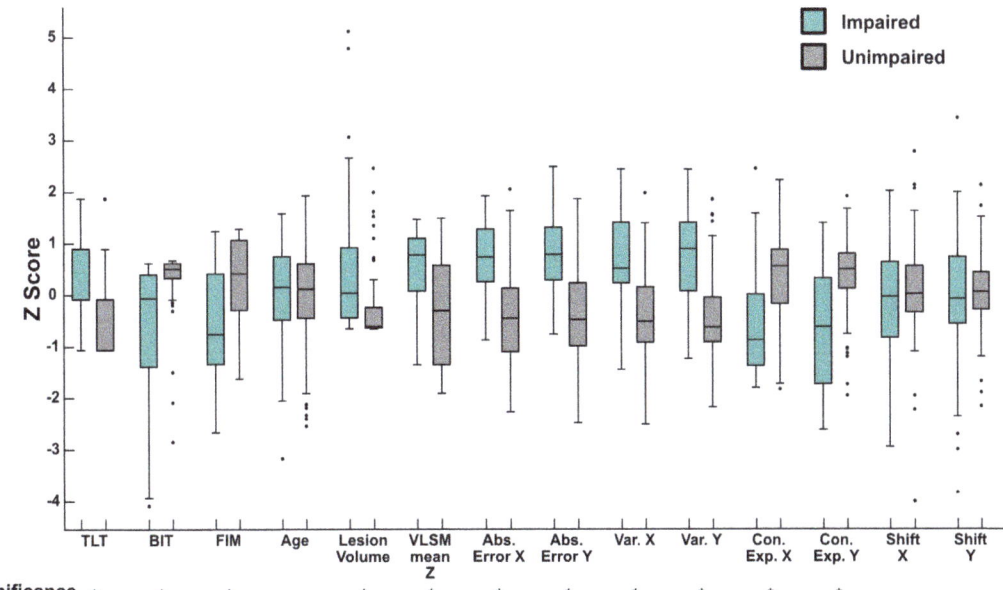

Figure 3. Group Level Differences in Clinical, Neuroimaging and Robotic Featuress Between Those Impaired and Unimpaired on the Arm Position Matching Task—Boxplots presenting features collected at two weeks post-stroke, for those impaired on the APM task (green) and those unimpaired (grey) at six months post-stroke. Given the varied scales each feature is scored on, scores are presented as z-scores for illustrative purposes. Boxes represent the median (centre line), 25th percentile (bottom line) and 75th percentile (top line), respectively. Whiskers extend to the highest and lowest data points, within 1.5 times the interquartile range from the top or bottom of the box. Individual data points displayed outside of this range signify outliers. Mann–Whitney U tests were conducted on the raw scores for each measure, between groups. * below each label indicates that feature had a significant difference between the impaired and unimpaired groups ($p < 0.0005$). Abs. Error = Absolute Error, Var = Variability, Con. Exp = Contraction Expansion.

3.4. Classification Models

3.4.1. Single Modality Models

Performance metrics of each classification model are presented in Table 3, with ROC curves for each model presented in Figure 4. When classifying impairments at six months post-stroke, using data collected two weeks post-stroke, all models containing single modality features (e.g., *Clinical*, *Imaging* and *Robotic* models) performed reasonably well (Table 3), with the exception of the *Basic model*. The most accurate model was the *Clinical model* (Accuracy = 78.95%, F1-score = 0.78), closely followed by the *Robotic model* (Accuracy = 77.44%, F1-score = 0.77) and then the *Imaging model* (Accuracy = 72.18%, F1-score = 0.71). With regard to the AUC metric, the highest performing single modality model was the *Robotic model* (AUC = 0.84), followed by the *Clinical model* (AUC = 0.79) and then the *Imaging model* (AUC = 0.74). The *Robotic model* also had the lowest AIC value (AIC = 120.07), compared with the *Clinical model* (AIC = 146.96) and *Imaging model* (148.43). The *Basic model* performed poorly on all metrics, except for specificity (Table 3). The highest contributing features for each model are presented in Supplemental Table S1. For the *Clinical model*, TLT scores (0.9513) and Affected arm (−0.6551) were the most important features of the model. For the *Imaging model*, Affected Arm (−0.7606) and VLSM mean Z (0.6665) were most important. For the *Robotic model*, the prediction was mostly driven by Affected Arm (−0.9762), Variability Y (0.8015) and Absolute Error X (0.4643).

Table 3. Predictive model performance—Performance metrics for each of the predictive models trained. For accuracy, sensitivity and specificity, values presented are percentages. * indicates the model(s) with the best performance for each given metric. For all metrics, except AIC, higher values indicate better performance. AUC = Area under the Receiver-Operator Characteristic curve, AIC = Akaike Information Criterion.

	Accuracy	F1-Score	AUC	Sensitivity	Specificity	AIC
Basic Model	63.16	0.49	0.45	0.00	98.82 *	176.94
Clinical model	78.95 *	0.78 *	0.79	62.50	88.24	146.96
Imaging model	72.18	0.71	0.74	47.92	85.88	148.43
Robotic model	77.44	0.77	0.84	68.75*	82.35	120.07 *
Augmented model	76.69	0.77	0.86*	64.58	83.53	126.07

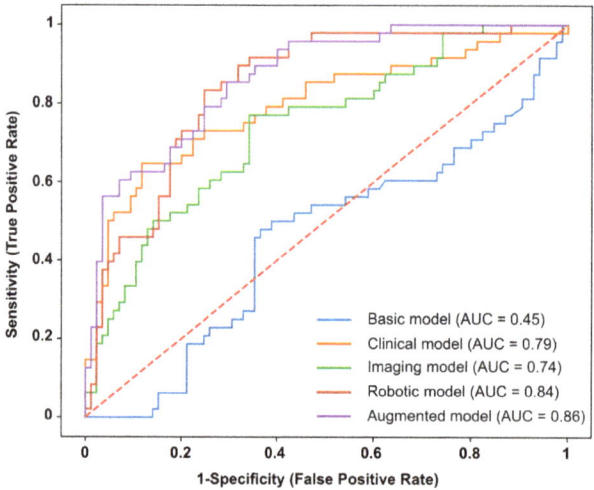

Figure 4. Receiver Operator Characteristic Curves (ROC curves)—Receiver Operator Characteristic (ROC) curves for the models predicting APM Task impairments at six months post-stroke. Each line represents the ROC curve for an individual model. Blue line = Basic model, orange line = Clinical model, green line = Imaging model, red line = Robotic model, purple line = Augmented model. Area under each curve (AUC) is reported in the figure legend. Dashed red line represents an AUC of 0.5 and a model that performs at random.

3.4.2. Augmented Model

When combining all demographic, clinical, neuroimaging and robotic features, the *Augmented model* also performed well, with an accuracy of 76.69%, F1-score of 0.77 and an AUC of 0.86. Of all the models trained, the *Augmented model* had the highest AUC (Table 3). With the exception of the *Robotic model*, the *Augmented model* also had a lower AIC than all other models. Upon closer inspection of the model coefficients (Figure 5, Supplemental Table S1), there were five features, in particular, that contributed the most towards the *Augmented model* predictions. The largest contributors to the model prediction were: Affected Arm (-0.857), Variability Y (0.755), Absolute Error X (0.441), VLSM mean Z (0.333) and Variability X (-0.330) (Figure 5, Supplemental Table S1). Contraction Expansion Y (-0.245) and TLT scores (0.233) were also relatively important features.

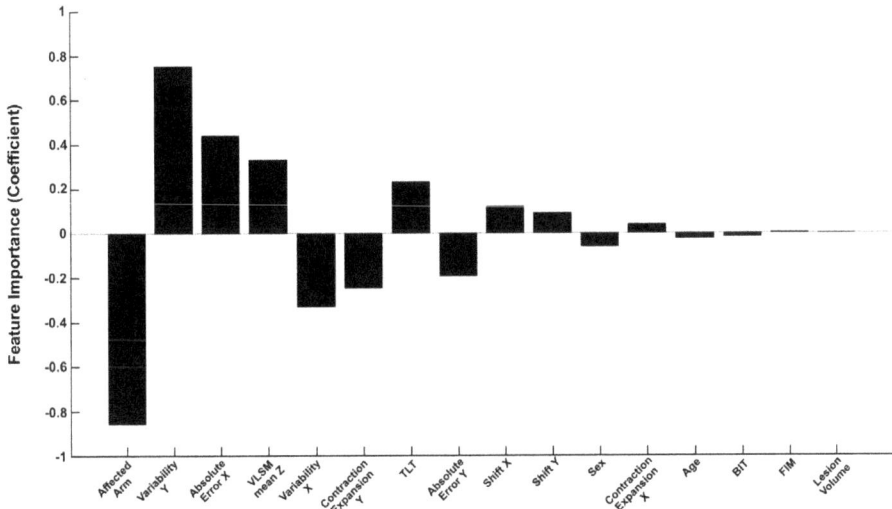

Figure 5. Augmented Model Feature Importance—Feature coefficients presented for the Augmented model. Features are ranked in order of absolute coefficient value. TLT = Thumb Localisation Task, BIT = Behavioural Inattention Test, FIM = Functional Independence Measure, VLSM = Voxel-based Lesion Symptom Mapping.

4. Discussion

The idea of predicting functional outcomes after a stroke is not new, as many studies have focused on predicting motor recovery and ADLs post-stroke [42–47]. Much less attention, however, has been placed on predicting sensory and proprioceptive recovery. This study demonstrated the utility of clinical, neuroimaging, and robotic measures, collected two weeks post-stroke, for predicting proprioceptive outcomes at six months post-stroke. Models which only contained a single modality of features (e.g., only clinical, neuroimaging or robotic features) resulted in prediction accuracies for long-term impairment that were greater than a model performing at chance, ranging from 72 to 79% (Table 3). Surprisingly, however, the combination of robotic features with clinical and neuroimaging features did not improve prediction accuracy or F1-score over the single modality models. When evaluating model performance based on AUC and AIC, there was, however, a clear advantage for models that utilized robotic features over those without (Table 3, Figure 4). The higher AUC, along with a relatively low AIC value, validates the use of models that are rich in features derived from robotic assessments when predicting long-term proprioceptive outcomes. Overall, this study advances our understanding of the predictors of proprioceptive recovery, something which has recently been called for in stroke recovery research [29]. Developing this understanding is important for identifying individuals who are at risk of long-term impairment, who could benefit from additional proprioceptive rehabilitation in the first six months post-stroke.

Independent of clinical and neuroimaging features, the use of robotic features resulted in a prediction accuracy of 77.44%. Although the accuracy and F1-score of the models containing robotic features were similar to those containing just clinical or neuroimaging features, the *Robotic* and *Augmented* models outperformed the *Clinical* and *Imaging* models in terms of AUC and AIC metrics. The relatively higher AUC suggests a greater ability of the models containing robotic features to separate those with proprioceptive impairments at six months from those without. Additionally, the lower AIC supports the use of the extra robotic features in these models. The improvements observed in AUC but not in accuracy are likely a reflection of what each metric measures. While accuracy is simply the proportion of correct predictions at a single model threshold, AUC measures the relationship between the True Positive Rate (Sensitivity) and the False Positive Rate (1-Specificity) at different threshold values. AUC is also biased towards the positive class (in this case, the impaired class). As seen in Figure 4, the *Robotic* and *Augmented model's* performance separates from the *Clinical* and *Imaging* models as the True Positive Rate exceeds 0.7 (i.e., a higher True Positive Rate/Sensitivity for a lower False Positive Rate), suggesting the greater ability for the models containing robotic features to correctly identify the impaired participants across a wide range of threshold values.

To date, the literature is limited when predicting and classifying sensory outcomes after stroke. Other classification studies have, however, attempted to predict functional outcomes post stroke [42,43,45,46,48] based on the Modified Rankin Scale or Barthel Index. Many of these have been deemed successful, reporting accuracies in the range of 56–85% [43,45] and AUC values in the range of 0.76–0.91 [42,48–50]. The *Clinical*, *Robotic* and *Augmented models* in the current study had comparable accuracies and AUC values, ranging between 76.69–79.95% and 0.79–0.86, respectively. Furthermore, in contrast to proprioception, there is a far deeper body of the literature aimed at predicting upper limb motor recovery, with a particular focus on clinical and physical markers such as finger extension and shoulder abduction, neurophysiological markers such as the presence of motor evoked potentials and neuroimaging markers such as corticospinal tract integrity [51–53] (for a comprehensive review of the literature, see [54]). That said, similarities are shared with those in the motor literature, whereby clinical and neuroimaging features contributed to successful prediction of proprioceptive outcomes in this study. In order to fully critique the performance of the models trained in this study, further research is required that attempts to predict sensory outcomes post-stroke. Doing so would allow the effectiveness of the models trained in this study to be compared with other suitable literature. As the body of literature grows surrounding sensory outcome prediction post-stroke, more tailored models can be trained that utilize a growing wealth of knowledge.

The present study has strong implications for stroke rehabilitation and promoting a more routine use of, and investments in, robotic technology in clinical practice. Being able to accurately assess proprioception and predict the likelihood of long-term impairments is an integral step towards developing better treatment plans for patients identified at risk of long-term impairments, who would otherwise have reduced independence in daily living and quality of life [7,55]. Robotics may be an important tool in improving both sensory prediction and assessment post-stroke.

Importantly, within the *Robotic* and *Augmented models*, this work has identified key components from a robotic assessment of proprioception that, when collected early post-stroke, are indicative of long-term proprioceptive problems for patients. In addition to the successful performance of the *Robotic model*, there were key features of the *Augmented model*, derived from robotic assessments, that were major contributors to predicting outcomes, for example, Variability Y, Absolute Error X and Variability X (Figure 5, Supplemental Table S1). This is of particular importance as rehabilitation looks towards a personalized medicine approach. Since robotics can identify key areas that predict long-term impairments, they have the capacity to inform the rehabilitation process by aiding the design of targeted interventions for these specific areas and mitigating long-term impairments. Robotics are advantageous for assessing proprioception as they provide an abundance of information about someone's performance and are far more precise than clinical assessments [31], collecting data every millisecond (in the case of the Kinarm Exoskeleton used in this study). As such, robotics are optimally suited to provide additional details about a person's particular proprioceptive impairment. Additionally, compared to the clinical assessments performed in this study (TLT, BIT and FIM), which can take up to 30 min to perform and require a trained clinician/rater, the APM task provides plentiful data in under four minutes of assessment time. Taken together, the present findings support the use of robotics to inform and improve the prediction of long-term patient outcomes, as well as inform rehabilitation.

Despite limited clinical uptake for the treatment of post-stroke proprioception, some potentially promising evidence comes from experimental interventions [12]. These studies, which are limited and only conducted in small samples, have been shown to increase proprioceptive acuity following stroke using a variety of treatment methods [56–65]. Many of these studies have utilized alternative treatments such as robotic therapy [57,59,60,63] including robotic mirror therapy [65] and assisted movement with enhanced sensation [58] but have also included more traditional tactile and proprioceptive discrimination training [56]. Interestingly, robotic therapy has also been proven to be beneficial for treating motor function after a stroke [66,67]. Given the capability of robotics to facilitate prediction of proprioceptive impairment, either alone or in conjunction with clinical assessments, the use of robotics in clinical settings in addition to their apparent benefit for proprioceptive rehabilitation should continue to be explored and considered.

It has previously been demonstrated that the ability to predict functional outcomes post-stroke, using clinical measures alone, hits a ceiling of prediction accuracy at around 80% [43,45], with the addition of specialized features (such as neuroimaging or robotics) potentially required to facilitate improvements in model performance [43]. Although it was anticipated that robotic features would result in higher prediction accuracy than clinical or neuroimaging features, unfortunately this was not found to be the case, with the *Robotic* and *Augmented models* performing similarly to the *Clinical and Imaging models*.

It must be noted, however, that the *Clinical model* still performed well, even in the absence of more specialized features such as neuroimaging or robotics. Within this model, TLT scores and the affected arm were the most informative features (Supplemental Table S1). The TLT was also amongst the more informative features of the *Augmented model* (Figure 5, Supplemental Table S1). The relative success of using clinical measures for long-term prediction corroborates the findings of Reid et al. [42], who demonstrated that outcome predictions, based on the Modified Rankin Scale, were just as good using simple clinical measures compared to more complex models which utilized neuroimaging measures. The ability of the clinical measures used in the current study to predict proprioceptive outcome also may not be surprising, considering the close associations that have previously been described between attentional deficits, the ability to perform ADLs and proprioception post-stroke [7,15,18]. The high prediction accuracy in this study may therefore reflect these tight relationships between clinical and robotic measures of proprioception (Supplemental Figure S2). While robotics provide distinct advantages over clinical assessments [31], they are not common in clinical sites. In sites where robotics are not accessible, it is important that clinicians recognize the associations between these types of clinical measures and the likelihood of long-term proprioceptive difficulties in their patients, when performing assessments early after stroke and prescribing rehabilitation.

Finally, within the *Augmented model*, the affected arm and VLSM mean Z also contributed to the model prediction (Figure 5, Supplemental Table S1). There is a growing body of evidence that suggests that proprioception is lateralized to the right hemisphere, with a distributed network of brain regions likely responsible for proprioception [16,68–76]. With APM Task Scores greater (worse) in left-arm affected individuals (Supplemental Figure S4) and greater VLSM mean Z scores in those with impairments at six months, the relative importance of these measures as predictors of long-term impairment likely reflects this lateralized neuroanatomy for proprioception.

Limitations

Like all studies, the current study has limitations. Given the size of the dataset, models were both trained and tested within samples and the test data were not necessarily unseen. While it is suggested that using the same data to train and test models might be useful from the standpoint of exploring potential predictive measures [77–79], in an ideal scenario a vastly larger dataset would be available, allowing these findings to be generalized to a wider sample. In this study stratified 10-fold cross-validation was used, which can protect against these biases. It must also be noted that there were slight imbalances in the number of participants with and without impairments in the sample (approximately 60–40% split), something which was maintained through each cross-validation sample. This imbalance may have the potential to bias the current findings and distort the perceived performance of each model trained. That said, all the models outperformed a single class model by 10–15% accuracy.

5. Conclusions

Predicting proprioceptive impairments out to six months post-stroke using clinical, neuroimaging and robotic measures, collected within the first two weeks post-stroke, is feasible. Considering the current clinical standard of care often does not focus on treating proprioceptive impairments, identifying those likely to have long-lasting impairments is a key step towards personalized approaches in the treatment of proprioception. Further studies are, however, needed to refine predictive models and increase the prediction accuracy of proprioceptive recovery post-stroke.

Supplementary Materials: The following supporting information can be downloaded at: https://www.mdpi.com/article/10.3390/brainsci13060953/s1, Supplementary Figure S1: Relationship between six-month BIT scores and APM Task Scores; Supplementary Figure S2: Examining the relationships between two-week clinical and neuroimaging measures and six-month Arm Position Matching Task Scores; Supplementary Figure S3: Examining the relationships between two-week robotic measures and six-month Arm Position Matching Task Scores; Supplementary Figure S4: Examining the relationships between demographic measures and six-month Arm Position Matching Task Scores; Supplementary Table S1: Predictive model coefficients.

Author Contributions: Conceptualization, M.J.C., T.A.L., D.R. and S.P.D.; methodology, M.J.C. and T.A.L.; software, M.J.C., T.A.L. and D.R.; validation, M.J.C.; formal analysis, M.J.C.; investigation, M.J.C.; resources, S.H.S. and S.P.D.; data curation, M.J.C.; writing—original draft preparation, M.J.C. and S.P.D.; writing—review and editing, M.J.C., T.A.L., D.R., S.H.S. and S.P.D.; visualization, M.J.C.; supervision, D.R. and S.P.D.; project administration, M.J.C. and S.P.D.; funding acquisition, S.P.D. and S.H.S. All authors have read and agreed to the published version of the manuscript.

Funding: This research was funded by a Canadian Institutes of Health Research Operating Grant (MOP106662), Heart and Stroke Foundation of Canada Grant-in-aid (G-13-0003029), Alberta Innovates Health Solutions Team Grant (201500788) and an Ontario Research Fund grant (ORF-RE 04-47).

Institutional Review Board Statement: The study was conducted in accordance with the Declaration of Helsinki and approved by the Institutional Review Board (or Ethics Committee) of The University of Calgary (REB15-1340).

Informed Consent Statement: Informed consent was obtained from all subjects involved in the study.

Data Availability Statement: The data presented in this study is not publicly available due to restrictions on data sharing without formal data sharing agreements in place, as determined by the Institutional Review Board. Those wishing to obtain the study data should contact the corresponding author (Sean Dukelow).

Acknowledgments: The authors would like to thank Mark Piitz and Janice Yajure for their assistance with recruitment and data collection.

Conflicts of Interest: S.H.S is co-founder and chief scientific officer of BKIN Technologies, the company that commercializes the Kinarm robot used in the current study. All other authors declare no conflict of interest.

References

1. Sherrington, C.S. On the proprioceptive system, especially in its reflex aspect. *Brain* **1906**, *29*, 467–482. [CrossRef]
2. Proske, U.; Gandevia, S.C. The proprioceptive senses: Their roles in signaling body shape, body position and movement, and muscle force. *Physiol. Rev.* **2012**, *92*, 1651–1697. [CrossRef]
3. Dukelow, S.P.; Herter, T.M.; Moore, K.D.; Demers, M.J.; Glasgow, J.I.; Bagg, S.D.; Norman, K.E.; Scott, S.H. Quantitative assessment of limb position sense following stroke. *Neurorehabilit. Neural Repair* **2010**, *24*, 178–187. [CrossRef]

4. Carey, L.M.; Oke, L.E.; Matyas, T.A. Impaired limb position sense after stroke: A quantitative test for clinical use. *Arch. Phys. Med. Rehabil.* **1996**, *77*, 1271–1278. [CrossRef] [PubMed]
5. Rand, D. Proprioception deficits in chronic stroke: Upper extremity function and daily living. *PLoS ONE* **2018**, *13*, e0195043. [CrossRef]
6. Tyson, S.F.; Hanley, M.; Chillala, J.; Selley, A.B.; Tallis, R.C. Sensory loss in hospital-admitted people with stroke: Characteristics, associated factors, and relationship with function. *Neurorehabil. Neural Repair* **2018**, *22*, 166–172. [CrossRef] [PubMed]
7. Dukelow, S.P.; Herter, T.M.; Bagg, S.D.; Scott, S.H. The independence of deficits in position sense and visually guided reaching following stroke. *J. Neuroeng. Rehabil.* **2012**, *9*, 1. [CrossRef]
8. Mostafavi, S.M.; Mousavi, P.; Dukelow, S.P.; Scott, S.H. Robot-based assessment of motor and proprioceptive function identifies biomarkers for prediction of functional independence measures. *J. Neuroeng. Rehabil.* **2015**, *12*, 105. [CrossRef] [PubMed]
9. Semrau, J.A.; Herter, T.M.; Scott, S.H.; Dukelow, S.P. Examining differences in patterns of sensory and motor recovery after stroke with robotics. *Stroke* **2015**, *46*, 3459–3469. [CrossRef] [PubMed]
10. Findlater, S.E.; Hawe, R.L.; Semrau, J.A.; Kenzie, J.M.; Yu, A.Y.; Scott, S.H.; Dukelow, S.P. Lesion locations associated with persistent proprioceptive impairment in the upper limbs after stroke. *Neuroimage Clin.* **2018**, *20*, 955–971. [CrossRef]
11. Findlater, S.E.; Dukelow, S.P. Upper Extremity Proprioception After Stroke: Bridging the Gap Between Neuroscience and Rehabilitation. *J. Mot. Behav.* **2017**, *49*, 27–34. [CrossRef] [PubMed]
12. Hughes, C.M.L.; Tommasino, P.; Budhota, A.; Campolo, D. Upper extremity proprioception in healthy aging and stroke populations, and the effects of therapist- and robot-based rehabilitation therapies on proprioceptive function. *Front. Hum. Neurosci.* **2015**, *9*, 120. [CrossRef] [PubMed]
13. Pumpa, L.U.; Cahill, L.S.; Carey, L.M. Somatosensory assessment and treatment after stroke: An evidence-practice gap. *Aust. Occup. J.* **2015**, *62*, 93–104. [CrossRef]
14. Otaka, E.; Otaka, Y.; Kasuga, S.; Nishimoto, A.; Yamazaki, K.; Kawakami, M.; Ushiba, J.; Liu, M. Reliability of the thumb localizing test and its validity against quantitative measures with a robotic device in patients with hemiparetic stroke. *PLoS ONE* **2020**, *15*, e0236437. [CrossRef]
15. Fisher, G.; De Oliveira, C.Q.; Verhagen, A.; Gandevia, S.; Kennedy, D. Proprioceptive impairment in unilateral neglect after stroke: A systematic review. *SAGE Open Med.* **2020**, *8*, 205031212095107. [CrossRef]
16. Chilvers, M.J.; Hawe, R.L.; Scott, S.H.; Dukelow, S.P. Investigating the neuroanatomy underlying proprioception using a stroke model. *J. Neurol. Sci.* **2021**, *430*, 120029. [CrossRef] [PubMed]
17. Meyer, S.; De Bruyn, N.; Lafosse, C.; Van Dijk, M.; Michielsen, M.; Thijs, L.; Truyens, V.; Oostra, K.; Krumlinde-Sundholm, L.; Peeters, A.; et al. Somatosensory impairments in the upper limb poststroke: Distribution and association with motor function and visuospatial neglect. *Neurorehabil. Neural Repair* **2016**, *30*, 731–742. [CrossRef]
18. Semrau, J.A.; Wang, J.C.; Herter, T.M.; Scott, S.H.; Dukelow, S.P. Relationship between visuospatial neglect and kinesthetic deficits after stroke. *Neurorehabil. Neural Repair* **2015**, *29*, 318–328. [CrossRef]
19. Hawe, R.L.; Findlater, S.E.; Kenzie, J.M.; Hill, M.D.; Scott, S.H.; Dukelow, S.P.; Sunderland, A.; Marquine, M.J.; Attix, D.K.; Goldstein, L.B.; et al. Differential impact of acute lesions versus white matter hyperintensities on stroke recovery. *J. Am. Heart Assoc.* **2018**, *7*, e009360. [CrossRef]
20. Kenzie, J.M.; Semrau, J.A.; Findlater, S.E.; Yu, A.Y.; Desai, J.A.; Herter, T.M.; Hill, M.D.; Scott, S.H.; Dukelow, S.P. Localization of impaired kinesthetic processing post-stroke. *Front. Hum. Neurosci.* **2016**, *10*, 505. [CrossRef]
21. Findlater, S.E.; Desai, J.A.; Semrau, J.A.; Kenzie, J.M.; Rorden, C.; Herter, T.M.; Scott, S.H.; Dukelow, S.P. Central perception of position sense involves a distributed neural network—Evidence from lesion-behavior analyses. *Cortex* **2016**, *79*, 42–56. [CrossRef]
22. Meyer, S.; Kessner, S.S.; Cheng, B.; Bönstrup, M.; Schulz, R.; Hummel, F.C.; De Bruyn, N.; Peeters, A.; Van Pesch, V.; Duprez, T.; et al. Voxel-based lesion-symptom mapping of stroke lesions underlying somatosensory deficits. *Neuroimage Clin.* **2016**, *10*, 257–266. [CrossRef]
23. Lin, L.; Ramsey, L.; Metcalf, N.V.; Rengachary, J.; Shulman, G.L.; Shimony, J.S.; Corbetta, M. Stronger prediction of motor recovery and outcome post-stroke by cortico-spinal tract integrity than functional connectivity. *PLoS ONE* **2018**, *13*, e0202504. [CrossRef] [PubMed]
24. Feys, H.; De Weerdt, W.; Nuyens, G.; Van De Winckel, A.; Selz, B.; Kiekens, C. Predicting motor recovery of the upper limb after stroke rehabilitation: Value of a clinical examination. *Physiother. Res. Int.* **2000**, *5*, 1–18. [CrossRef]
25. Chen, C.-L.; Tang, F.-T.; Chen, H.-C.; Chung, C.-Y.; Wong, M.-K. Brain lesion size and location: Effects on motor recovery and functional outcome in stroke patients. *Arch. Phys. Med. Rehabil.* **2000**, *81*, 447–452. [CrossRef] [PubMed]
26. Kwakkel, G.; Kollen, B. Predicting improvement in the upper paretic limb after stroke: A longitudinal prospective study. *Restor. Neurol. Neurosci.* **2007**, *25*, 453–460. [PubMed]
27. DeVetten, G.; Coutts, S.B.; Hill, M.D.; Goyal, M.; Eesa, M.; O'Brien, B.; Demchuk, A.M.; Kirton, A. Acute corticospinal tract wallerian degeneration is associated with stroke outcome. *Stroke* **2010**, *41*, 751–756. [CrossRef] [PubMed]
28. Stinear, C. Prediction of recovery of motor function after stroke. *Lancet Neurol.* **2010**, *9*, 1228–1232. [CrossRef]
29. Boyd, L.A.; Hayward, K.S.; Ward, N.S.; Stinear, C.M.; Rosso, C.; Fisher, R.J.; Carter, A.R.; Leff, A.P.; Copland, D.A.; Carey, L.M.; et al. Biomarkers of stroke recovery: Consensus-based core recommendations from the stroke recovery and rehabilitation roundtable. *Int. J. Stroke* **2017**, *12*, 480–493. [CrossRef]

30. van Heugten, C.M.; Dekker, J.; Deelman, B.G.; De Stehmann-Saris, A.K. A diagnostic test for apraxia in stroke patients: Internal consistency and diagnostic value. *Clin. Neuropsychol.* **1999**, *13*, 182–192. [CrossRef]
31. Scott, S.H.; Dukelow, S.P. Potential of robots as next-generation technology for clinical assessment of neurological disorders and upper-limb therapy. *J. Rehabil. Res. Dev.* **2011**, *48*, 335–353. [CrossRef] [PubMed]
32. *Kinarm Dexterit-E 3.9*; Addendum: Kinarm Standard Tests Summary. BKIN Technologies Ltd.: Kingston, ON, Canada, 2021. Available online: https://kinarm.com/download/kst-summary-analysis-version-3-9/ (accessed on 4 June 2022).
33. Scott, S.H.; Lowrey, C.R.; Brown, I.E.; Dukelow, S.P. Assessment of neurological impairment and recovery using statistical models of neurologically healthy behavior. *Neurorehabilit. Neural Repair* **2022**, 1–15. [CrossRef] [PubMed]
34. Simmatis, L.E.R.; Early, S.; Moore, K.D.; Appaqaq, S.; Scott, S.H. Statistical measures of motor, sensory and cognitive performance across repeated robot-based testing. *J. Neuroeng. Rehabil.* **2020**, *17*, 86. [CrossRef] [PubMed]
35. Hirayama, K.; Fukutake, T.; Kawamura, M. "Thumb localizing test" for detecting a lesion in the posterior column-medial lemniscal system. *J. Neurol. Sci.* **1999**, *167*, 45–49. [CrossRef] [PubMed]
36. Wilson, B.; Cockburn, J.; Halligan, P. Development of a behavioral test of visuospatial neglect. *Arch. Phys. Med. Rehabil.* **1987**, *68*, 98–102.
37. Keith, R.A.; Granger, C.V.; Hamilton, B.B.; Sherwin, F.S. The functional independence measure: A new tool for rehabilitation. *Adv. Clin. Rehabil.* **1987**, *1*, 6–18.
38. Rorden, C.; Bonilha, L.; Fridriksson, J.; Bender, B.; Karnath, H.O. Age-specific CT and MRI templates for spatial normalization. *Neuroimage* **2012**, *61*, 957–965. [CrossRef]
39. Bates, E.; Wilson, S.M.; Saygin, A.P. Voxel-Based Lesion-Symptom Mapping. *Nat. Neurosci.* **2003**, *6*, 448–450. [CrossRef]
40. Geva, S.; Jones, P.S.; Crinion, J.T.; Price, C.J.; Baron, J.-C.; Warburton, E.A. The neural correlates of inner speech defined by voxel-based lesion-symptom mapping. *Brain* **2011**, *134*, 3071–3082. [CrossRef]
41. Kalénine, S.; Buxbaum, L.J.; Coslett, H.B. Critical brain regions for action recognition: Lesion symptom mapping in left hemisphere stroke. *Brain* **2010**, *133*, 3269–3280. [CrossRef]
42. Reid, J.M.; Gubitz, G.J.; Dai, D.; Kydd, D.; Eskes, G.; Reidy, Y.; Christian, C.; Counsell, C.E.; Dennis, M.; Phillips, S.J. Predicting functional outcome after stroke by modelling baseline clinical and CT variables. *Age Ageing* **2010**, *39*, 360–366. [CrossRef]
43. Forkert, N.D.; Verleger, T.; Cheng, B.; Thomalla, G.; Hilgetag, C.C.; Fiehler, J. Multiclass support vector machine-based lesion mapping predicts functional outcome in ischemic stroke patients. *PLoS ONE* **2015**, *10*, e0129569. [CrossRef]
44. Meijer, R.; Ihnenfeldt, D.S.; De Groot, I.J.M.; Van Limbeek, J.; Vermeulen, M.; De Haan, R.J. Prognostic factors for ambulation and activities of daily living in the subacute phase after stroke. A systematic review of the literature. *Clin. Rehabil.* **2003**, *17*, 119–129. [CrossRef] [PubMed]
45. Weimar, C.; Ziegler, A.; König, I.R.; Diener, H.C. Predicting functional outcome and survival after acute ischemic stroke. *J. Neurol.* **2002**, *249*, 888–895. [CrossRef]
46. Thijs, V.N.; Lansberg, M.G.; Beaulieu, C.; Marks, M.P.; Moseley, M.E.; Albers, G.W. Is early ischemic lesion volume on diffusion-weighted imaging an independent predictor of stroke outcome? A multivariable analysis. *Stroke* **2000**, *31*, 2597–2602. [CrossRef] [PubMed]
47. Kwakkel, G.; Wagenaar, R.C.; Kollen, B.J.; Lankhorst, G.J. Predicting disability in stroke—A critical review of the literature. *Age Ageing* **1996**, *25*, 479–489. [CrossRef]
48. Johnston, K.C.; Barrett, K.M.; Ding, Y.H.; Wagner, D.P. Clinical and imaging data at 5 days as a surrogate for 90-day outcome in ischemic stroke. *Stroke* **2009**, *40*, 1332–1333. [CrossRef]
49. Scrutinio, D.; Lanzillo, B.; Guida, P.; Mastropasqua, F.; Monitillo, V.; Pusineri, M.; Formica, R.; Russo, G.; Guarnaschelli, C.; Ferretti, C.; et al. Development and validation of a predictive model for functional outcome after stroke rehabilitation: The Maugeri model. *Stroke* **2017**, *48*, 3308–3315. [CrossRef]
50. Kent, D.M.; Selker, H.P.; Ruthazer, R.; Bluhmki, E.; Hacke, W. The stroke-thrombolytic predictive instrument: A predictive instrument for intravenous thrombolysis in acute ischemic stroke. *Stroke* **2006**, *37*, 2957–2962. [CrossRef] [PubMed]
51. Nijland, R.H.M.; Van Wegen, E.E.H.; Harmeling-Van Der Wel, B.C.; Kwakkel, G. Presence of finger extension and shoulder abduction within 72 hours after stroke predicts functional recovery: Early prediction of functional outcome after stroke: The EPOS cohort study. *Stroke* **2010**, *41*, 745–750. [CrossRef]
52. Stinear, C.M.; Barber, P.A.; Petoe, M.; Anwar, S.; Byblow, W.D. The PREP algorithm predicts potential for upper limb recovery after stroke. *Brain* **2012**, *135*, 2527–2535. [CrossRef]
53. Stinear, C.M.; Barber, P.A.; Smale, P.R.; Coxon, J.P.; Fleming, M.K.; Byblow, W.D. Functional potential in chronic stroke patients depends on corticospinal tract integrity. *Brain* **2007**, *130*, 170–180. [CrossRef]
54. Stinear, C.M. Prediction of motor recovery after stroke: Advances in biomarkers. *Lancet Neurol.* **2017**, *16*, 826–836. [CrossRef]
55. Meyer, S.; Karttunen, A.H.; Thijs, V.; Feys, H.; Verheyden, G. How do somatosensory deficits in the arm and hand relate to upper limb impairment, activity, and participation problems after stroke? A systematic review. *Phys. Ther.* **2014**, *94*, 1220–1231. [CrossRef]
56. Carey, L.M.; Matyas, T.A.; Oke, L.E. Sensory loss in stroke patients: Effective training of tactile and proprioceptive discrimination. *Arch. Phys. Med. Rehabil.* **1993**, *74*, 602–611. [CrossRef]
57. Cuppone, A.V.; Squeri, V.; Semprini, M.; Masia, L.; Konczak, J. Robot-assisted proprioceptive training with added vibro-tactile feedback enhances somatosensory and motor performance. *PLoS ONE* **2016**, *11*, e0164511. [CrossRef]

58. Cordo, P.; Lutsep, H.; Cordo, L.; Wright, W.G.; Cacciatore, T.; Skoss, R. Assisted movement with enhanced sensation (AMES): Coupling motor and sensory to remediate motor deficits in chronic stroke patients. *Neurorehabil. Neural Repair* **2009**, *23*, 67–77. [CrossRef] [PubMed]
59. Casadio, M.; Morasso, P.; Sanguineti, V.; Giannoni, P. Minimally assistive robot training for proprioception enhancement. *Exp. Brain Res.* **2009**, *194*, 219–231. [CrossRef] [PubMed]
60. Santis, D.E.; Ezenzeri, J.; Ecasadio, M.; Emasia, L.; Eriva, A.; Emorasso, P.; Esqueri, V. Robot-assisted training of the kinesthetic sense: Enhancing proprioception after stroke. *Front. Hum. Neurosci.* **2015**, *8*, 1037. [CrossRef] [PubMed]
61. Aman, J.E.; Elangovan, N.; Yeh, I.-L.; Konczak, J. The effectiveness of proprioceptive training for improving motor function: A systematic review. *Front. Hum. Neurosci.* **2015**, *8*, 1075. [CrossRef] [PubMed]
62. Schabrun, S.M.; Hillier, S. Evidence for the retraining of sensation after stroke: A systematic review. *Clin. Rehabil.* **2009**, *23*, 27–39. [CrossRef] [PubMed]
63. Elangovan, N.; Yeh, I.L.; Holst-Wolf, J.; Konczak, J. A Robot-Assisted Sensorimotor Training Program can Improve Proprioception and Motor Function in Stroke Survivors. In Proceedings of the 2019 IEEE 16th International Conference on Rehabilitation Robotics (ICORR), Toronto, ON, Canada, 24–28 June 2019.
64. Cho, S.; Ku, J.; Cho, Y.K.; Kim, I.Y.; Kang, Y.J.; Jang, D.P.; Kim, S.I. Development of virtual reality proprioceptive rehabilitation system for stroke patients. *Comput. Methods Programs Biomed.* **2014**, *113*, 258–265. [CrossRef]
65. Nam, H.S.; Koh, S.; Beom, J.; Kim, Y.J.; Park, J.W.; Koh, E.-S.; Chung, S.G.; Kim, S. Recovery of proprioception in the upper extremity by robotic mirror therapy: A clinical pilot study for proof of concept. *J. Korean Med. Sci.* **2017**, *32*, 1568. [CrossRef] [PubMed]
66. Dukelow, S.P. The potential power of robotics for upper extremity stroke rehabilitation. *Int. J. Stroke* **2017**, *12*, 7–8. [CrossRef] [PubMed]
67. Mehrholz, J.; Pohl, M.; Platz, T.; Kugler, J.; Elsner, B. Electromechanical and robot-assisted arm training for improving activities of daily living, arm function, and arm muscle strength after stroke. *Cochrane Database Syst. Rev.* **2018**, *9*, CD006876. [CrossRef] [PubMed]
68. Sainburg, R.L. Evidence for a dynamic-dominance hypothesis of handedness. *Exp. Brain Res.* **2002**, *142*, 241–258. [CrossRef]
69. Sainburg, R.L.; Kalakanis, D. Differences in control of limb dynamics during dominant and nondominant arm reaching. *J. Neurophysiol.* **2000**, *83*, 2661–2675. [CrossRef]
70. Bagesteiro, L.B.; Sainburg, R.L. Nondominant arm advantages in load compensation during rapid elbow joint movements. *J. Neurophysiol.* **2003**, *90*, 1503–1513. [CrossRef]
71. Bagesteiro, L.B.; Sainburg, R.L. Handedness: Dominant arm advantages in control of limb dynamics. *J. Neurophysiol.* **2002**, *88*, 2408–2421. [CrossRef]
72. Wang, J.; Sainburg, R.L. The dominant and nondominant arms are specialized for stabilizing different features of task performance. *Exp. Brain Res.* **2007**, *178*, 565–570. [CrossRef]
73. Amemiya, K.; Naito, E. Importance of human right inferior frontoparietal network connected by inferior branch of superior longitudinal fasciculus tract in corporeal awareness of kinesthetic illusory movement. *Cortex* **2016**, *78*, 15–30. [CrossRef] [PubMed]
74. Naito, E.; Nakashima, T.; Kito, T.; Aramaki, Y.; Okada, T.; Sadato, N. Human limb-specific and non-limb-specific brain representations during kinesthetic illusory movements of the upper and lower extremities. *Eur. J. Neurosci.* **2007**, *25*, 3476–3487. [CrossRef] [PubMed]
75. Naito, E.; Morita, T.; Saito, D.N.; Ban, M.; Shimada, K.; Okamoto, Y.; Kosaka, H.; Okazawa, H.; Asada, M. Development of right-hemispheric dominance of inferior parietal lobule in proprioceptive illusion task. *Cereb. Cortex* **2017**, *27*, 5385–5397. [CrossRef]
76. Naito, E.; Roland, P.E.; Grefkes, C.; Choi, H.J.; Eickhoff, S.B.; Geyer, S.; Zilles, K.; Ehrsson, H.H.; Proske, U.; Gandevia, S.C.; et al. Dominance of the right hemisphere and role of area 2 in human kinesthesia. *J. Neurophysiol.* **2005**, *93*, 1020–1034. [CrossRef] [PubMed]
77. Bonkhoff, A.K.; Grefkes, C. Precision medicine in stroke: Towards personalized outcome predictions using artificial intelligence. *Brain* **2022**, *145*, 457–475. [CrossRef]
78. Shmueli, G. To explain or to predict? *Stat. Sci.* **2010**, *25*, 289–310. [CrossRef]
79. Bzdok, D.; Engemann, D.; Thirion, B. Inference and Prediction Diverge in Biomedicine. *Patterns* **2020**, *1*, 100119. [CrossRef] [PubMed]

Disclaimer/Publisher's Note: The statements, opinions and data contained in all publications are solely those of the individual author(s) and contributor(s) and not of MDPI and/or the editor(s). MDPI and/or the editor(s) disclaim responsibility for any injury to people or property resulting from any ideas, methods, instructions or products referred to in the content.

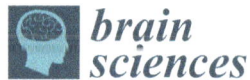

Review

Remapping and Reconnecting the Language Network after Stroke

Victoria Tilton-Bolowsky [†], Melissa D. Stockbridge [†] and Argye E. Hillis *

Departments of Neurology, Physical Medicine & Rehabilitation, and Cognitive Science, Johns Hopkins University School of Medicine, Baltimore, MD 21287, USA; vbolows1@jhmi.edu (V.T.-B.); md.stockbridge@jhmi.edu (M.D.S.)
* Correspondence: argye@jhmi.edu; Tel.: +1-443-287-4610
† These authors contributed equally to this work.

Abstract: Here, we review the literature on neurotypical individuals and individuals with post-stroke aphasia showing that right-hemisphere regions homologous to language network and other regions, like the right cerebellum, are activated in language tasks and support language even in healthy people. We propose that language recovery in post-stroke aphasia occurs largely by potentiating the right hemisphere network homologous to the language network and other networks that previously supported language to a lesser degree and by modulating connection strength between nodes of the right-hemisphere language network and undamaged nodes of the left-hemisphere language network. Based on this premise (supported by evidence we review), we propose that interventions should be aimed at potentiating the right-hemisphere language network through Hebbian learning or by augmenting connections between network nodes through neuroplasticity, such as non-invasive brain stimulation and perhaps modulation of neurotransmitters involved in neuroplasticity. We review aphasia treatment studies that have taken this approach. We conclude that further aphasia rehabilitation with this aim is justified.

Keywords: stroke; aphasia; mechanisms of recovery; language networks; connectivity

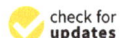

Citation: Tilton-Bolowsky, V.; Stockbridge, M.D.; Hillis, A.E. Remapping and Reconnecting the Language Network after Stroke. *Brain Sci.* **2024**, *14*, 419. https://doi.org/10.3390/brainsci14050419

Academic Editors: Noureddin Nakhostin Ansari, Gholamreza Hassanzadeh and Ardalan Shariat

Received: 22 March 2024
Revised: 22 April 2024
Accepted: 23 April 2024
Published: 24 April 2024

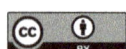

Copyright: © 2024 by the authors. Licensee MDPI, Basel, Switzerland. This article is an open access article distributed under the terms and conditions of the Creative Commons Attribution (CC BY) license (https:// creativecommons.org/licenses/by/ 4.0/).

1. Introduction

Aphasia refers to deficits in language (comprehension and production, written and spoken) following damage to the brain. It is distinct from deficits in broader cognition or articulation (dysarthria, apraxia). Recovery of language function after a stroke causing aphasia is thought to take place in part through "reorganization" of structure–function relationships or "take-over" (by undamaged) tissue of functions that are impaired by damaged tissue. One interpretation of this concept is that neurons are sufficiently pluripotent; that is, they can change the type of stimulus they are tuned to or that a functional network can change the type of computation it carries out. Makin and Krakauer [1] review extensive evidence from animal and human studies against this interpretation of reorganization. They argue instead that remapping occurs through potentiation (i.e., increases in synaptic efficacy or strengthening of synapses through activity) of preexisting networks or circuits that have the necessary representational and computational capacity prior to stroke. Potentiation of preexisting networks that may have been supportive of function such as language can be facilitated via Hebbian learning and other neuroplasticity mechanisms. Hebbian learning mechanisms are engaged through repeated patterns of neuronal firing, which is thought to strengthen these pathways and make them more efficient [2]. Neuroplasticity refers to the brain's ability to form new connections and/or reorganize to restore or regain function after some disruption in function. While Makin and Krakauer mention language recovery, their paper focuses on motor and sensory recovery after injury.

In this paper, we similarly propose that language recovery takes place largely through remapping language networks by potentiating the right-hemisphere network homologous to the language network (hereafter referred to as the "right-hemisphere language network") and by modulating connection strength between nodes of the right-hemisphere language network and undamaged nodes of the left-hemisphere language network. Based on this premise (supported by evidence we review), we propose that interventions should be aimed at potentiating the right-hemisphere language network through Hebbian learning or by augmenting connections between network nodes through neuroplasticity (such as non-invasive brain stimulation and perhaps modulation of neurotransmitters involved in neuroplasticity). The aim of our discussion focuses on evidence from the most common patterns of hemispheric functional dominance observed in the population. In the majority of healthy people, functional representations unique to higher-level language processing are predominantly left-lateralized, while lower-level processing underpinning language, such as sound identification, is more commonly associated with a bilateral representation [3].

First, we review a representative sample of evidence from neurotypical control participants for the existence of a reliable language network in the left hemisphere as well as a homologous right-hemisphere language network that together support virtually all language functions, including phonological (sound based), orthographic (writing based), semantic (meaning based), and syntactic (grammar based) processes involved in understanding and producing spoken and written language. Certainly, an exhaustive review is impossible in a single paper. However, we review illustrative studies using various functional resting state and task-related imaging approaches. These networks each include ventral (sound to meaning [3]) and dorsal (meaning to production [4]) streams [5] composed of cortical regions and their connections as well as the contralateral cerebellum [6]. Although these networks are modulated by subcortical structures such as the basal ganglia and thalamus, the role of subcortical structures in post-stroke aphasia is likely through diaschisis (i.e., dysfunction in distant areas of cortex that are otherwise spared but occurs due to their connections with damaged structures), and recovery from damage to these subcortical regions may reflect the resolution of diaschisis [7].

Then, we review evidence from functional imaging studies of people with aphasia indicating that recovery occurs through remapping and change in connection strength between nodes of the right- and left-hemisphere language networks as we have defined them. We include studies of positron emission tomography (PET), resting state and task-related functional magnetic resonance imaging (fMRI), and functional near-infrared spectroscopy (fNIRS), although there are also data from electroencephalography (EEG) that are relevant to the discussion.

Finally, we discuss the types of interventions that have been used in aphasia that might be utilized to potentiate networks that are supportive of language, including right-hemisphere language network and right cerebellar–cortical connections. We review interventions focused on enhancing the supportive roles of the right hemisphere in language processing through music, drawing, prosody, and manipulations to attention and intention. Although there is scant evidence that these interventions actually have potentiated, that is, increased, synaptic strength and efficiency via activity in the right-hemisphere language network, we provide directions for future studies to evaluate this hypothesis. We also review studies of treatments aimed at increasing neuroplasticity and connectivity between language network nodes, including connections between the right cerebellum and language network. Some of these studies have, in fact, demonstrated changes in connection strength as predicted by our proposals.

2. The Language Network and Supporting Areas in Neurotypical Controls

2.1. The Left-Hemisphere Language Network

One of the most remarkable findings from functional imaging of language processing is that the same cortical regions are activated in nearly every language task, even though damage to distinct regions causes very different deficits. Although "subtraction" designs, those selected to reveal distinct areas activated for two different language tasks (e.g., reading aloud irregular words minus reading aloud regular words), can show differences, virtually all language tasks activate the same regions of left hemisphere when contrasted with low level tasks that are primarily attentional or perceptual (e.g., fixation, counting, saying "skip" to scrambled pictures or scrambled words). Nodes of the language network generally include the posterior superior temporal cortex (pSTG, often referred to as "Wernike's area"), middle temporal gyrus (MTG), inferior temporal gyrus or fusiform gyrus (FuG), posterior inferior frontal gyrus (pIFG, often referred to as "Broca's area"), dorsolateral prefrontal cortex (DLPFC), and inferior parietal cortex (IPC), which includes the supramarginal gyrus (SMG) and angular gyrus (AG) (list of frequently-occurring abbreviations provided below). Importantly, recent authors have argued against viewing the language network as a set of discrete, specialized, regions each contributing a constituent function toward the emergence of language. Instead, it may be better understood as a synergistic network acting together [5,8,9].

Activation of this language network is observed in fMRI studies across clinical and healthy populations with tasks as divergent as word generation/letter fluency [10], word retrieval (naming and oral reading compared to counting) [11], comprehension and production of syntactically complex sentences [12], passive viewing and listening to discourse [13], detecting sensible vs. not sensible sentences [14], and reading [15]. Early PET studies first revealed activation in these areas during most language tasks, although PET studies also frequently showed activation of the cingulate cortex (see [16] and [17] for review). Occipital areas are activated consistently when visual stimuli are included as part of the task unless compared to a baseline condition that includes comparable visual demands.

This "language network" is among the networks revealed by task-free ("resting state") fMRI. The best known (and first described) network of brain regions that show highly correlated blood oxygen level-dependent (BOLD) activation at rest is the Default Mode Network [18]. However, several other networks defined by their "connectivity" (correlated BOLD activity at rest) have been described, including the language network [19], which includes the network nodes described above, as well as superior frontal cortex.

Other types of studies have evaluated the interplay between nodes of the language network during specific tasks. For example, one study of concurrent transcranial magnetic stimulation and electroencephalography (TMS-EEG) revealed time- and region-specific causal evidence for a bidirectional flow of activation from the left pSTG/superior temporal sulcus (STS) to the left posterior inferior frontal gyrus (pIFG) and back during auditory sentence processing, as well as interplay between left pSTG/STS and left AG [20].

Structural imaging studies, for example, using diffusion tensor imaging (DTI), also have revealed the major white matter tracts that connect the nodes of the left-hemisphere language network [21,22]. In the dorsal stream of language processing (meaning to production), the three segments of the arcuate fasciculus with distinct connections and the frontal aslant tract provide the main connections within the language network. In the ventral stream, the connections are provided by the inferior longitudinal fasciculus, inferior fronto-occipital fasciculus, middle longitudinal fasciculus, uncinate fasciculus, and temporo-frontal extreme capsule fasciculus. The frontal aslant tract is a recently described short monosynaptic association tract connecting the lateral IFG to the superior frontal gyrus, an area that may have a supportive role in language, along with the cingulate cortex.

2.2. The Right-Hemisphere (Homologous) Language Cortex

The language network, as defined by task-free fMRI connectivity, also includes the right pSTG [19]. This finding fits well with current models of language processing that propose left-dominant dorsal and ventral streams of language processing, but also more bilateral processing of phonology in right and left pSTG. Virtually all fMRI studies of language processing by neurotypical controls show activation of at least some of the right hemisphere homologues of the language networks, although these areas are rarely discussed. For example, control participants presented with sensible sentences versus not sensible sentences activated right IFG, DLPFC, and MTG, as well as the left-hemisphere language network. Generally, activation of the right-hemisphere language network is lower than the left hemisphere homologues or may not include all of the language network [16,23]. While this may contribute to the trend of not acknowledging when bilateral activation is observed, it seems likely that a prepotent belief about hemispheric dominance also discourages investigators from interpreting right hemisphere activation as truly necessary to healthy language processing. When discussed, right hemisphere activation has sometimes been attributed to processing the prosody of language stimuli (e.g., emotional prosody [24]), recognizing multiple meanings of words (e.g., [25–27]), extracting the main idea or "gist" of discourse [28], or auditory processing of either the stimuli or one's own spoken output.

Other studies have specifically evaluated the role of the right hemisphere in language tasks. For example, Patel and colleagues carried out an fMRI study of neurotypical participants producing and listening to discourse on a variety of topics [29]. They identified regions where similar neural activity was predicted by semantic similarity. They found that spoken discourse on similar topics elicited similar activation patterns in a widely distributed and bilateral brain network. This bilateral network was more extensive but overlapped with regions where similar activation was associated with similar topics during comprehension. Semantic similarity effects were bilateral, even while univariate activation contrasts of these data were left-lateralized. This result suggests that the right hemisphere homologues of the language network encode semantic properties even when they do not show significant activation over baseline. The authors concluded that right hemisphere homologues have a supportive role in processing the meaning of discourse during comprehension and production.

Another study evaluated inter- and intra-hemispheric connectivity in processing unambiguous versus semantically ambiguous words (homophonic homographs, such as bark on a tree and bark of a dog, and heterophonic homographs, such as bass the fish vs. bass the instrument) in neurotypical adults. For heterophonic homographs, they observed increased connectivity within the left hemisphere, indicating top-down re-activation of orthographic representations by phonological representations to process alternative meanings. For homophonic homographs, they showed bidirectional flow of information from left to right and from right to left, indicating a greater role of the right hemisphere in understanding these words [30].

2.3. The Role of the Cerebellum

Several recent reviews have discussed neuroanatomical and functional imaging evidence for a strongly lateralized involvement of the right cerebellum in a variety of nonmotor (as well as motor) language functions through functional and structural connections between the right cerebellum and language cortex [31–33]. The right cerebellum is at least involved in monitoring and coordinating functions of the cortical language network. Many functional imaging studies of language show activation of the right or bilateral cerebellum as well as the right hemisphere homologues of the language network, although these areas are often not mentioned in the text [34]. A recent coordinate-based meta-analysis of the language processing of 403 experiments found that language primarily engaged the bilateral fronto-temporal cortices, with the highest activation in the left pIFG but also the left fusiform gyrus (FuG), bilateral auditory, and left postcentral regions. Importantly, they also found strong bilateral subcortical and cerebellar contributions. The right cerebellum was activated during a variety of speech production and visual and phonological language tasks [35].

2.4. The Language Networks and Supporting Areas: Summary

This brief review of evidence from language processing in neurotypical individuals supports the view that there exists a reliable left-hemisphere cortical language network that includes the superior, middle, and inferior temporal cortex, Fu, pIFG, DLPFC, and IPC and their connections. Additionally, there are left hemisphere areas that seem to be frequently engaged in language that may have a supportive role, including the superior frontal gyrus (which includes the supplementary motor area (SMA) and the pre-supplementary motor area (pre-SMA)), the cingulate gyrus, and their connections, especially with the IFG. Additionally, both right hemisphere homologues of the language network and the right cerebellum play critical supporting roles in neurotypical individuals. We propose that these areas and their connections might be potentiated to help recover language after stroke. Furthermore, connections between undamaged language network nodes and these supporting regions can be strengthened to support recovery. In the next section, we review imaging studies of language recovery in post-stroke recovery that provide some support for this type of remapping underlying aphasia recovery.

3. Imaging Recovery via the Pre-Existing Right-Hemisphere Language Network

The dominant underlying mechanisms driving aphasia recovery are thought to shift over time after stroke. Acute functional recovery is attributable to restoration of local blood flow in perilesional (i.e., surrounding) tissue [36–38]. Over time, the mechanisms of recovery shift. Subacute recovery is supported by increased activation of the right-hemisphere language network [39] and driven by lesion extent and location within the left hemisphere [7]. That is, while spared ipsilateral perilesional tissue plays a key role [40,41] where left-hemisphere language network tissue is damaged, homologous contralateral regions are engaged to a greater degree. If the entire left hemisphere is damaged, the right MTG, SMG, and AG become most active in language [42].

More selective lesions are associated with more restricted right hemisphere engagement. For example, a meta-analysis contrasting those with and without lesions in the left IFG demonstrated that in those for whom the left IFG was preserved, activation of the right frontal areas was limited to the anterior pars triangularis and MTG [9]. However, in those for whom the left IFG was damaged, right-sided activation extended from the pars triangularis to the dorsal pars opercularis, pars orbitalis, and pre- and post-central gyrus. Irrespective of IFG lesion, activation of the right ventral pars opercularis and left MFG was noted. Sebastian et al. longitudinally examined four participants with naming deficits following stroke in the posterior cerebral artery (PCA, which does not supply the traditional language network, so these areas were structurally intact) using task-based and resting-state functional MRI [43]. During language tasks, participants generally demonstrated robust activation of the bilateral language network, even when measured acutely. Language recovery from the acute to chronic phase was associated with greater balance of left- and right-dominant activation within the language network and its homologues.

Language recovery in aphasia is supported further by domain-general processes that arise from a bilateral network [44–46]. Because language tasks are presumably more difficult for people with disordered language than those without, there may be greater activation of regions supporting attention and cognitive control during language tasks in people with aphasia than in those without. This can lead to ambiguity about how to best interpret bilateral frontal activation in people with aphasia. However, taken together, there is relative consensus that recovery of language involves the right STG and likely the right SMA, middle frontal gyrus, precentral gyrus, AG, MTG, temporal pole, pSTS, precuneus, insula, and anterior cingulate cortex [41], reflecting both domain-specific and domain-general regions.

Multiple studies have observed changes in bilateral and right hemisphere homologous network connectivity associated with functional improvement following treatment of aphasia. For example, in one trial, naming impairment was associated with poor coherence of low frequency BOLD fluctuations within and across the ipsilesional left and contralesional right language cortex at the acute stage after PCA stroke, and functional connectivity improved over time only in participants who showed good naming recovery [43]. Another trial contrasted pre- and post-treatment connectivity and found that pre-treatment fluctuations in BOLD signal and synchrony of fluctuations across regions (amplitude of low-frequency fluctuations) measured in the right MTG were associated with greater treatment response [47]. In the same sample, post-treatment fluctuations in the left MTG and STG and right IFG were associated with greater treatment response. Treatment was associated with restored connectivity between the left MTG and STG and between the right and left IFG. Connectivity of the right pars triangularis [48] and bidirectionally between the right pars triangularis and left fusiform gyrus [49] have been associated more specifically with recovery of concrete words.

However, sustained, greater than normal interhemispheric connectivity is not a positive sign for all individuals when considering all paired regions and functions. The complex landscape of changing function and changing activation is only beginning to be disentangled [50]. However, the granular knowledge of these systems will be crucial to individualizing treatment and predicting outcomes in future individuals. Predictably, it is the extent to which connectivity is preserved at baseline that significantly predicts treatment outcomes (in fMRI [51], EEG [52–54], and in functional near-infrared spectroscopy [55]). While acute interhemispheric connectivity in stroke survivors with language deficits is below that of normal age-matched adults, the magnitude of change can reflect an over-correction or "hyper-normalization" and can be negatively correlated with functional improvement. For example, greater magnitude of increased functional connectivity between the right and left dorsal frontoparietal and dorsal prefrontal areas has been associated with *poorer* response to treatment of spelling [56]. However, the authors note that connectivity after treatment was not associated with poorer accuracy (just a smaller change in accuracy), arguing against a maladaptation interpretation of their findings. In an electroencephalographic dynamic causal modeling study, *reduced* coupling between the right IFG and pSTG was associated with the best recovery [53]. Consistently, normal-like levels of connectivity within a left-dominant language network result in optimal levels of function and the greatest improvement [14,57,58]. This association is also found when examining global measures of network fidelity [59,60] and dynamics [61,62].

These observations add nuance to our understanding of the right-hemisphere language network's role in functional recovery. Studies converge in showing that the best recovery is generally seen when the normal, left-hemisphere language network is adequately spared such that enhanced dependence on the right homologous network is not needed. However, when the normal left-hemisphere language network is sufficiently damaged such that normal or compensatory intrahemispheric connectivity cannot be restored, at least part of the right homologous network is often recruited to support language recovery.

4. Treatments Aimed to Engage Supportive Areas or Connections to Promote Recovery

4.1. Treatments Thought to Engage Right Homologous Network

Various intervention strategies for aphasia are thought to stimulate the right-hemisphere language network, such as those that incorporate music, musical techniques, and drawing. Often, multimodal approaches are introduced in combination to provide communication intervention and support for people with aphasia. Studies have also explored methods involving experimental manipulations to attention and intention, as well as neurostimulation of the right cerebellum, with the aim of improving outcomes. While not all of these approaches have been employed sufficiently broadly and diversely to generate the highest quality evidence of their efficacy (e.g., clinical trials of individual strategies and subsequent meta-analyses), taken together, they provide an important line of evidence for the utility of incorporating right-hemisphere dominant tasks in language treatment.

4.2. Music-Based Treatments

Music-based approaches incorporate such elements as intoned speech, melodic contour, metrical timing, rhythmic tapping, and unison production and are broadly aimed at facilitating speech output by improving one's speech fluency [63,64]. Treatment protocols for aphasia involving music and musical techniques include Melodic Intonation Therapy (MIT [65]), Speech Music Therapy for Aphasia [66], SIPARI® [67], and other music-based methods that incorporate singing, melody, and rhythm [64,68]. MIT—which has the largest research evidence base of the music-based intervention approaches for aphasia— integrates melody via varied intonation and rhythm via left-hand tapping during verbal expression [69]. During MIT, the participant is guided to produce a slower rate of articulation with continuous voicing, which is thought to reduce dependence on the left hemisphere and engage the right hemisphere. The participant is also guided to tap their left hand, which is thought to provide pacing and continuous cueing for syllable production and to engage the sensorimotor network in the right hemisphere [69,70]. Treatment progresses along hierarchies of token complexity and clinician support, initially beginning with two-syllable words/phrases and greater clinician support and advancing to longer phrases with less or no clinician support [70].

In terms of behavioral outcomes in people with aphasia, reviews of MIT report positive effects on participants' word and sentence repetition ability, story retelling, and phrase length, with smaller effects seen in measures of functional, everyday communication and variable effects seen in measures of comprehension [71–73] One group [73] conducted a review of MIT clinical trials that included imaging and found that the right hemisphere brain regions activated by MIT included areas of the frontal motor cortex, including the pIFG, auditory cortex (including the STG and MTG), and the parietal cortex (including the angular gyrus and gyrus). Another study [63] found evidence of changes in activation in various right hemisphere regions, including the pSTG, pIFG, inferior pre-central gyrus, postcentral gyrus, pre-SMA, and SMG, following participation in MIT. In reviews of other music-based interventions, improvements in speech outcomes, such as word and sentence repetition, and language outcomes, such as improved conversational informativeness, are noted [74,75]. Interestingly, individuals with co-occurring aphasia and motor speech deficits seem to benefit more from music-based interventions compared to participants with aphasia without co-occurring motor speech deficit. This may suggest a motor-speech-based mechanism of improvement [64].

4.3. Drawing

Drawing is another modality used in aphasia interventions that is thought to engage the right hemisphere. While drawing often serves as an alternative, compensatory means of communication for people with aphasia (i.e., in lieu of verbal speech in moments of anomia), it is also used as a treatment element in multimodal, restorative treatment approaches designed to facilitate improvements in verbal speech. Drawing is thought to facilitate a different level of semantic processing and a different approach to accessing one's semantic system by increasing the person's attention to an object's structural and perceptual characteristics—or in other words, its visual features [76,77]. This differs from other modalities such as writing, which relies on a lexical route to phonological output and engages the left hemisphere [78]. Drawing has been found to increase accurate naming in significantly more instances than writing [76,78]. Relatedly, fMRI studies have shown that in a group of people with aphasia, drawing produces stronger activation in the right hemisphere compared to writing, indicating that drawing differentially engages the brain compared to a linguistically-based task like writing [76,79]. When drawing an object, its semantic features are activated, which is thought to potentially eliminate semantic competitors that do not share semantic features with the target and to subsequently facilitate target retrieval and production [78]. Additionally, it has been proposed that the fixed nature of drawn symbols may facilitate success in retrieving or activating an object's name by serving as a non-transient representation of the underlying concept [80].

Systematic reviews assessing the effectiveness of drawing in improving language outcomes are limited in number, primarily because drawing is typically integrated as one of several components within multimodal treatments for aphasia. Consequently, these reviews cannot parse out the unique contributions of drawing on improvements seen in language outcomes following such multi-modal treatment approaches. Alongside gesturing and writing, drawing is one of the modalities included in Multi-Modality Aphasia Therapy [81], Promoting Aphasics' Communicative Effectiveness [82], and the ongoing clinical trial for treating subacute-chronic post-stroke aphasia via telemedicine, PICTURE IT (NCT05845047). Reports examining the effectiveness of multimodal approaches that include drawing combined with semantic feature cueing and other communicative modalities (e.g., gesturing) generally report improvements in naming [83]. Case reports and treatment studies that have isolated drawing as the sole element of treatment, such as Back to the Drawing Board [84] and Functional Drawing Training [85], primarily aim to increase people with aphasia's use of drawing as a means of communication (e.g., in the case of severe expressive aphasia) or to improve their drawing ability/quality, and thus, the extent to which such approaches result in improvements in the more standardized, impairment-based language outcomes is not clear.

4.4. Attention and Intention Treatments

Manipulations to attention and intention have also emerged as promising strategies to engage the right hemisphere during language tasks. Manipulating spatial attention during naming/treatment activities, by directing attention to the left visual space, is hypothesized to transfer language function to the right hemisphere [86]. Several studies have demonstrated that placing stimuli in the left hemispace, which may be engaging spatial attention mechanisms in the intact right hemisphere, can improve people with aphasia's language performance [86–88]. Intention treatments aim to shift the lateralization of language production to right frontal structures by incorporating complex left-hand movements that engage the pre-SMA area [89]. A number of studies have reported that performing complex, multi-stage movements with the left-hand during naming tasks results in improved naming accuracy and can lead to higher concentrations of activity in the right frontal lobe following the treatment [90–92]. In one study [93], the investigators compared naming outcomes in a cohort of 34 people with moderate to profound aphasia following both attention and intention treatment conditions. They found that all participants showed significant improvements in naming following both treatment conditions; however, the rate of improvement was greater in the intention treatment condition for those with moderate and severe aphasia. These findings underscore the potential that attention and intention manipulations can enhance recovery outcomes.

4.5. Non-Invasive Brain Stimulation

Non-invasive brain stimulation (NIBS) techniques most commonly refer to the application of repetitive transcranial magnetic stimulation (rTMS) or transcranial direct current stimulation (tDCS), though transcranial alternating current stimulation (tACS) has also been explored [94]. In contrast to the behavioral approaches to aphasia rehabilitation reviewed thus far, NIBS may be applied concurrently with (theoretically) any behavioral approach in the hope of enhancing the therapeutic benefit due to the physiological effects of neurostimulation on synaptic plasticity (that is, generating or inhibiting action potentials). While TMS and tDCS are applied using differing devices and, subsequently, have differing safety profiles, the underlying physiological mechanism of proposed augmentation is comparable. One way in which strategies for applying NIBS differ beyond stimulation site is in whether they apply inhibitory stimulation to the homologous regions in the right hemisphere or excitatory stimulation to the ipsilateral, ideally preserved regions. There are multiple systematic reviews of the literature on the efficacy of NIBS in the treatment of aphasia [95–98]. These meta-analyses generally conclude that there is a small but measurable augmentative effect of NIBS, though it may vary due to individual factors (e.g., genetics, age) and lesion characteristics [99,100].

An example application of neurostimulation that provides unique insight into the present discussion of the right-hemisphere language network is the application of tDCS to the right cerebellum. Two studies investigating the efficacy of neuromodulation to the right cerebellum have demonstrated that pairing right cerebellar transcranial direct current stimulation (tDCS) with behavioral treatment may be a promising avenue through which to augment behavioral treatment outcomes. In one study, a participant who had sustained bilateral strokes and was experiencing anarthria participated in a course of therapy in which right cerebellar tDCS (initially a sham condition followed by an active condition) was coupled with behavioral spelling therapy [101]. Results included significant improvements in the participant's spelling accuracy (to dictation) for both trained and untrained words following both conditions; however, improvements were greater in the active tDCS condition compared to the sham condition. Notably, improvements in spelling accuracy for untrained words and generalization to written picture naming were exclusively observed following the active tDCS condition [101]. Furthermore, imaging results indicated increased cerebro-cerebellar resting state functional connectivity following treatment, suggesting potential modifications to the underlying networks supporting spelling as a result of right cerebellar tDCS. In another study, a group of 21 participants with chronic post-stroke aphasia participated in a randomized, double-blind, sham-controlled, within-subject crossover design experiment in which the right cerebellar tDCS (again, either sham or active) was coupled with a computerized program of word picture matching [102]. Similar to the findings from the case study, improvements in the outcome for untrained targets were only seen following the active condition. These findings suggest that tDCS over the right cerebellum (with concomitant behavioral treatment) enhances language recovery compared to sham stimulation. Additionally, it appears to increase connectivity between the right cerebellum and the right and left language networks as well as within the right and left language networks.

5. Conclusions

Here we have reviewed studies that have shown that a network of right hemisphere areas homologous to the language network and the right cerebellum have a supportive role in language in neurotypical individuals. We have also reviewed evidence that some people with aphasia remap language to these supportive areas or show increased functional connections between these areas and left-hemisphere language network as they recover language. Finally, we discussed behavioral interventions designed to engage the right hemisphere to promote language recovery using music, drawing, gesture, attention, or pragmatics. Other studies have shown the benefit of stimulating the right cerebellum to increase connections between the cerebellum and language network areas in both hemispheres to augment aphasia recovery. Together, these studies indicate that one successful approach to language improvement is to augment remapping of language to the right hemisphere, or right cerebellar–cortical connections.

Author Contributions: Conceptualization, A.E.H.; Investigation, V.T.-B., M.D.S. and A.E.H.; Writing—original draft preparation, V.T.-B., M.D.S. and A.E.H.; Writing—review and editing, V.T.-B., M.D.S. and A.E.H.; Funding acquisition, A.E.H. All authors have read and agreed to the published version of the manuscript.

Funding: This work is supported by NIH/National Institute on Deafness and Other Communication Disorders (NIH/NIDCD) R01 DC05375 (V.T.-B., M.D.S., A.E.H.), R01 DC015466 (A.E.H.), and P50 DC014664 (M.D.S., A.E.H.). The content is solely the responsibility of the authors and does not necessarily represent the official views of the National Institutes of Health.

Acknowledgments: We are grateful to the members of the Stroke Cognitive Outcomes and Recovery (SCORE) Lab for their ongoing efforts and dedication to our participants. We gratefully acknowledge our clinical research participants with stroke whose commitment makes this work possible.

Conflicts of Interest: Argye Hillis receives compensation from the American Heart Association as Editor-in-Chief of Stroke and from Elsevier as Associate Editor of PracticeUpdate Neurology. All authors receive salary support from NIH (NIDCD) through grants.

Abbreviations

AG	Angular gyrus
DLPFC	Dorso-lateral prefrontal cortex
FuG	Fusiform gyrus
IFG	Inferior frontal gyrus
IPC	Inferior parietal cortex
MTG	Middle temporal gyrus
Pre-SMA	Pre-supplementary motor area
SMA	Supplementary motor area
SMG	Supramarginal gyrus
STG	Superior temporal cortex
STS	Superior temporal sulcus

References

1. Makin, T.R.; Krakauer, J.W. Against Cortical Reorganisation. *eLife* **2023**, *12*, e84716. [CrossRef] [PubMed]
2. Nunn, K.; Vallila-Rohter, S. Theory-Driven Treatment Modifications: A Discussion on Meeting the Linguistic, Cognitive, and Psychosocial Needs of Individual Clients with Aphasia. *J. Commun. Disord.* **2023**, *103*, 106327. [CrossRef]
3. Hickok, G.; Poeppel, D. The Cortical Organization of Speech Processing. *Nat. Rev. Neurosci.* **2007**, *8*, 393–402. [CrossRef] [PubMed]
4. Rauschecker, J.P. Cortical Processing of Complex Sounds. *Curr. Opin. Neurobiol.* **1998**, *8*, 516–521. [CrossRef] [PubMed]
5. Saur, D.; Kreher, B.W.; Schnell, S.; Kümmerer, D.; Kellmeyer, P.; Vry, M.-S.; Umarova, R.; Musso, M.; Glauche, V.; Abel, S.; et al. Ventral and Dorsal Pathways for Language. *Proc. Natl. Acad. Sci. USA* **2008**, *105*, 18035–18040. [CrossRef] [PubMed]
6. Silveri, M.C.; Leggio, M.G.; Molinari, M. The Cerebellum Contributes to Linguistic Production: A Case of Agrammatic Speech Following a Right Cerebellar Lesion. *Neurology* **1994**, *44*, 2047–2050. [CrossRef] [PubMed]
7. Jarso, S.; Li, M.; Faria, A.; Davis, C.; Leigh, R.; Sebastian, R.; Tsapkini, K.; Mori, S.; Hillis, A.E. Distinct Mechanisms and Timing of Language Recovery after Stroke. *Cogn. Neuropsychol.* **2013**, *30*, 454–475. [CrossRef] [PubMed]
8. Fedorenko, E.; Thompson-Schill, S.L. Reworking the Language Network. *Trends Cogn. Sci.* **2014**, *18*, 120–126. [CrossRef]
9. Turken, A.U.; Dronkers, N.F. The Neural Architecture of the Language Comprehension Network: Converging Evidence from Lesion and Connectivity Analyses. *Front. Syst. Neurosci.* **2011**, *5*, 1. [CrossRef]
10. Prabhakaran, V.; Raman, S.P.; Grunwald, M.R.; Mahadevia, A.; Hussain, N.; Lu, H.; Van Zijl, P.C.M.; Hillis, A.E. Neural Substrates of Word Generation during Stroke Recovery: The Influence of Cortical Hypoperfusion. *Behav. Neurol.* **2007**, *18*, 45–52. [CrossRef]
11. Parker Jones, O.; Green, D.W.; Grogan, A.; Pliatsikas, C.; Filippopolitis, K.; Ali, N.; Lee, H.L.; Ramsden, S.; Gazarian, K.; Prejawa, S.; et al. Where, When and Why Brain Activation Differs for Bilinguals and Monolinguals during Picture Naming and Reading Aloud. *Cereb. Cortex* **2012**, *22*, 892–902. [CrossRef]
12. Segaert, K.; Menenti, L.; Weber, K.; Petersson, K.M.; Hagoort, P. Shared Syntax in Language Production and Language Comprehension—an FMRI Study. *Cereb. Cortex* **2012**, *22*, 1662–1670. [CrossRef]
13. Bartels, A.; Zeki, S. Brain Dynamics during Natural Viewing Conditions—A New Guide for Mapping Connectivity In Vivo. *Neuroimage* **2005**, *24*, 339–349. [CrossRef]
14. Saur, D.; Lange, R.; Baumgaertner, A.; Schraknepper, V.; Willmes, K.; Rijntjes, M.; Weiller, C. Dynamics of Language Reorganization after Stroke. *Brain* **2006**, *129*, 1371–1384. [CrossRef]
15. Turkeltaub, P.E.; Eden, G.F.; Jones, K.M.; Zeffiro, T.A. Meta-Analysis of the Functional Neuroanatomy of Single-Word Reading: Method and Validation. *Neuroimage* **2002**, *16*, 765–780. [CrossRef]
16. Démonet, J.F.; Wise, R.; Frackowiak, R.S.J. Language Functions Explored in Normal Subjects by Positron Emission Tomography: A Critical Review. *Hum. Brain Mapp.* **1993**, *1*, 39–47. [CrossRef]
17. Price, C.J. A Review and Synthesis of the First 20 Years of PET and FMRI Studies of Heard Speech, Spoken Language and Reading. *Neuroimage* **2012**, *62*, 816–847. [CrossRef]
18. Shirer, W.R.; Ryali, S.; Rykhlevskaia, E.; Menon, V.; Greicius, M.D. Decoding Subject-Driven Cognitive States with Whole-Brain Connectivity Patterns. *Cereb. Cortex* **2012**, *22*, 158–165. [CrossRef]
19. Branco, P.; Seixas, D.; Castro, S.L. Mapping Language with Resting-state Functional Magnetic Resonance Imaging: A Study on the Functional Profile of the Language Network. *Hum. Brain Mapp.* **2020**, *41*, 545–560. [CrossRef] [PubMed]
20. Schroën, J.A.M.; Gunter, T.C.; Numssen, O.; Kroczek, L.O.H.; Hartwigsen, G.; Friederici, A.D. Causal Evidence for a Coordinated Temporal Interplay within the Language Network. *Proc. Natl. Acad. Sci. USA* **2023**, *120*, e2306279120. [CrossRef] [PubMed]
21. Kargar, Y.; Jalilian, M. Anatomo-Functional Profile of White Matter Tracts in Relevance to Language: A Systematic Review. *J. Neurolinguist.* **2024**, *69*, 101175. [CrossRef]
22. Smits, M.; Jiskoot, L.C.; Papma, J.M. White Matter Tracts of Speech and Language. *Semin. Ultrasound CT MRI* **2014**, *35*, 504–516. [CrossRef] [PubMed]
23. Frith, C.D.; Friston, K.J.; Liddle, P.F.; Frackowiak, R.S.J. A PET Study of Word Finding. *Neuropsychologia* **1991**, *29*, 1137–1148. [CrossRef] [PubMed]

24. Ross, E.D.; Mesulam, M.M. Dominant Language Functions of the Right Hemisphere? Prosody and Emotional Gesturing. *Arch. Neurol.* **1979**, *36*, 144–148. [CrossRef] [PubMed]
25. Mason, R.A.; Just, M.A. Lexical Ambiguity in Sentence Comprehension. *Brain Res.* **2007**, *1146*, 115–127. [CrossRef]
26. Peleg, O.; Eviatar, Z. Semantic Asymmetries Are Modulated by Phonological Asymmetries: Evidence from the Disambiguation of Homophonic versus Heterophonic Homographs. *Brain Cogn.* **2009**, *70*, 154–162. [CrossRef] [PubMed]
27. Peleg, O.; Eviatar, Z. Hemispheric Sensitivities to Lexical and Contextual Information: Evidence from Lexical Ambiguity Resolution. *Brain Lang.* **2008**, *105*, 71–82. [CrossRef]
28. Myers, P. Discourse Deficits. In *Right Hemisphere Damage*; Singular Publishing Group: San Diego, CA, USA, 1999; pp. 101–134.
29. Patel, T.; Morales, M.; Pickering, M.J.; Hoffman, P. A Common Neural Code for Meaning in Discourse Production and Comprehension. *Neuroimage* **2023**, *279*, 120295. [CrossRef] [PubMed]
30. Mizrachi, N.; Eviatar, Z.; Peleg, O.; Bitan, T. Inter- and Intra- Hemispheric Interactions in Reading Ambiguous Words. *Cortex* **2023**, *171*, 257–271. [CrossRef]
31. Mariën, P.; Ackermann, H.; Adamaszek, M.; Barwood, C.H.S.; Beaton, A.; Desmond, J.; De Witte, E.; Fawcett, A.J.; Hertrich, I.; Küper, M.; et al. Consensus Paper: Language and the Cerebellum: An Ongoing Enigma. *Cerebellum* **2013**, *13*, 386–410. [CrossRef]
32. Mariën, P.; Borgatti, R. Language and the Cerebellum. In *Handbook of Clinical Neurology*; Manto, M., Huisman, T.A.G.M., Eds.; Elsevier: New York, NY, USA, 2018; Volume 154, pp. 181–202.
33. van Dun, K.; Manto, M.; Mariën, P. The Language of the Cerebellum. *Aphasiology* **2016**, *30*, 1378–1398. [CrossRef]
34. Xiong, J.; Rao, S.; Jerabek, P.; Zamarripa, F.; Woldorff, M.; Lancaster, J.; Fox, P.T. Intersubject Variability in Cortical Activations during a Complex Language Task. *Neuroimage* **2000**, *12*, 326–339. [CrossRef]
35. Turker, S.; Kuhnke, P.; Eickhoff, S.B.; Caspers, S.; Hartwigsen, G. Cortical, Subcortical, and Cerebellar Contributions to Language Processing: A Meta-Analytic Review of 403 Neuroimaging Experiments. *Psychol. Bull.* **2023**, *149*, 699–723. [CrossRef]
36. Marsh, E.B.; Hillis, A.E. Chapter 9 Recovery from Aphasia Following Brain Injury: The Role of Reorganization. *Prog. Brain Res.* **2006**, *157*, 143–156.
37. Hillis, A.E.; Kleinman, J.T.; Newhart, M.; Heidler-Gary, J.; Gottesman, R.; Barker, P.B.; Aldrich, E.; Llinas, R.; Wityk, R.; Chaudhry, P. Restoring Cerebral Blood Flow Reveals Neural Regions Critical for Naming. *J. Neurosci.* **2006**, *26*, 8069–8073. [CrossRef]
38. Motta, M.; Ramadan, A.; Hillis, A.E.; Gottesman, R.F.; Leigh, R. Diffusion-Perfusion Mismatch: An Opportunity for Improvement in Cortical Function. *Front. Neurol.* **2015**, *6*, 280. [CrossRef]
39. Wilson, S.M.; Schneck, S.M. Neuroplasticity in Post-Stroke Aphasia: A Systematic Review and Meta-Analysis of Functional Imaging Studies of Reorganization of Language Processing. *Neurobiol. Lang.* **2021**, *2*, 22–82. [CrossRef]
40. Heiss, W.-D.; Thiel, A. A Proposed Regional Hierarchy in Recovery of Post-Stroke Aphasia. *Brain Lang.* **2006**, *98*, 118–123. [CrossRef]
41. Kiran, S.; Meier, E.L.; Johnson, J.P. Neuroplasticity in Aphasia: A Proposed Framework of Language Recovery. *J. Speech Lang. Hear. Res.* **2019**, *62*, 3973–3985. [CrossRef] [PubMed]
42. Sims, J.A.; Kapse, K.; Glynn, P.; Sandberg, C.; Tripodis, Y.; Kiran, S. The Relationships between the Amount of Spared Tissue, Percent Signal Change, and Accuracy in Semantic Processing in Aphasia. *Neuropsychologia* **2016**, *84*, 113–126. [CrossRef] [PubMed]
43. Sebastian, R.; Long, C.; Purcell, J.J.; Faria, A.V.; Lindquist, M.; Jarso, S.; Race, D.; Davis, C.; Posner, J.; Wright, A.; et al. Imaging Network Level Language Recovery after Left PCA Stroke. *Restor. Neurol. Neurosci.* **2016**, *34*, 473–489. [CrossRef] [PubMed]
44. Geranmayeh, F.; Brownsett, S.L.E.; Wise, R.J.S. Task-Induced Brain Activity in Aphasic Stroke Patients: What Is Driving Recovery? *Brain* **2014**, *137*, 2632–2648. [CrossRef] [PubMed]
45. Geranmayeh, F.; Chau, T.W.; Wise, R.J.S.; Leech, R.; Hampshire, A. Domain-General Subregions of the Medial Prefrontal Cortex Contribute to Recovery of Language after Stroke. *Brain* **2017**, *140*, 1947–1958. [CrossRef] [PubMed]
46. Turkeltaub, P.E.; Messing, S.; Norise, C.; Hamilton, R.H. Are Networks for Residual Language Function and Recovery Consistent across Aphasic Patients? *Neurology* **2011**, *76*, 1726–1734. [CrossRef] [PubMed]
47. van Hees, S.; McMahon, K.; Angwin, A.; de Zubicaray, G.; Copland, D.A. Neural Activity Associated with Semantic versus Phonological Anomia Treatments in Aphasia. *Brain Lang.* **2014**, *129*, 47–57. [CrossRef] [PubMed]
48. Kiran, S.; Meier, E.L.; Kapse, K.J.; Glynn, P.A. Changes in Task-Based Effective Connectivity in Language Networks Following Rehabilitation in Post-Stroke Patients with Aphasia. *Front. Hum. Neurosci.* **2015**, *9*, 316. [CrossRef] [PubMed]
49. Stockbridge, M.D.; Faria, A.V.; Fridriksson, J.; Rorden, C.; Bonilha, L.; Hillis, A.E. Subacute Aphasia Recovery Is Associated with Resting-State Connectivity within and beyond the Language Network. *Ann. Clin. Transl. Neurol.* **2023**, *10*, 1525–1532. [CrossRef] [PubMed]
50. Stefaniak, J.D.; Geranmayeh, F.; Lambon Ralph, M.A. The Multidimensional Nature of Aphasia Recovery Post-Stroke. *Brain* **2022**, *145*, 1354–1367. [CrossRef] [PubMed]
51. Falconer, I.; Varkanitsa, M.; Kiran, S. Resting-State Brain Network Connectivity Is an Independent Predictor of Responsiveness to Language Therapy in Chronic Post-Stroke Aphasia. *Cortex* **2024**, *173*, 296–312. [CrossRef]
52. Vatinno, A.A.; Simpson, A.; Ramakrishnan, V.; Bonilha, H.S.; Bonilha, L.; Seo, N.J. The Prognostic Utility of Electroencephalography in Stroke Recovery: A Systematic Review and Meta-Analysis. *Neurorehabil. Neural Repair* **2022**, *36*, 255–268. [CrossRef]
53. Iyer, K.K.; Angwin, A.J.; Van Hees, S.; McMahon, K.L.; Breakspear, M.; Copland, D.A. Alterations to Dual Stream Connectivity Predicts Response to Aphasia Therapy Following Stroke. *Cortex* **2020**, *125*, 30–43. [CrossRef] [PubMed]

54. Johnson, L.; Yourganov, G.; Basilakos, A.; Newman-Norlund, R.D.; Thors, H.; Keator, L.; Rorden, C.; Bonilha, L.; Fridriksson, J. Functional Connectivity and Speech Entrainment Speech Entrainment Improves Connectivity between Anterior and Posterior Cortical Speech Areas in Non-Fluent Aphasia. *Neurorehabil. Neural Repair* **2022**, *36*, 164–174. [CrossRef] [PubMed]
55. Meier, E.; Bunker, L.; Kim, H.; Hillis, A.E. Connectivity in Acute and Subacute PostStroke Aphasia: A Functional Near-Infrared Spectroscopy Pilot Study. *Brain Connect.* **2023**, *13*, 441–452. [CrossRef] [PubMed]
56. Tao, Y.; Rapp, B. How Functional Network Connectivity Changes as a Result of Lesion and Recovery: An Investigation of the Network Phenotype of Stroke. *Cortex* **2020**, *131*, 17–41. [CrossRef]
57. Nenert, R.; Allendorfer, J.B.; Martin, A.M.; Banks, C.; Vannest, J.; Holland, S.K.; Hart, K.W.; Lindsell, C.J.; Szaflarski, J.P. Longitudinal FMRI Study of Language Recovery after a Left Hemispheric Ischemic Stroke. *Restor. Neurol. Neurosci.* **2018**, *36*, 359–385. [CrossRef] [PubMed]
58. Stockert, A.; Wawrzyniak, M.; Klingbeil, J.; Wrede, K.; Kümmerer, D.; Hartwigsen, G.; Kaller, C.P.; Weiller, C.; Saur, D. Dynamics of Language Reorganization after Left Temporo-Parietal and Frontal Stroke. *Brain* **2020**, *143*, 844–861. [CrossRef] [PubMed]
59. Bonilha, L.; Gleichgerrcht, E.; Nesland, T.; Rorden, C.; Fridriksson, J. Success of Anomia Treatment in Aphasia Is Associated with Preserved Architecture of Global and Left Temporal Lobe Structural Networks. *Neurorehabil. Neural Repair* **2016**, *30*, 266–279. [CrossRef]
60. Duncan, E.S.; Small, S.L. Changes in Dynamic Resting State Network Connectivity Following Aphasia Therapy. *Brain Imaging Behav.* **2018**, *12*, 1141–1149. [CrossRef]
61. Fan, H.; Su, P.; Lin, D.D.M.; Goldberg, E.B.; Walker, A.; Leigh, R.; Hillis, A.E.; Lu, H. Simultaneous Hemodynamic and Structural Imaging of Ischemic Stroke with Magnetic Resonance Fingerprinting Arterial Spin Labeling. *Stroke* **2022**, *53*, 2016–2025. [CrossRef] [PubMed]
62. Guo, J.; Biswal, B.B.; Han, S.; Li, J.; Yang, S.; Yang, M.; Chen, H. Altered Dynamics of Brain Segregation and Integration in Poststroke Aphasia. *Hum. Brain Mapp.* **2019**, *40*, 3398–3409. [CrossRef]
63. Marchina, S.; Norton, A.; Schlaug, G. Effects of Melodic Intonation Therapy in Patients with Chronic Nonfluent Aphasia. *Ann. N. Y. Acad. Sci.* **2023**, *1519*, 173–185. [CrossRef] [PubMed]
64. Zumbansen, A.; Tremblay, P. Music-Based Interventions for Aphasia Could Act through a Motor-Speech Mechanism: A Systematic Review and Case–Control Analysis of Published Individual Participant Data. *Aphasiology* **2019**, *33*, 466–497. [CrossRef]
65. Albert, M.L.; Sparks, R.W.; Helm, N.A. Melodic Intonation Therapy for Aphasia. *Arch. Neurol.* **1973**, *29*, 130–131. [CrossRef] [PubMed]
66. De Bruijn, M.; Hurkmans, J.; Zielman, T. *Speech-Music Therapy for Aphasia (SMTA)*; Beetsterzwaag: Revalidatie, Friesland, 2011.
67. Jungblut, M. SIPARI(R): A Music Therapy Intervention for Patients Suffering with Chronic, Nonfluent Aphasia. *Music. Med.* **2009**, *1*, 102–105. [CrossRef]
68. Leonardi, S.; Cacciola, A.; De Luca, R.; Aragona, B.; Andronaco, V.; Milardi, D.; Bramanti, P.; Calabrò, R.S. The Role of Music Therapy in Rehabilitation: Improving Aphasia and Beyond. *Int. J. Neurosci.* **2018**, *128*, 90–99. [CrossRef] [PubMed]
69. Norton, A.; Zipse, L.; Marchina, S.; Schlaug, G. Melodic Intonation Therapy. *Ann. N. Y. Acad. Sci.* **2009**, *1169*, 431–436. [CrossRef] [PubMed]
70. Schlaug, G.; Marchina, S.; Norton, A. From Singing to Speaking: Why Singing May Lead to Recovery of Expressive Language Function in Patients with Broca's Aphasia. *Music. Percept.* **2008**, *25*, 315–323. [CrossRef]
71. Haro-Martínez, A.; Pérez-Araujo, C.M.; Sanchez-Caro, J.M.; Fuentes, B.; Díez-Tejedor, E. Melodic Intonation Therapy for Post-Stroke Non-Fluent Aphasia: Systematic Review and Meta-Analysis. *Front. Neurol.* **2021**, *12*, 700115. [CrossRef] [PubMed]
72. Popescu, T.; Stahl, B.; Wiernik, B.M.; Haiduk, F.; Zemanek, M.; Helm, H.; Matzinger, T.; Beisteiner, R.; Fitch, W.T. Melodic Intonation Therapy for Aphasia: A Multi-level Meta-analysis of Randomized Controlled Trials and Individual Participant Data. *Ann. N. Y. Acad. Sci.* **2022**, *1516*, 76–84. [CrossRef]
73. Zhang, X.; Li, J.; Du, Y. Melodic Intonation Therapy on Non-Fluent Aphasia after Stroke: A Systematic Review and Analysis on Clinical Trials. *Front. Neurosci.* **2022**, *15*, 753356. [CrossRef]
74. Hurkmans, J.; Jonkers, R.; de Bruijn, M.; Boonstra, A.M.; Hartman, P.P.; Arendzen, H.; Reinders-Messelink, H.A. The Effectiveness of Speech–Music Therapy for Aphasia (SMTA) in Five Speakers with Apraxia of Speech and Aphasia. *Aphasiology* **2015**, *29*, 939–964. [CrossRef]
75. Zumbansen, A.; Peretz, I.; HÃ©bert, S. The Combination of Rhythm and Pitch Can Account for the Beneficial Effect of Melodic Intonation Therapy on Connected Speech Improvements in Broca's Aphasia. *Front. Hum. Neurosci.* **2014**, *8*, 592. [CrossRef]
76. Farias, D.; Davis, C.; Harrington, G. Drawing: Its Contribution to Naming in Aphasia. *Brain Lang.* **2006**, *97*, 53–63. [CrossRef]
77. Pierce, J.E.; Menahemi-Falkov, M.; O'Halloran, R.; Togher, L.; Rose, M.L. Constraint and Multimodal Approaches to Therapy for Chronic Aphasia: A Systematic Review and Meta-Analysis. *Neuropsychol. Rehabil.* **2019**, *29*, 1005–1041. [CrossRef] [PubMed]
78. Hung, P.-F.; Ostergren, J. A Comparison of Drawing and Writing on Facilitating Word Retrieval in Individuals with Aphasia. *Aphasiology* **2019**, *33*, 1462–1481. [CrossRef]
79. Harrington, G.S.; Farias, D.; Davis, C.H.; Buonocore, M.H. Comparison of the Neural Basis for Imagined Writing and Drawing. *Hum. Brain Mapp.* **2007**, *28*, 450–459. [CrossRef]
80. Lyon, J.G.; Sims, E. Drawing: Its Use as a Communicative Aid with Aphasic and Normal Adults. In *Aphasia Treatment: World Perspectives*; Holland, A., Forbes, M.M., Eds.; Springer: New York, NY, USA, 1989; Volume 18, pp. 339–355.
81. Rose, M.; Attard, M. *Multi-Modality Aphasia Therapy: A Treatment Manual*; La Trobe University: Melbourne, Australia, 2011.

82. Davis, G.A.; Wilcox, M.J. *Adult Aphasia Rehabilitation: Applied Pragmatics*; Singular: San Diego, CA, USA, 1985.
83. Kinney, J.; Wallace, S.E.; Schreiber, J.B. The Relationship between Word Retrieval, Drawing, and Semantics in People with Aphasia. *Aphasiology* **2020**, *34*, 254–274. [CrossRef]
84. Morgan, A.L.; Helm-Estabrooks, N. Back to the Drawing Board: A Treatment Program for Nonverbal Aphasic Patients. *Clin. Aphasiol.* **1987**, *17*, 64–72.
85. Ward-Lonergan, J.M.; Nicholas, M. Drawing to Communicate: A Case Report of an Adult with Global Aphasia. *Int. J. Lang. Commun. Disord.* **1995**, *30*, 475–491. [CrossRef]
86. Dotson, V.M.; Singletary, F.; Fuller, R.; Koehler, S.; Moore, A.B.; Gonzalez Rothi, L.J.; Crosson, B. Treatment of Word-finding Deficits in Fluent Aphasia through the Manipulation of Spatial Attention: Preliminary Findings. *Aphasiology* **2008**, *22*, 103–113. [CrossRef]
87. Anderson, B. Semantic Neglect? *J. Neurol. Neurosurg. Psychiatry* **1996**, *60*, 349–350. [CrossRef] [PubMed]
88. Coslett, H. Spatial Influences on Motor and Language Function. *Neuropsychologia* **1999**, *37*, 695–706. [CrossRef] [PubMed]
89. Picard, N.; Strick, P.L. Motor Areas of the Medial Wall: A Review of Their Location and Functional Activation. *Cereb. Cortex* **1996**, *6*, 342–353. [CrossRef] [PubMed]
90. Crosson, B.; Moore, A.B.; McGregor, K.M.; Chang, Y.-L.; Benjamin, M.; Gopinath, K.; Sherod, M.E.; Wierenga, C.E.; Peck, K.K.; Briggs, R.W.; et al. Regional Changes in Word-Production Laterality after a Naming Treatment Designed to Produce a Rightward Shift in Frontal Activity. *Brain Lang.* **2009**, *111*, 73–85. [CrossRef]
91. Crosson, B.; Moore, A.B.; Gopinath, K.; White, K.D.; Wierenga, C.E.; Gaiefsky, M.E.; Fabrizio, K.S.; Peck, K.K.; Soltysik, D.; Milsted, C.; et al. Role of the Right and Left Hemispheres in Recovery of Function during Treatment of Intention in Aphasia. *J. Cogn. Neurosci.* **2005**, *17*, 392–406. [CrossRef] [PubMed]
92. Richards, K.; Singletary, F.; Rothi, L.J.G.; Koehler, S.; Crosson, B. Activation of Intentional Mechanisms through Utilization of Nonsymbolic Movements in Aphasia Rehabilitation. *J. Rehabil. Res. Dev.* **2002**, *39*, 445–454. [PubMed]
93. Crosson, B.; Fabrizio, K.S.; Singletary, F.; Cato, M.A.; Wierenga, C.E.; Parkinson, R.B.; Sherod, M.E.; Moore, A.B.; Ciampitti, M.; Holiway, B.; et al. Treatment of Naming in Nonfluent Aphasia through Manipulation of Intention and Attention: A Phase 1 Comparison of Two Novel Treatments. *J. Int. Neuropsychol. Soc.* **2007**, *13*, 582–594. [CrossRef]
94. Keator, L.M. Transcranial Alternating Current Stimulation as an Adjuvant for Nonfluent Aphasia Therapy: A Proof-Of-Concept Study. Ph.D. Thesis, University of South Carolina, Columbia, SC, USA, 2022.
95. Marangolo, P. The Potential Effects of Transcranial Direct Current Stimulation (TDCS) on Language Functioning: Combining Neuromodulation and Behavioral Intervention in Aphasia. *Neurosci. Lett.* **2020**, *719*, 133329. [CrossRef] [PubMed]
96. Elsner, B.; Kugler, J.; Pohl, M.; Mehrholz, J. Transcranial Direct Current Stimulation (TDCS) for Improving Aphasia in Patients after Stroke. *Cochrane Database Syst. Rev.* **2013**, CD009760. [CrossRef]
97. Ren, C.-L.; Zhang, G.-F.; Xia, N.; Jin, C.-H.; Zhang, X.-H.; Hao, J.-F.; Guan, H.-B.; Tang, H.; Li, J.-A.; Cai, D.-L. Effect of Low-Frequency RTMS on Aphasia in Stroke Patients: A Meta-Analysis of Randomized Controlled Trials. *PLoS ONE* **2014**, *9*, e102557. [CrossRef]
98. Otal, B.; Olma, M.C.; Flöel, A.; Wellwood, I. Inhibitory Non-Invasive Brain Stimulation to Homologous Language Regions as an Adjunct to Speech and Language Therapy in Post-Stroke Aphasia: A Meta-Analysis. *Front. Hum. Neurosci.* **2015**, *9*, 236. [CrossRef]
99. Stockbridge, M.D.; Elm, J.; Teklehaimanot, A.A.; Cassarly, C.; Spell, L.-A.; Fridriksson, J.; Hillis, A.E. Individual Differences in Response to Transcranial Direct Current Stimulation with Language Therapy in Subacute Stroke. *Neurorehabil. Neural Repair* **2023**, *37*, 519–529. [CrossRef]
100. Fridriksson, J.; Elm, J.; Stark, B.C.; Basilakos, A.; Rorden, C.; Sen, S.; George, M.S.; Gottfried, M.; Bonilha, L. BDNF Genotype and TDCS Interaction in Aphasia Treatment. *Brain Stimul.* **2018**, *11*, 1276–1281. [CrossRef]
101. Sebastian, R.; Saxena, S.; Tsapkini, K.; Faria, A.V.; Long, C.; Wright, A.; Davis, C.; Tippett, D.C.; Mourdoukoutas, A.P.; Bikson, M.; et al. Cerebellar TDCS: A Novel Approach to Augment Language Treatment Post-Stroke. *Front. Hum. Neurosci.* **2017**, *10*, 695. [CrossRef]
102. Sebastian, R.; Kim, J.H.; Brenowitz, R.; Tippett, D.C.; Desmond, J.E.; Celnik, P.A.; Hillis, A.E. Cerebellar Neuromodulation Improves Naming in Post-Stroke Aphasia. *Brain Commun.* **2020**, *2*, fcaa179. [CrossRef]

Disclaimer/Publisher's Note: The statements, opinions and data contained in all publications are solely those of the individual author(s) and contributor(s) and not of MDPI and/or the editor(s). MDPI and/or the editor(s) disclaim responsibility for any injury to people or property resulting from any ideas, methods, instructions or products referred to in the content.

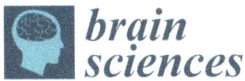

Review

Exploring the Prospects of Transcranial Electrical Stimulation (tES) as a Therapeutic Intervention for Post-Stroke Motor Recovery: A Narrative Review

Hao Meng [1,*], Michael Houston [2], Yingchun Zhang [3] and Sheng Li [1,4,*]

1. Department of Physical Medicine & Rehabilitation, McGovern Medical School, University of Texas Health Science Center at Houston, Houston, TX 77030, USA
2. Department of Biomedical Engineering, University of Houston, Houston, TX 77204, USA; mjhousto@cougarnet.uh.edu
3. Department of Biomedical Engineering, University of Miami, Coral Gables, FL 33146, USA; y.zhang@miami.edu
4. TIRR Memorial Hermann Hospital, Houston, TX 77030, USA
* Correspondence: hao.meng@uth.tmc.edu (H.M.); sheng.li@uth.tmc.edu (S.L.)

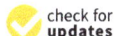

Citation: Meng, H.; Houston, M.; Zhang, Y.; Li, S. Exploring the Prospects of Transcranial Electrical Stimulation (tES) as a Therapeutic Intervention for Post-Stroke Motor Recovery: A Narrative Review. *Brain Sci.* **2024**, *14*, 322. https://doi.org/10.3390/brainsci14040322

Academic Editors: Noureddin Nakhostin Ansari, Gholamreza Hassanzadeh and Ardalan Shariat

Received: 8 February 2024
Revised: 12 March 2024
Accepted: 23 March 2024
Published: 27 March 2024

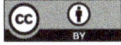

Copyright: © 2024 by the authors. Licensee MDPI, Basel, Switzerland. This article is an open access article distributed under the terms and conditions of the Creative Commons Attribution (CC BY) license (https://creativecommons.org/licenses/by/4.0/).

Abstract: Introduction: Stroke survivors often have motor impairments and related functional deficits. Transcranial Electrical Stimulation (tES) is a rapidly evolving field that offers a wide range of capabilities for modulating brain function, and it is safe and inexpensive. It has the potential for widespread use for post-stroke motor recovery. Transcranial Direct Current Stimulation (tDCS), Transcranial Alternating Current Stimulation (tACS), and Transcranial Random Noise Stimulation (tRNS) are three recognized tES techniques that have gained substantial attention in recent years but have different mechanisms of action. tDCS has been widely used in stroke motor rehabilitation, while applications of tACS and tRNS are very limited. The tDCS protocols could vary significantly, and outcomes are heterogeneous. Purpose: the current review attempted to explore the mechanisms underlying commonly employed tES techniques and evaluate their prospective advantages and challenges for their applications in motor recovery after stroke. Conclusion: tDCS could depolarize and hyperpolarize the potentials of cortical motor neurons, while tACS and tRNS could target specific brain rhythms and entrain neural networks. Despite the extensive use of tDCS, the complexity of neural networks calls for more sophisticated modifications like tACS and tRNS.

Keywords: tES; tDCS; tACS; tRNS; stroke; motor recovery

1. Introduction

Stroke results from damage to the central nervous system [1]. The typical symptoms caused by stroke can include motor deficits like muscle weakness, impaired coordination, and spasticity; cognitive impairments affecting memory, attention, and problem-solving; speech and language difficulties; and emotional disturbances, such as depression and anxiety [2]. Transcranial Electrical Stimulation (tES) is a rapidly developing field that has gained considerable attention for its potential in post-stroke motor recovery over the past two decades. This technique applies an electric field to the scalp surface to modulate brain activity. In fact, instead of using high-intensity stimulation current in the early efforts, contemporary tES applies a weak electric current (1~2 mA) to the scalp to modulate the cortical excitability [3]. tES can be classified into Transcranial Direct Current Stimulation (tDCS), Transcranial Alternating Current Stimulation (tACS), and Transcranial Random Noise Stimulation (tRNS) [4]. Compared to other Non-Invasive Brain Stimulation (NIBS) techniques like Transcranial Magnetic Stimulation (TMS), the popularity of tES arises from several factors. First, when applied within guidelines, it is non-invasive and relatively safe, with minimal side effects and risks. Second, its low cost and portability make it accessible for various research and therapeutic purposes. Finally, it offers ease of operation and customization, allowing researchers and clinicians to tailor its use to meet specific goals [5]. However, various tES techniques have limitations that challenge their clinical efficacy and the replication of research findings.

Recent reviews suggest that tDCS can modulate cortical excitability and potentially benefit motor recovery in stroke survivors [6–9]. However, when combined with physical therapy, several other reviews have indicated that tDCS might not consistently augment the effects [10–13]. While tDCS has been widely studied for stroke motor recovery, research on tACS in this field is still comparatively limited. Takeuchi and Izumi [14] reviewed the potential of tACS to enhance motor function and concluded that, although targeting brain oscillations with tACS shows promise for improving motor learning, further research is necessary to provide more conclusive evidence. The review also highlights the potential for a synergistic effect on motor learning when combining tACS with other neurorehabilitation methods. Yang et al. [15] also reviewed relevant tACS studies in stroke recovery, finding that tACS is linked to improvements in overall functional recovery, sensorimotor impairment, aphasia, and hemispatial neglect. Despite the common advantages, emerging tES methods employ distinct mechanisms to modulate cortical excitability, and the paradigms for applying tES are continually evolving. However, the efficacy of tES in stroke motor recovery presents challenges, and there is not yet a definitive conclusion regarding which technique could optimize the benefits of stroke neurorehabilitation. This review aims to explore the potential of tES for improving upper-limb motor recovery in stroke survivors. We will compare the mechanisms and neuromodulatory effects of tDCS, tACS, and tRNS in both healthy individuals and stroke patients. Additionally, we'll analyze the advantages and disadvantages of each technique, suggesting future applications of tES in stroke motor recovery. The findings of this review will provide researchers with a deeper understanding of the mechanisms, paradigms, and potential future applications of tES in this important area.

2. Literature Search

We conducted a PubMed literature search using keywords "tDCS/tACS/tRNS", "primary motor cortex", "cortical excitability", and "healthy/stroke" to identify relevant studies published between 2014 and 2024. We excluded studies that did not apply stimulation over the primary motor cortex. After applying these criteria, 79 studies were included: 54 investigating tDCS, 16 investigating tACS, and 9 investigating tRNS.

3. Stroke Upper Limb Motor Recovery

Muscle weakness or paralysis on one side of the body can severely impact upper limb function in stroke survivors. This impairment may present as difficulty performing simple movements or a complete inability to use the affected arm and hand. These motor deficits can significantly disrupt activities of daily living—dressing, feeding, and personal care—thus substantially diminishing the stroke survivor's autonomy and life quality [16]. A previous review has indicated that approximately 80% of individuals post-stroke experience upper limb impairments early in the recovery process, with a minority achieving full functional restoration by six months [17]. Abnormal motor synergies can often be observed in the upper limb functions of stroke survivors, such as abnormal reaching movements characterized by shoulder abduction and elbow flexion instead of the normal shoulder flexion and elbow extension. Additionally, adaptations in reaching and grasping movements may occur due to sensory impairments [16]. In clinical settings, a well-accepted three-stage motor recovery framework has been proposed: flaccid, spastic, and recovered [18]. Recovery from stroke is a long journey; for some stroke survivors, it could last a lifetime. The success of stroke recovery requires collaboration among patients, doctors, therapists, and family members [19]. Current consensus indicates that rehabilitative interventions are most effective when they provide early, intensive, task-specific, and multisensory stimulation.

Integrating both bottom-up and top-down processes is advantageous for promoting brain plasticity [20].

4. Transcranial Direct Current Stimulation (tDCS)

In the early 2000s, Nitsche and Paulus [21] proposed an approach to modulating cortical excitability by applying an anodal electrode that delivers constant current to the motor cortex and a cathodal electrode to the contralateral forehead (Figure 1A). They discovered that this specific electrode arrangement enhanced motor cortex excitability, attributed to the anodal stimulation depolarizing the motor neuron membrane, thereby potentiating action potentials. Conversely, cathodal stimulation results in the hyperpolarization of the membrane. This initial experiment with tDCS laid the groundwork for tES neuromodulation, leading studies to apply tDCS across various fields. Furthermore, at the molecular and cellular levels, the modulation associated with tDCS may be linked to activity in various neurotransmitter systems, including glutamatergic, GABAergic, dopaminergic, serotonergic, and cholinergic pathways [22]. In fact, the mechanism of tDCS can be interpreted in two parts: the acute effect (online effect) and the plastic effect (offline effect). In the acute phase, the action potential of the neuronal membrane is determined by afferent activity via electrical and chemical synapses and also by extra-synaptic substances, which activate specific ion channels and receptors [23–25]. On the other hand, neuroplasticity can also be observed following tDCS. Neuroplasticity refers to the brain's ability to change its structure and function at the level of individual neurons or throughout entire neuronal networks [26]. When the membrane of glutamatergic synapses is depolarized or hyperpolarized, tDCS may increase or decrease the amount of calcium flow through the N-methyl-D-aspartate (NMDA) receptor and calcium channels. Depending on the changes in intraneuronal calcium levels, glutamatergic α-amino-3-hydroxy-5-methyl-4-isoxazolepropionic acid (AMPA) receptors can be inserted into or removed from the subsynaptic membrane, consequently improving or reducing synaptic connectivity [23,25,27]. Furthermore, changes in intracellular calcium levels can contribute to long-term potentiation (LTP) or long-term depression (LTD), which are further influenced by the intensity and varying protocols of tDCS [23,28].

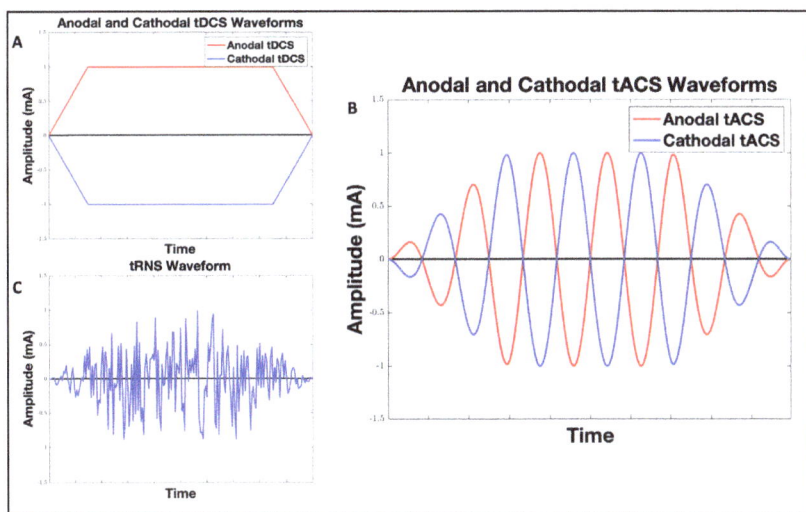

Figure 1. Demonstration of Transcranial Direct Current Stimulation (tDCS) (**A**), Transcranial Alternating Current Stimulation (tACS) (**B**), and Transcranial Random Noise Stimulation (tRNS) (**C**) waveforms.

The red waveform represents the anodal current, and the blue waveform represents the cathodal current in tDCS and tACS. tDCS features a constant, flat waveform, while the waveform of tACS varies according to its frequency, and tRNS exhibits a waveform with a randomized frequency. In tDCS, the anode increases neural excitability while the cathode decreases it. However, tACS uses a sinusoidal waveform, meaning the current alternates between positive and negative values, minimizing the distinction between anodal and cathodal effects [29]

Despite the diverse mechanisms proposed, tDCS has been extensively studied for its ability to modulate excitability in the motor cortex. Owing to its polarity feature, conventional tDCS applications involve placing the anodal electrode over the primary motor cortex (M1) and the cathodal electrode over the supraorbital region of the prefrontal cortex. In healthy subjects, applying the anodal electrode over M1 has shown modulation effects in numerous studies, employing a wide range of outcome measures. Notturno et al. [30] applied tDCS with an intensity of 1 mA for 20 min at the M1 area and observed an increase in cortical low alpha-band power and beta-band brain connectivity following anodal tDCS. Romero Lauro et al. [31] explored the broader effects of tDCS on cortical excitability, finding significant shifts in global excitability and increased cortical activity during and after anodal tDCS application. However, they also reported that both anodal and cathodal tDCS resulted in widespread changes in regional cerebral blood flow (CBF) compared to sham tDCS. Similarly, Jamil et al. [32] reported that anodal tDCS over M1 increased CBF, and more so at higher intensities. In addition, more recent studies have demonstrated increased Motor Evoked Potentials (MEPs) following a specific period of time and intensity of anodal tDCS stimulation over M1 [33–38].

In stroke survivors, damage to the motor cortex can lead to impaired motor function and muscle weakness. Given its ability to modulate cortical excitability, tDCS is increasingly applied in the rehabilitation of motor function in stroke survivors. In studies focusing on unilateral tDCS application with therapy, Allman et al. [39] combined anodal tDCS at the M1 ipsilesional site with the Graded Repetitive Arm Supplementary Program (GRASP) for 9 days. They reported significant improvements in the Action Research Arm Test (ARAT) and the Wolf Motor Function Test (WMFT) among the anodal tDCS group, along with increased cortical activity in the ipsilesional premotor and motor areas from fMRI and longer retention of benefits compared to the sham group. Halakoo et al. [40] evaluated the impact of anodal tDCS on spasticity and muscle activity in sub-acute stroke patients' wrists. They reported significant reductions in wrist flexor spasticity and increased activity in both wrist flexor and extensor muscles immediately and one-month post-intervention in the tDCS group compared to controls. Llorens et al. [41] examined the effects of combining tDCS with virtual reality (VR)-based therapy for chronic stroke patients. The result indicated that this approach significantly enhanced upper limb motor function, surpassing the outcomes of conventional physical therapy. Additionally, Kashoo et al. [42] investigated the benefits of combining tDCS with motor imagery (MI) and upper-limb motor training in chronic stroke rehabilitation. In conjunction with MI and functional training, they discovered that anodal tDCS stimulation applied to the affected M1 effectively reduced impairment and enhanced recovery in upper limb function. Furthermore, Ehsani et al. [43] applied anodal tDCS over the M1 of the ankle muscles with physical therapy. The group receiving the combined intervention showed improved EMG activity and more sustained clinical improvements. In addition, unilateral tDCS shows promise in enhancing physical therapy for lower limb recovery in stroke survivors. Seo et al. [44] observed enhanced walking function with anodal-tDCS and robotic-assisted gait training, with improvements in Functional Ambulatory Category (FAC) scores and the 6 min walk test four weeks post-treatment. Ehsani, Mortezanejad, Yosephi, Daniali, and Jaberzadeh [43] reported that anodal-tDCS reduced spasticity and improved muscle activity and balance, with lasting effects for a month. Qurat Ul et al. [45] showed that tDCS targeting the cerebellum or motor cortex, combined with virtual reality training, improved balance, gait, and cognition without significant differences between target areas. Interestingly, Duan et al. [46] demonstrated that even cathodal-tDCS with rehabilitation significantly improved lower limb function, as evidenced by FMA-LE scores and gait measures in subacute stroke patients.

Following a stroke, both the ipsilesional and contralesional hemispheres undergo significant changes. While the ipsilesional hemisphere's alterations are directly linked to motor deficits, the contralesional hemisphere plays a more complex role in recovery. The contralesional hemisphere can support recovery by compensating for lost functions in the ipsilesional hemisphere [47]. However, its increased activity can also become maladaptive, hindering recovery by disrupting relearning processes in the damaged hemisphere [47–49]. Therefore, recent studies have modified their protocols by applying bi-hemispheric stimulation, aiming to regulate the imbalance between the hemispheres. In this approach, the anode is placed over the ipsilesional M1, and the cathode is positioned over the contralesional M1. Goodwill et al. [50] investigated the effects of a 3-week dual-tDCS combined with upper limb rehabilitation in chronic stroke survivors. The findings revealed that real-tDCS improved motor function and maintained these gains at a 3-week follow-up. Additionally, real-tDCS led to increased MEP amplitudes and enhanced corticospinal plasticity. Lefebvre et al. [51] reported that combining motor learning with dual-tDCS in stroke survivors increased functional brain connectivity, particularly in motor and premotor regions, suggesting improved cortical network efficiency. Kuo et al. [52] combined dual-tDCS with paretic hand exercise in subacute stroke survivors, and they reported that dual-tDCS successfully modulated ipsilesional M1 excitability and inter-hemispheric balance. Moreover, Garrido et al. [53] observed significant motor function improvements in acute and subacute stroke patients using dual-tDCS with constraint-induced movement therapy.

In addition, Andrade et al. [54] explored the impact of different tDCS montages on fall prevention and lower limb function in acute stroke patients, applying anodal, cathodal, bilateral, and sham tDCS across ten sessions over two weeks. The findings revealed that all active tDCS groups experienced reduced fall risks and improved lower limb function, with dual-tDCS stimulation showing the most significant benefits. Youssef et al. [55] compared the efficacy of dual-tDCS to anodal-tDCS in boosting motor function in sub-acute ischemic stroke survivors, finding substantial improvements in motor skills for both upper and lower limbs in both groups, with no discernible difference in effectiveness between the two tDCS approaches. Moreover, studies have also shown that combining dual-tDCS with physical therapy significantly enhances outcomes [56,57].

5. Transcranial Alternating Current Stimulation (tACS)

Brain activity exhibits rhythmic patterns that oscillate at specific frequencies. Unlike tDCS, which delivers a constant direct current, tACS applies weak sinusoidal currents at a fixed frequency, aiming to entrain the brain's endogenous oscillations (Figure 1B). tACS does not significantly alter the overall rate of action potentials. Instead, it modulates the timing of neuronal spikes, resulting in a phase shift in endogenous oscillations, i.e., entrainment [58,59]. The modulation effect of tACS can also be explained through the concept of the Arnold tongue, which represents a triangular relationship between stimulation frequency and amplitude. This triangular area is centered at the frequency of the endogenous oscillation, illustrating how the effectiveness of tACS is influenced by the alignment of external stimulation parameters with the brain's natural frequencies [58,60,61]. In addition, Ali, Sellers, and Frohlich [61] utilized large-scale simulations of cortical networks to investigate how tACS modifies these networks. They discovered that tACS entrainment can be mediated by the resonance dynamics of the brain. Liu, Voroslakos, Kronberg, Henin, Krause, Huang, Opitz, Mehta, Pack, Krekelberg, Berenyi, Parra, Melloni, Devinsky, and Buzsaki [3] also summarized that stochastic resonance, rhythm resonance, temporal biasing of neuronal spikes, entrainment of network patterns, and imposed patterns could affect the effect of tACS. In general, tACS's widespread effects are attributed to two synergistic mechanisms: entrainment and neuroplasticity. Entrainment occurs when an external rhythm influences another system, causing it to synchronize its frequency and phase. Neuroplasticity, involving LTP/LTD processes, reinforces these online effects by either strengthening or weakening neural connections based on their activity levels [62,63].

As anticipated, tACS has demonstrated its capability of modulating cortical excitability when applied over M1 with various frequencies. Fresnoza et al. [64] observed that individual alpha frequency tACS increased MEP amplitudes post-stimulation in both young and old individuals, with a stronger effect in the young. The same group later also found that tACS improved old adults' gross motor sequence scores [65]. Suzuki et al. [66] applied 10 Hz and 20 Hz tACS to the hand motor area for 20 min. Their findings revealed increased corresponding oscillatory activity at both frequencies in magnetic resonance images, demonstrating frequency-specific effects on motor cortex function. In addition, Guerra et al. [67] investigated the effects of beta and gamma tACS applied over M1 on repetitive finger tapping in healthy subjects. Their findings revealed that beta tACS decreased movement amplitude while gamma tACS increased it. However, other movement parameters and MEPs remained unchanged, suggesting a specific role for beta and gamma brain oscillations in the control of repetitive finger movements. Similarly, Miyaguchi et al. [68] explored the impact of beta and gamma tACS on motor performance by applying them to the M1 and cerebellar cortex in healthy adults. The study found no impact of beta-oscillation tACS on motor performance. However, gamma-tACS applied to M1 and the cerebellum significantly improved motor performance. Later, the same group investigated the impact of gamma-tACS on motor learning. They found that gamma-tACS significantly enhanced motor learning retention compared to sham stimulation. However, there were no differences in initial learning efficiency or the ability to re-learn between the gamma-tACS and sham groups [69]. Conflicting outcomes have also been reported. Geffen et al. [70] assessed the effects of slow oscillatory tACS (0.75 Hz) on motor cortex responsiveness in healthy subjects. Their results showed a significant increase in MEP amplitude following tACS. However, the study found no phase-dependent changes in excitability, suggesting that entrainment of endogenous neural oscillations might not be the primary mechanism underlying the observed effects. Pozdniakov et al. [71] reported that applying tACS at alpha and beta frequencies over M1 can increase cortical excitability during stimulation, especially at the beta frequency of 20 Hz. However, these excitability enhancements did not persist after the stimulation had ceased, indicating a lack of lasting offline effects. Therefore, applying tACS over the M1 region shows promise for modulating cortical activity, as demonstrated by changes in MEPs and cortical coherence. Importantly, different stimulation frequencies likely yield distinct modulation effects. However, direct evidence demonstrating that neural entrainment causes the observed changes in cortical excitability remains elusive.

Despite the extensive body of literature on applying tDCS to stroke survivors, the implementation of tACS on individuals with stroke remains considerably restricted. Chen et al. [72] investigated the effects of tACS at different frequencies on brain network integration and segregation in chronic stroke patients. The findings indicated that 20 Hz tACS might facilitate local segregation in motor-related regions and global integration at the whole-brain level. Naros and Gharabaghi [73] demonstrated that individualized tACS improved neurofeedback intervention accuracy in chronic stroke patients. Schuhmann et al. [74] found that high-definition tACS (HD-tACS) at alpha frequency effectively ameliorated hemi-spatial neglect symptoms in stroke patients by shifting attentional resources towards the contralesional hemifield. Wu et al. [75] reported significant neurological improvements in subacute stroke patients treated with tACS, as evidenced by reduced National Institutes of Health Stroke Scale scores. Later, Xie et al. [76] explored the benefits of 6 Hz tACS for chronic post-stroke aphasia, noting significant enhancements in various aspects of language performance, specifically in patients receiving active tACS targeted at the supplementary motor area.

6. Transcranial Random Stimulation (tRNS)

tRNS can be regarded as an adaptation of tACS, characterized by its delivery of stimulation across a wide frequency range instead of a single, fixed frequency (Figure 1C). Even if the exact physiological mechanisms of tRNS are not fully understood, following the mechanisms of tACS, former studies suggest that the modulation effects of tRNS may be enhanced by stochastic resonance and by repetitive activation of sodium channels that occur due to rectification when high-frequency stimulation is applied [77–79]. Interestingly, studies by Terney et al. [80] and Moret et al. [81] have found that the modulatory effects of tRNS are most pronounced within a wide-range high-frequency spectrum (100–700 Hz). This observation could be attributed to insufficient noise levels failing to adequately influence the activity of Na+ channels, thereby affecting their modulation [81]. In addition, Chaieb et al. [82] explored the effects of tRNS (101–640 Hz) on M1 cortical excitability and found that a 5 min application of tRNS led to a significant increase in excitability. Abe et al. [83] explored how tRNS (0.1–640 Hz) affects corticospinal excitability and motor performance. The study found that tRNS significantly increased MEP amplitudes and motor performance in healthy participants. Similarly, a recent review suggested that tRNS has the potential to increase motor cortex excitability, and this excitability enhancement is found to be dependent on the width of the frequency range used, the stimulation intensity, and duration [84].

In stroke motor recovery, a study investigating the combined effects of tRNS and upper limb training in stroke patients revealed that participants in the tRNS group exhibited significantly improved outcomes than the sham group [85]. Hayward et al. [86] explored whether tRNS applied over M1 can enhance upper limb recovery during reaching training in four stroke survivors with severe arm paresis. Participants underwent 12 training sessions, receiving either active or sham tRNS. They reported no adverse events and notable clinical improvements in motor outcomes in the active and sham groups. Moreover, Anwer, Waris, Gilani, Iqbal, Shaikh, Pujari, and Niazi [6] examined the combination of tRNS and functional electrical stimulation (FES) for improving upper extremity function in individuals with moderate-to-severe stroke for 18 sessions. Results showed significant improvements were observed in upper extremity impairment and function in the tRNS group, with no significant differences in motor function or grip strength between the groups.

7. Challenges in Transcranial Electrical Stimulation (tES)

Nevertheless, it is crucial to recognize that challenges in replication can arise, potentially impacting the reliability of conclusions drawn about the efficacy of tES techniques. In tDCS, Horvath et al. [87] pointed out that inter-subject variability, intra-subject reliability, challenges with sham stimulation and blinding, the impact of motor and cognitive activities on tDCS effects, and factors influencing electric current flow like hair thickness and electrode attachment methods should be carefully considered in the tDCS studies. In fact, a few recent studies have suggested that tDCS may not enhance cortical connectivity in healthy participants. Jonker et al. [88] investigated the impact of anodal tDCS applied over the M1 on cortical excitability in healthy participants, using MEPs as the measure. Despite previous findings suggesting that anodal tDCS can increase cortical excitability, this double-blind, placebo-controlled trial found no significant effect of tDCS on cortical excitability, nor did it find any interaction with individual-specific factors. Kudo et al. [89] investigated the effects of tDCS on corticomuscular coherence (CMC) and MEPs. CMC represents a measure of functional connectivity between cortical activity and muscular activity. However, their study found that tDCS did not significantly modulate either measure. Apsvalka et al. [90] investigated if anodal tDCS applied to M1 could enhance motor skill acquisition. The results indicated no significant benefit of active stimulation over sham in observing keypress sequences. Moreover, Gardi et al. [91] investigated the impact of tDCS device type and electrode size on cortical excitability. They reported that no significant differences were found in cortical excitability changes between different devices or electrode sizes, nor was there a significant effect of anodal tDCS alone.

Similar findings have also been reported in stroke rehabilitation concerning tDCS efficacy in augmenting stroke rehabilitation. In contrast to healthy individuals, the challenges of applying tDCS to stroke survivors can arise from the interhemispheric inhibition model and montage, optimal dose and safety concerns, interindividual variability, subject selection, outcome measures, or medication use [92]. Despite the positive outcomes from above, Rossi et al. [93] applied anodal tDCS to the affected M1 hemisphere in acute stroke patients. The motor deficits were evaluated using the Fugl-Meyer motor scale (FM) and the National Institute of Health Stroke Scale (NIHSS). The study found that both active and sham groups showed significant improvements in NIHSS and FM scores over time, but there was no significant difference in clinical outcomes between the anodal TDCS and sham groups. Similarly, Au-Yeung et al. [94] found that a 20 min session of cathodal tDCS applied to the contralesional M1 in chronic stroke survivors significantly improves hand dexterity. However, no significant hand dexterity improvements were observed with anodal tDCS targeting the lesioned hemisphere's M1. Hamoudi et al. [95] explored the impact of anodal tDCS on motor skill learning in chronic stroke patients. They reported that while tDCS augmented motor skill learning during the online phase, these improvements were limited to the specific skills learned and did not generalize to broader motor functions.

Moreover, when combining tDCS with physical therapy in clinical practice, some studies have shown that tDCS does not augment the effectiveness of physical therapy. Straudi et al. [96] examined the effects of combining dual-tDCS with Robotic Assisted Training (RAT) for upper extremities in stroke survivors. Participants received either real or sham tDCS along with robotic therapy for 10 sessions. The results indicated that dual-tDCS might enhance the benefits of robotic therapy, but only when adjusted with stroke duration and type. Triccas et al. [97] explored the impact of anodal tDCS along with unilateral and three-dimensional RAT on the impaired upper limb in people with sub-acute and chronic stroke for 18 sessions. They found that the addition of tDCS showed no extra benefits, and RAT might be more advantageous in the sub-acute phase of stroke than the chronic phase. Moreover, Morone, Capone, Iosa, Cruciani, Paolucci, Martino Cinnera, Musumeci, Brunelli, Costa, Paolucci, and Di Lazzaro [10] examined dual-tDCS combined with exoskeleton RAT on upper limb motor functions in chronic stroke patients after 10 sessions of repetitive training. They reported that dual-tDCS combined with RAT did not further enhance recovery compared to controls. Bernal-Jimenez et al. [98] explored the effects of combining tDCS with RAT on the rehabilitation of upper limb function in chronic stroke patients for 20 sessions. They reported that the combination did not lead to significant improvements in the Fugl-Meyer Upper Limb Motor Score (mFM-UL), the Action Research Arm Test (ARAT), or the Functional Independence Measure (FIM) among the stroke patients. Moreover, two recent review articles [12,99] examined the effectiveness of integrating tDCS with RAT for upper limb function recovery after stroke. They concluded that while tDCS might enhance the effects of RAT on lower limb function, the combination does not appear to improve upper limb function, strength, spasticity, functional independence, or velocity of movement after stroke.

While the primary focus of this review is not on lower limb motor recovery, it's pertinent to acknowledge that similar challenges have been observed regarding the effects of tDCS on lower limb recovery in stroke survivors. van Asseldonk and Boonstra [100] explored the impact of tDCS on walking in both healthy subjects and chronic stroke survivors, noting slight improvements in force production during walking among healthy participants with dual-tDCS, but no significant benefits for stroke survivors. Concurrently, Leon et al. [101] investigated the combination of tDCS with robotic gait training, finding no substantial difference in walking ability between those who received tDCS during training and those who underwent robotic training alone. Similarly, Kindred et al. [102] assessed the effects of high-definition tDCS (HD-tDCS) on gait and corticomotor response in post-stroke individuals, concluding that a single HD-tDCS session, regardless of being anodal or cathodal, failed to significantly alter gait kinematics, walking speed, or corticomotor responses. In addition, a research group conducted multiple studies on tDCS for lower-limb recovery in stroke survivors. Klomjai et al. [103] explored the effects of a single session of dual-tDCS combined with conventional physical therapy on lower limb function and gait, finding significant improvements in the Five-Times-Sit-To-Stand (FTSTS) test in the real tDCS group but no significant muscle strength changes. Subsequently, Klomjai et al. [104] assessed various tDCS setups over five days, noting that dual-tDCS offered the most significant lower limb motor function improvements. In contrast, Aneksan et al. [105] did not observe enhanced outcomes from five sessions of dual-tDCS with task-specific training. Similarly, Klomjai and Aneksan [106] found no significant lower limb performance improvements when dual-tDCS was applied during physical therapy. Additionally, recent reviews showed that tDCS had limited effects in an isolated treatment environment, but it is possible to improve lower limb functions when combined with other therapies [106–109].

Stimulation intensity and duration in tDCS significantly influence its modulation effects. However, there is no consensus on the optimal settings for either intensity or duration. Chew et al. [110] examined cortical excitability in healthy subjects with different anodal-tDCS intensities; significant MEP variations were observed between individuals across different current intensities, with 2 mA and 0.2 mA tDCS proving to be more effective in eliciting a clear response compared to 0.5 mA and 1 mA intensities. Additionally, notable variations were also seen within individuals across repeated sessions of identical tDCS. Vignaud et al. [111] compared the effects of tDCS's duration (20 vs. 30 min) and intensity (1 vs. 2 mA) on cortical excitability. The findings revealed that a 20 min session of anodal-tDCS, irrespective of the intensity used, enhanced MEP responses. Conversely, a 30 min tDCS session did not alter cortical excitability. Esmaeilpour et al. [112] discussed whether increasing the electric current in tDCS improves its effectiveness under different models. However, their findings suggest a lack of clear understanding regarding the dose–response relationship in tDCS. Interestingly, another recent study explored individualized dose-control of tDCS to examine variability among healthy individuals. Their findings suggest that individualized dose-control of tDCS has the potential to reduce variance in cortical excitability [113]. In addition to the challenges mentioned above, the challenges of tDCS might be due to the complexity of motor skills, which involve both cortical and spinal and peripheral mechanisms. The task-specific effects of tDCS imply that its neuromodulation impact is closely associated with the neural circuits activated during specific training, indicating a lack of broad influence on other motor areas or unrelated skills [13,96,114]. These findings highlight the need for further studies to confirm these results and better understand the varying effects of tDCS in stroke rehabilitation.

However, due to the heterogeneity across studies, directly comparing the motor recovery effects between tDCS, tACS, and tRNS is challenging, as they do not adhere to the same stimulation paradigms or protocols or involve identical populations. To address the challenges of understanding the relative effectiveness of different tES techniques, several studies have endeavored to compare the efficacy of conventionally used tDCS with the more recently developed tACS and tRNS within the same population. In a study comparing the efficacy of tDCS, tACS, and tRNS on altering cortical excitability, each type of stimulation was applied over the M1 area in the same healthy adults at an intensity of 1.0 mA for 10 min on separate days. The findings revealed that tACS and tRNS led to an increase in MEPs compared to sham stimulation, while tDCS did not produce similar effects [115]. Krause et al. [116] investigated the effects of tACS and tDCS on motor sequence retrieval and reacquisition during early motor consolidation. Both tACS and tDCS showed facilitatory effects on motor sequence retrieval, with 20 Hz tACS being particularly effective in enhancing reaction times. Unfortunately, direct comparisons between tDCS, tACS, and tRNS in the motor cortex were quite limited. Although some comparisons did not specifically target the motor cortex, their findings merit consideration. Rohner et al. [117] aimed to directly compare the effects of theta-tACS and anodal tDCS on working memory (WM) performance. Their results revealed that tACS resulted in a greater improvement in reaction time for correct hits than tDCS. Moreover, Kim et al. [118] explored the efficacy of tACS and tDCS in enhancing cognitive function in patients with mild cognitive impairment. Participants received both gamma-tACS (40 Hz) and tDCS at the same intensity applied to the dorsolateral prefrontal cortex. The study found that gamma-tACS improved cognitive performance compared to tDCS and sham treatments. In contrast, tDCS did not demonstrate significant differences from sham in any of the cognitive test scores. In addition, a recent review by Senkowski et al. [119] compared the effects of tDCS and tACS on working memory (WM) in healthy adults, drawing from 43 studies. Results indicated a limited impact of single-session tDCS on WM, while tACS demonstrated frequency-dependent effects, particularly with frontoparietal stimulation. However, to the best of my knowledge, no study has directly compared the effectiveness of tDCS, tACS, and tRNS in stroke motor recovery.

8. Advantages of Using tACS/tRNS in Cortical Excitability Modulation and Motor Recovery

After a stroke, the brain's neural oscillation patterns change based on lesion location and severity. Alpha waves, known for their role in relaxation and information processing, slow down and become more synchronized. Conversely, beta waves, associated with motor control, exhibit increased activity in both hemispheres. Additionally, gamma waves, crucial for sensory integration and information binding, experience disruption [120]. However, brain oscillations begin to show different characteristics associated with improved outcomes in the chronic stroke recovery phase. Studies have shown that a decrease in the synchronization of alpha waves is linked to better motor function [121]. Furthermore, increased coherence between beta waves in the motor cortex and other brain regions during the acute phase has been associated with improved functionality later [122]. Interestingly, the role of beta waves appears to be hemisphere-specific, with higher power in the affected hemisphere correlating with better motor recovery, while the opposite is true for the unaffected hemisphere. Finally, an increase in gamma wave power in the affected hemisphere emerges as a promising target for stroke rehabilitation, as it has been linked to positive outcomes [120,121,123].

To address why tACS/tRNS might have potential in stroke motor recovery, it is reasonable to have the hypothesis that the entrainment of neurons could achieve better performance than simply depolarization or hyperpolarization of neurons. In contrast to tDCS, Wischnewski et al. [124] reported in a review that beta-tACS significantly increases M1 excitability. A notable finding was that tACS intensities above 1 mA peak-to-peak robustly increased M1 excitability. A potential advantage of tACS lies in the selection of stimulation frequency, aimed at modulating task-relevant physiological processes. In contrast to tDCS, whose effects are primarily contingent upon electrode placement and current intensity, tACS introduces an additional dimension through the manipulation of the stimulation frequency [119]. The effects of stroke on neural oscillations depend on the damage's severity and location. Stroke survivors typically experience a reduction in low-frequency wave power, with alpha oscillations showing decreased frequency and increased synchronization. On the other hand, beta oscillation power usually increases across both hemispheres [125]. Therefore, simply depolarizing and hyperpolarizing the motor cortex might not precisely address the changes in neural oscillations, suggesting that tDCS may not effectively modify neural oscillations in a frequency-specific way.

Moreover, unlike fixed-frequency protocols, tACS can be adjusted to match an individual's endogenous frequency. Fresnoza, Christova, Feil, Gallasch, Korner, Zimmer, and Ischebeck [64] applied individual alpha frequency tACS to the motor cortex in both young and older groups, observing increased cortical excitability post-stimulation in both. Similarly, Schilberg et al. [126] demonstrated that tACS set to individual beta band frequencies can modulate MEPs. Therefore, tailoring tACS to individual frequencies may enhance its effectiveness, potentially aligning more closely with the brain's intrinsic neuronal oscillations. This suggests that individualized tACS protocols could play a significant role in stroke patient motor recovery in the future. Finally, the modulation effect of tACS can be state-dependent. Alagapan et al. [127] applied tACS across different behavioral states: eyes open, eyes closed, and during a task. They found that the effect of tACS was dependent on the behavioral state. The complexity and dependency of brain activity upon the current behavioral state demonstrate the strength of tACS to accommodate more variable applications over the limitations of other tools. Therefore, tACS/tRNS may be a good tool to augment the intervention outcomes.

9. Limitations

The current review was primarily focused on upper-limb motor recovery. The neural oscillation patterns associated with lower limb movements (such as walking) or balance control might differ significantly from those of the upper limb, potentially complicating the interpretation of tES modulation effects. However, future reviews should specifically address lower limb recovery in stroke, exploring how various tES techniques influence motor functions in this area. In addition, although there is a growing body of research on tACS in motor recovery, the existing literature on both tACS and tRNS remains too scarce to draw definitive conclusions about their modulatory effects on stroke survivors.

10. Conclusions

In this review, we primarily focused on studies published within the past 10 years examining tES modulation of healthy motor cortical excitability and stroke upper limb motor recovery. The field of tES modulation has gained tremendous attention, as evidenced by the increasing number of publications. However, despite its emergence as a promising technique with advantages for research and clinical settings, replicating the benefits of tES remains challenging due to variability in study designs, participant characteristics, and stimulation protocols. While tDCS is the most frequently used tES technique in stroke motor recovery, its efficacy in augmenting the effects of physical therapy remains uncertain. In contrast, emerging tES techniques like tACS and tRNS, with distinct mechanisms from tDCS, show potential in preliminary stroke motor recovery studies. The complexity of neural networks suggests that more sophisticated approaches capable of targeting specific neural oscillations may offer an alternative for stroke motor rehabilitation and enhance the effects of physical therapy. Therefore, future progress hinges on understanding neural mechanisms and refining tES techniques for consistent, therapeutically valuable results. As the field develops, modified tES holds the potential to become a powerful neuromodulatory tool, enhancing stroke upper limb motor rehabilitation.

Author Contributions: Conceptualization, H.M. and S.L.; methodology, H.M.; software, H.M.; validation, S.L., M.H. and Y.Z.; formal analysis, H.M.; investigation, H.M.; resources, H.M.; data curation, H.M.; writing—original draft preparation, H.M.; writing—review and editing, S.L., M.H. and Y.Z.; visualization, H.M.; supervision, S.L.; project administration, S.L.; funding acquisition, S.L. All authors have read and agreed to the published version of the manuscript.

Funding: This research received no external funding.

Data Availability Statement: This narrative review article synthesizes and analyzes findings from existing literature. No new data were generated for this study. All referenced materials and sources are publicly available and can be accessed through PubMed. Since this work involved the aggregation and interpretation of existing public data, no specific datasets were created.

Conflicts of Interest: The authors declare no conflicts of interest.

References

1. Murphy, S.J.; Werring, D.J. Stroke: Causes and clinical features. *Medicine* **2020**, *48*, 561–566. [CrossRef] [PubMed]
2. Beal, C.C. Gender and stroke symptoms: A review of the current literature. *J. Neurosci. Nurs.* **2010**, *42*, 80–87. [CrossRef]
3. Liu, A.; Voroslakos, M.; Kronberg, G.; Henin, S.; Krause, M.R.; Huang, Y.; Opitz, A.; Mehta, A.; Pack, C.C.; Krekelberg, B.; et al. Immediate neurophysiological effects of transcranial electrical stimulation. *Nat. Commun.* **2018**, *9*, 5092. [CrossRef] [PubMed]
4. Paulus, W. Transcranial electrical stimulation (tES—tDCS; tRNS, tACS) methods. *Neuropsychol. Rehabil.* **2011**, *21*, 602–617. [CrossRef] [PubMed]

5. Polania, R.; Nitsche, M.A.; Ruff, C.C. Studying and modifying brain function with non-invasive brain stimulation. *Nat. Neurosci.* **2018**, *21*, 174–187. [CrossRef]
6. Anwer, S.; Waris, A.; Gilani, S.O.; Iqbal, J.; Shaikh, N.; Pujari, A.N.; Niazi, I.K. Rehabilitation of Upper Limb Motor Impairment in Stroke: A Narrative Review on the Prevalence, Risk Factors, and Economic Statistics of Stroke and State of the Art Therapies. *Healthcare* **2022**, *10*, 190. [CrossRef] [PubMed]
7. Bao, S.C.; Khan, A.; Song, R.; Kai-Yu Tong, R. Rewiring the Lesioned Brain: Electrical Stimulation for Post-Stroke Motor Restoration. *J. Stroke* **2020**, *22*, 47–63. [CrossRef] [PubMed]
8. Ahmed, I.; Mustafaoglu, R.; Rossi, S.; Cavdar, F.A.; Agyenkwa, S.K.; Pang, M.Y.C.; Straudi, S. Non-invasive Brain Stimulation Techniques for the Improvement of Upper Limb Motor Function and Performance in Activities of Daily Living After Stroke: A Systematic Review and Network Meta-analysis. *Arch. Phys. Med. Rehabil.* **2023**, *104*, 1683–1697. [CrossRef] [PubMed]
9. Lee, J.H.; Jeun, Y.J.; Park, H.Y.; Jung, Y.J. Effect of Transcranial Direct Current Stimulation Combined with Rehabilitation on Arm and Hand Function in Stroke Patients: A Systematic Review and Meta-Analysis. *Healthcare* **2021**, *9*, 1705. [CrossRef]
10. Morone, G.; Capone, F.; Iosa, M.; Cruciani, A.; Paolucci, M.; Martino Cinnera, A.; Musumeci, G.; Brunelli, N.; Costa, C.; Paolucci, S.; et al. May Dual Transcranial Direct Current Stimulation Enhance the Efficacy of Robot-Assisted Therapy for Promoting Upper Limb Recovery in Chronic Stroke? *Neurorehabil. Neural Repair.* **2022**, *36*, 800–809. [CrossRef]
11. Van Hoornweder, S.; Vanderzande, L.; Bloemers, E.; Verstraelen, S.; Depestele, S.; Cuypers, K.; Dun, K.V.; Strouwen, C.; Meesen, R. The effects of transcranial direct current stimulation on upper-limb function post-stroke: A meta-analysis of multiple-session studies. *Clin. Neurophysiol.* **2021**, *132*, 1897–1918. [CrossRef]
12. Comino-Suarez, N.; Moreno, J.C.; Gomez-Soriano, J.; Megia-Garcia, A.; Serrano-Munoz, D.; Taylor, J.; Alcobendas-Maestro, M.; Gil-Agudo, A.; Del-Ama, A.J.; Avendano-Coy, J. Transcranial direct current stimulation combined with robotic therapy for upper and lower limb function after stroke: A systematic review and meta-analysis of randomized control trials. *J. Neuroeng. Rehabil.* **2021**, *18*, 148. [CrossRef]
13. Chow, A.D.; Shin, J.; Wang, H.; Kellawan, J.M.; Pereira, H.M. Influence of Transcranial Direct Current Stimulation Dosage and Associated Therapy on Motor Recovery Post-stroke: A Systematic Review and Meta-Analysis. *Front. Aging Neurosci.* **2022**, *14*, 821915. [CrossRef]
14. Takeuchi, N.; Izumi, S.I. Motor Learning Based on Oscillatory Brain Activity Using Transcranial Alternating Current Stimulation: A Review. *Brain Sci.* **2021**, *11*, 1095. [CrossRef]
15. Yang, S.; Yi, Y.G.; Chang, M.C. The effect of transcranial alternating current stimulation on functional recovery in patients with stroke: A narrative review. *Front. Neurol.* **2023**, *14*, 1327383. [CrossRef] [PubMed]
16. Raghavan, P. Upper Limb Motor Impairment After Stroke. *Phys. Med. Rehabil. Clin. N. Am.* **2015**, *26*, 599–610. [CrossRef]
17. Hayward, K.S.; Kramer, S.F.; Thijs, V.; Ratcliffe, J.; Ward, N.S.; Churilov, L.; Jolliffe, L.; Corbett, D.; Cloud, G.; Kaffenberger, T.; et al. A systematic review protocol of timing, efficacy and cost effectiveness of upper limb therapy for motor recovery post-stroke. *Syst. Rev.* **2019**, *8*, 187. [CrossRef] [PubMed]
18. Li, S. Spasticity, Motor Recovery, and Neural Plasticity after Stroke. *Front. Neurol.* **2017**, *8*, 120. [CrossRef] [PubMed]
19. Li, S. Stroke Recovery Is a Journey: Prediction and Potentials of Motor Recovery after a Stroke from a Practical Perspective. *Life* **2023**, *13*, 2061. [CrossRef]
20. Masiero, S.; Poli, P.; Rosati, G.; Zanotto, D.; Iosa, M.; Paolucci, S.; Morone, G. The value of robotic systems in stroke rehabilitation. *Expert. Rev. Med. Devices* **2014**, *11*, 187–198. [CrossRef]
21. Nitsche, M.A.; Paulus, W. Excitability changes induced in the human motor cortex by weak transcranial direct current stimulation. *J. Physiol.* **2000**, *527 Pt 3*, 633–639. [CrossRef]
22. Medeiros, L.F.; de Souza, I.C.; Vidor, L.P.; de Souza, A.; Deitos, A.; Volz, M.S.; Fregni, F.; Caumo, W.; Torres, I.L. Neurobiological effects of transcranial direct current stimulation: A review. *Front. Psychiatry* **2012**, *3*, 110. [CrossRef] [PubMed]
23. Stagg, C.J.; Antal, A.; Nitsche, M.A. Physiology of Transcranial Direct Current Stimulation. *J. ECT* **2018**, *34*, 144–152. [CrossRef]
24. Roche, N.; Geiger, M.; Bussel, B. Mechanisms underlying transcranial direct current stimulation in rehabilitation. *Ann. Phys. Rehabil. Med.* **2015**, *58*, 214–219. [CrossRef] [PubMed]
25. Pelletier, S.J.; Cicchetti, F. Cellular and molecular mechanisms of action of transcranial direct current stimulation: Evidence from in vitro and in vivo models. *Int. J. Neuropsychopharmacol.* **2014**, *18*, pyu047. [CrossRef]
26. Warraich, Z.; Kleim, J.A. Neural plasticity: The biological substrate for neurorehabilitation. *PM R* **2010**, *2*, S208–S219. [CrossRef] [PubMed]
27. Yamada, Y.; Sumiyoshi, T. Neurobiological Mechanisms of Transcranial Direct Current Stimulation for Psychiatric Disorders; Neurophysiological, Chemical, and Anatomical Considerations. *Front. Hum. Neurosci.* **2021**, *15*, 631838. [CrossRef]
28. Monai, H.; Hirase, H. Astrocytic calcium activation in a mouse model of tDCS-Extended discussion. *Neurogenesis* **2016**, *3*, e1240055. [CrossRef]
29. Herrmann, C.S.; Rach, S.; Neuling, T.; Struber, D. Transcranial alternating current stimulation: A review of the underlying mechanisms and modulation of cognitive processes. *Front. Hum. Neurosci.* **2013**, *7*, 279. [CrossRef]
30. Notturno, F.; Marzetti, L.; Pizzella, V.; Uncini, A.; Zappasodi, F. Local and remote effects of transcranial direct current stimulation on the electrical activity of the motor cortical network. *Hum. Brain Mapp.* **2014**, *35*, 2220–2232. [CrossRef]
31. Romero Lauro, L.J.; Rosanova, M.; Mattavelli, G.; Convento, S.; Pisoni, A.; Opitz, A.; Bolognini, N.; Vallar, G. TDCS increases cortical excitability: Direct evidence from TMS-EEG. *Cortex* **2014**, *58*, 99–111. [CrossRef] [PubMed]

32. Jamil, A.; Batsikadze, G.; Kuo, H.I.; Meesen, R.L.J.; Dechent, P.; Paulus, W.; Nitsche, M.A. Current intensity- and polarity-specific online and aftereffects of transcranial direct current stimulation: An fMRI study. *Hum. Brain Mapp.* **2020**, *41*, 1644–1666. [CrossRef] [PubMed]
33. Agboada, D.; Mosayebi Samani, M.; Jamil, A.; Kuo, M.F.; Nitsche, M.A. Expanding the parameter space of anodal transcranial direct current stimulation of the primary motor cortex. *Sci. Rep.* **2019**, *9*, 18185. [CrossRef] [PubMed]
34. Agboada, D.; Mosayebi-Samani, M.; Kuo, M.F.; Nitsche, M.A. Induction of long-term potentiation-like plasticity in the primary motor cortex with repeated anodal transcranial direct current stimulation—Better effects with intensified protocols? *Brain Stimul.* **2020**, *13*, 987–997. [CrossRef] [PubMed]
35. Farnad, L.; Ghasemian-Shirvan, E.; Mosayebi-Samani, M.; Kuo, M.F.; Nitsche, M.A. Exploring and optimizing the neuroplastic effects of anodal transcranial direct current stimulation over the primary motor cortex of older humans. *Brain Stimul.* **2021**, *14*, 622–634. [CrossRef] [PubMed]
36. Song, P.; Li, S.; Hao, W.; Wei, M.; Liu, J.; Lin, H.; Hu, S.; Dai, X.; Wang, J.; Wang, R.; et al. Corticospinal excitability enhancement with simultaneous transcranial near-infrared stimulation and anodal direct current stimulation of motor cortex. *Clin. Neurophysiol.* **2021**, *132*, 1018–1024. [CrossRef] [PubMed]
37. Strube, W.; Bunse, T.; Nitsche, M.A.; Nikolaeva, A.; Palm, U.; Padberg, F.; Falkai, P.; Hasan, A. Bidirectional variability in motor cortex excitability modulation following 1 mA transcranial direct current stimulation in healthy participants. *Physiol. Rep.* **2016**, *4*, e12884. [CrossRef] [PubMed]
38. Yamaguchi, T.; Moriya, K.; Tanabe, S.; Kondo, K.; Otaka, Y.; Tanaka, S. Transcranial direct-current stimulation combined with attention increases cortical excitability and improves motor learning in healthy volunteers. *J. Neuroeng. Rehabil.* **2020**, *17*, 23. [CrossRef]
39. Allman, C.; Amadi, U.; Winkler, A.M.; Wilkins, L.; Filippini, N.; Kischka, U.; Stagg, C.J.; Johansen-Berg, H. Ipsilesional anodal tDCS enhances the functional benefits of rehabilitation in patients after stroke. *Sci. Transl. Med.* **2016**, *8*, 330re1. [CrossRef]
40. Halakoo, S.; Ehsani, F.; Masoudian, N.; Zoghi, M.; Jaberzadeh, S. Does anodal trans-cranial direct current stimulation of the damaged primary motor cortex affects wrist flexor muscle spasticity and also activity of the wrist flexor and extensor muscles in patients with stroke?: A Randomized Clinical Trial. *Neurol. Sci.* **2021**, *42*, 2763–2773. [CrossRef]
41. Llorens, R.; Fuentes, M.A.; Borrego, A.; Latorre, J.; Alcaniz, M.; Colomer, C.; Noe, E. Effectiveness of a combined transcranial direct current stimulation and virtual reality-based intervention on upper limb function in chronic individuals post-stroke with persistent severe hemiparesis: A randomized controlled trial. *J. Neuroeng. Rehabil.* **2021**, *18*, 108. [CrossRef] [PubMed]
42. Kashoo, F.Z.; Al-Baradie, R.S.; Alzahrani, M.; Alanazi, A.; Manzar, M.D.; Gugnani, A.; Sidiq, M.; Shaphe, M.A.; Sirajudeen, M.S.; Ahmad, M.; et al. Effect of Transcranial Direct Current Stimulation Augmented with Motor Imagery and Upper-Limb Functional Training for Upper-Limb Stroke Rehabilitation: A Prospective Randomized Controlled Trial. *Int. J. Environ. Res. Public Health* **2022**, *19*, 5199. [CrossRef] [PubMed]
43. Ehsani, F.; Mortezanejad, M.; Yosephi, M.H.; Daniali, S.; Jaberzadeh, S. The effects of concurrent M1 anodal tDCS and physical therapy interventions on function of ankle muscles in patients with stroke: A randomized, double-blinded sham-controlled trial study. *Neurol. Sci.* **2022**, *43*, 1893–1901. [CrossRef] [PubMed]
44. Seo, H.G.; Lee, W.H.; Lee, S.H.; Yi, Y.; Kim, K.D.; Oh, B.M. Robotic-assisted gait training combined with transcranial direct current stimulation in chronic stroke patients: A pilot double-blind, randomized controlled trial. *Restor. Neurol. Neurosci.* **2017**, *35*, 527–536. [CrossRef] [PubMed]
45. Qurat Ul, A.; Ahmad, Z.; Ilyas, S.; Ishtiaq, S.; Tariq, I.; Nawaz Malik, A.; Liu, T.; Wang, J. Comparison of a single session of tDCS on cerebellum vs. motor cortex in stroke patients: A randomized sham-controlled trial. *Ann. Med.* **2023**, *55*, 2252439. [CrossRef] [PubMed]
46. Duan, Q.; Liu, W.; Yang, J.; Huang, B.; Shen, J. Effect of Cathodal Transcranial Direct Current Stimulation for Lower Limb Subacute Stroke Rehabilitation. *Neural Plast.* **2023**, *2023*, 1863686. [CrossRef]
47. Dodd, K.C.; Nair, V.A.; Prabhakaran, V. Role of the Contralesional vs. Ipsilesional Hemisphere in Stroke Recovery. *Front. Hum. Neurosci.* **2017**, *11*, 469. [CrossRef] [PubMed]
48. Grefkes, C.; Fink, G.R. Reorganization of cerebral networks after stroke: New insights from neuroimaging with connectivity approaches. *Brain* **2011**, *134*, 1264–1276. [CrossRef] [PubMed]
49. Hoyer, E.H.; Celnik, P.A. Understanding and enhancing motor recovery after stroke using transcranial magnetic stimulation. *Restor. Neurol. Neurosci.* **2011**, *29*, 395–409. [CrossRef]
50. Goodwill, A.M.; Teo, W.P.; Morgan, P.; Daly, R.M.; Kidgell, D.J. Bihemispheric-tDCS and Upper Limb Rehabilitation Improves Retention of Motor Function in Chronic Stroke: A Pilot Study. *Front. Hum. Neurosci.* **2016**, *10*, 258. [CrossRef]
51. Lefebvre, S.; Dricot, L.; Laloux, P.; Desfontaines, P.; Evrard, F.; Peeters, A.; Jamart, J.; Vandermeeren, Y. Increased functional connectivity one week after motor learning and tDCS in stroke patients. *Neuroscience* **2017**, *340*, 424–435. [CrossRef] [PubMed]
52. Kuo, I.J.; Tang, C.W.; Tsai, Y.A.; Tang, S.C.; Lin, C.J.; Hsu, S.P.; Liang, W.K.; Juan, C.H.; Zich, C.; Stagg, C.J.; et al. Neurophysiological signatures of hand motor response to dual-transcranial direct current stimulation in subacute stroke: A TMS and MEG study. *J. Neuroeng. Rehabil.* **2020**, *17*, 72. [CrossRef] [PubMed]
53. Garrido, M.M.; Alvarez, E.E.; Acevedo, P.F.; Moyano, V.A.; Castillo, N.N.; Cavada Ch, G. Early transcranial direct current stimulation with modified constraint-induced movement therapy for motor and functional upper limb recovery in hospitalized patients with stroke: A randomized, multicentre, double-blind, clinical trial. *Brain Stimul.* **2023**, *16*, 40–47. [CrossRef] [PubMed]

54. Andrade, S.M.; Ferreira, J.J.A.; Rufino, T.S.; Medeiros, G.; Brito, J.D.; da Silva, M.A.; Moreira, R.N. Effects of different montages of transcranial direct current stimulation on the risk of falls and lower limb function after stroke. *Neurol. Res.* **2017**, *39*, 1037–1043. [CrossRef] [PubMed]
55. Youssef, H.; Mohamed, N.A.E.; Hamdy, M. Comparison of bihemispheric and unihemispheric M1 transcranial direct current stimulations during physical therapy in subacute stroke patients: A randomized controlled trial. *Neurophysiol. Clin.* **2023**, *53*, 102895. [CrossRef]
56. Prathum, T.; Piriyaprasarth, P.; Aneksan, B.; Hiengkaew, V.; Pankhaew, T.; Vachalathiti, R.; Klomjai, W. Effects of home-based dual-hemispheric transcranial direct current stimulation combined with exercise on upper and lower limb motor performance in patients with chronic stroke. *Disabil. Rehabil.* **2022**, *44*, 3868–3879. [CrossRef] [PubMed]
57. Salameh, A.; McCabe, J.; Skelly, M.; Duncan, K.R.; Chen, Z.; Tatsuoka, C.; Bikson, M.; Hardin, E.C.; Daly, J.J.; Pundik, S. Stance Phase Gait Training Post Stroke Using Simultaneous Transcranial Direct Current Stimulation and Motor Learning-Based Virtual Reality-Assisted Therapy: Protocol Development and Initial Testing. *Brain Sci.* **2022**, *12*, 701. [CrossRef] [PubMed]
58. Elyamany, O.; Leicht, G.; Herrmann, C.S.; Mulert, C. Transcranial alternating current stimulation (tACS): From basic mechanisms towards first applications in psychiatry. *Eur. Arch. Psychiatry Clin. Neurosci.* **2021**, *271*, 135–156. [CrossRef]
59. He, Y.; Liu, S.; Chen, L.; Ke, Y.; Ming, D. Neurophysiological mechanisms of transcranial alternating current stimulation. *Front. Neurosci.* **2023**, *17*, 1091925. [CrossRef]
60. Huang, W.A.; Stitt, I.M.; Negahbani, E.; Passey, D.J.; Ahn, S.; Davey, M.; Dannhauer, M.; Doan, T.T.; Hoover, A.C.; Peterchev, A.V.; et al. Transcranial alternating current stimulation entrains alpha oscillations by preferential phase synchronization of fast-spiking cortical neurons to stimulation waveform. *Nat. Commun.* **2021**, *12*, 3151. [CrossRef]
61. Ali, M.M.; Sellers, K.K.; Frohlich, F. Transcranial alternating current stimulation modulates large-scale cortical network activity by network resonance. *J. Neurosci.* **2013**, *33*, 11262–11275. [CrossRef] [PubMed]
62. Vogeti, S.; Boetzel, C.; Herrmann, C.S. Entrainment and Spike-Timing Dependent Plasticity—A Review of Proposed Mechanisms of Transcranial Alternating Current Stimulation. *Front. Syst. Neurosci.* **2022**, *16*, 827353. [CrossRef] [PubMed]
63. Korai, S.A.; Ranieri, F.; Di Lazzaro, V.; Papa, M.; Cirillo, G. Neurobiological After-Effects of Low Intensity Transcranial Electric Stimulation of the Human Nervous System: From Basic Mechanisms to Metaplasticity. *Front. Neurol.* **2021**, *12*, 587771. [CrossRef] [PubMed]
64. Fresnoza, S.; Christova, M.; Feil, T.; Gallasch, E.; Korner, C.; Zimmer, U.; Ischebeck, A. The effects of transcranial alternating current stimulation (tACS) at individual alpha peak frequency (iAPF) on motor cortex excitability in young and elderly adults. *Exp. Brain Res.* **2018**, *236*, 2573–2588. [CrossRef] [PubMed]
65. Fresnoza, S.; Christova, M.; Bieler, L.; Korner, C.; Zimmer, U.; Gallasch, E.; Ischebeck, A. Age-Dependent Effect of Transcranial Alternating Current Stimulation on Motor Skill Consolidation. *Front. Aging Neurosci.* **2020**, *12*, 25. [CrossRef]
66. Suzuki, M.; Tanaka, S.; Gomez-Tames, J.; Okabe, T.; Cho, K.; Iso, N.; Hirata, A. Nonequivalent After-Effects of Alternating Current Stimulation on Motor Cortex Oscillation and Inhibition: Simulation and Experimental Study. *Brain Sci.* **2022**, *12*, 195. [CrossRef] [PubMed]
67. Guerra, A.; Suppa, A.; Bologna, M.; D'Onofrio, V.; Bianchini, E.; Brown, P.; Di Lazzaro, V.; Berardelli, A. Boosting the LTP-like plasticity effect of intermittent theta-burst stimulation using gamma transcranial alternating current stimulation. *Brain Stimul.* **2018**, *11*, 734–742. [CrossRef] [PubMed]
68. Miyaguchi, S.; Otsuru, N.; Kojima, S.; Saito, K.; Inukai, Y.; Masaki, M.; Onishi, H. Transcranial Alternating Current Stimulation with Gamma Oscillations Over the Primary Motor Cortex and Cerebellar Hemisphere Improved Visuomotor Performance. *Front. Behav. Neurosci.* **2018**, *12*, 132. [CrossRef] [PubMed]
69. Miyaguchi, S.; Inukai, Y.; Matsumoto, Y.; Miyashita, M.; Takahashi, R.; Otsuru, N.; Onishi, H. Effects on motor learning of transcranial alternating current stimulation applied over the primary motor cortex and cerebellar hemisphere. *J. Clin. Neurosci.* **2020**, *78*, 296–300. [CrossRef]
70. Geffen, A.; Bland, N.; Sale, M.V. Effects of Slow Oscillatory Transcranial Alternating Current Stimulation on Motor Cortical Excitability Assessed by Transcranial Magnetic Stimulation. *Front. Hum. Neurosci.* **2021**, *15*, 726604. [CrossRef]
71. Pozdniakov, I.; Vorobiova, A.N.; Galli, G.; Rossi, S.; Feurra, M. Online and offline effects of transcranial alternating current stimulation of the primary motor cortex. *Sci. Rep.* **2021**, *11*, 3854. [CrossRef]
72. Chen, C.; Yuan, K.; Chu, W.C.; Tong, R.K. The Effects of 10 Hz and 20 Hz tACS in Network Integration and Segregation in Chronic Stroke: A Graph Theoretical fMRI Study. *Brain Sci.* **2021**, *11*, 377. [CrossRef] [PubMed]
73. Naros, G.; Gharabaghi, A. Physiological and behavioral effects of beta-tACS on brain self-regulation in chronic stroke. *Brain Stimul.* **2017**, *10*, 251–259. [CrossRef] [PubMed]
74. Schuhmann, T.; Duecker, F.; Middag-van Spanje, M.; Gallotto, S.; van Heugten, C.; Schrijnemaekers, A.C.; van Oostenbrugge, R.; Sack, A.T. Transcranial alternating current stimulation at alpha frequency reduces hemispatial neglect symptoms in stroke patients. *Int. J. Clin. Health Psychol.* **2022**, *22*, 100326. [CrossRef]
75. Wu, J.F.; Wang, H.J.; Wu, Y.; Li, F.; Bai, Y.L.; Zhang, P.Y.; Chan, C.C. Efficacy of transcranial alternating current stimulation over bilateral mastoids (tACS(bm)) on enhancing recovery of subacute post-stroke patients. *Top. Stroke Rehabil.* **2016**, *23*, 420–429. [CrossRef]
76. Xie, X.; Hu, P.; Tian, Y.; Wang, K.; Bai, T. Transcranial alternating current stimulation enhances speech comprehension in chronic post-stroke aphasia patients: A single-blind sham-controlled study. *Brain Stimul.* **2022**, *15*, 1538–1540. [CrossRef] [PubMed]

77. Antal, A.; Herrmann, C.S. Transcranial Alternating Current and Random Noise Stimulation: Possible Mechanisms. *Neural Plast.* **2016**, *2016*, 3616807. [CrossRef]
78. Antal, A.; Boros, K.; Poreisz, C.; Chaieb, L.; Terney, D.; Paulus, W. Comparatively weak after-effects of transcranial alternating current stimulation (tACS) on cortical excitability in humans. *Brain Stimul.* **2008**, *1*, 97–105. [CrossRef]
79. Potok, W.; van der Groen, O.; Bachinger, M.; Edwards, D.; Wenderoth, N. Transcranial Random Noise Stimulation Modulates Neural Processing of Sensory and Motor Circuits, from Potential Cellular Mechanisms to Behavior: A Scoping Review. *eNeuro* **2022**, *9*, 5. [CrossRef]
80. Terney, D.; Chaieb, L.; Moliadze, V.; Antal, A.; Paulus, W. Increasing human brain excitability by transcranial high-frequency random noise stimulation. *J. Neurosci.* **2008**, *28*, 14147–14155. [CrossRef]
81. Moret, B.; Donato, R.; Nucci, M.; Cona, G.; Campana, G. Transcranial random noise stimulation (tRNS): A wide range of frequencies is needed for increasing cortical excitability. *Sci. Rep.* **2019**, *9*, 15150. [CrossRef] [PubMed]
82. Chaieb, L.; Paulus, W.; Antal, A. Evaluating aftereffects of short-duration transcranial random noise stimulation on cortical excitability. *Neural Plast.* **2011**, *2011*, 105927. [CrossRef] [PubMed]
83. Abe, T.; Miyaguchi, S.; Otsuru, N.; Onishi, H. The effect of transcranial random noise stimulation on corticospinal excitability and motor performance. *Neurosci. Lett.* **2019**, *705*, 138–142. [CrossRef] [PubMed]
84. Brancucci, A.; Rivolta, D.; Nitsche, M.A.; Manippa, V. The effects of transcranial random noise stimulation on motor function: A comprehensive review of the literature. *Physiol. Behav.* **2023**, *261*, 114073. [CrossRef] [PubMed]
85. Arnao, V.; Riolo, M.; Carduccio, F.; Tuttolomondo, A.; D'Amelio, M.; Brighina, F.; Gangitano, M.; Salemi, G.; Ragonese, P.; Aridon, P. Effects of transcranial random noise stimulation combined with Graded Repetitive Arm Supplementary Program (GRASP) on motor rehabilitation of the upper limb in sub-acute ischemic stroke patients: A randomized pilot study. *J. Neural Transm.* **2019**, *126*, 1701–1706. [CrossRef] [PubMed]
86. Hayward, K.S.; Brauer, S.G.; Ruddy, K.L.; Lloyd, D.; Carson, R.G. Repetitive reaching training combined with transcranial Random Noise Stimulation in stroke survivors with chronic and severe arm paresis is feasible: A pilot, triple-blind, randomised case series. *J. Neuroeng. Rehabil.* **2017**, *14*, 46. [CrossRef] [PubMed]
87. Horvath, J.C.; Carter, O.; Forte, J.D. Transcranial direct current stimulation: Five important issues we aren't discussing (but probably should be). *Front. Syst. Neurosci.* **2014**, *8*, 2. [CrossRef] [PubMed]
88. Jonker, Z.D.; Gaiser, C.; Tulen, J.H.M.; Ribbers, G.M.; Frens, M.A.; Selles, R.W. No effect of anodal tDCS on motor cortical excitability and no evidence for responders in a large double-blind placebo-controlled trial. *Brain Stimul.* **2021**, *14*, 100–109. [CrossRef]
89. Kudo, D.; Koseki, T.; Katagiri, N.; Yoshida, K.; Takano, K.; Jin, M.; Nito, M.; Tanabe, S.; Yamaguchi, T. Individualized beta-band oscillatory transcranial direct current stimulation over the primary motor cortex enhances corticomuscular coherence and corticospinal excitability in healthy individuals. *Brain Stimul.* **2022**, *15*, 46–52. [CrossRef]
90. Apsvalka, D.; Ramsey, R.; Cross, E.S. Anodal tDCS over Primary Motor Cortex Provides No Advantage to Learning Motor Sequences via Observation. *Neural Plast.* **2018**, *2018*, 1237962. [CrossRef]
91. Gardi, A.Z.; Vogel, A.K.; Dharia, A.K.; Krishnan, C. Effect of conventional transcranial direct current stimulation devices and electrode sizes on motor cortical excitability of the quadriceps muscle. *Restor. Neurol. Neurosci.* **2021**, *39*, 379–391. [CrossRef] [PubMed]
92. Feng, W.; Kautz, S.A.; Schlaug, G.; Meinzer, C.; George, M.S.; Chhatbar, P.Y. Transcranial Direct Current Stimulation for Poststroke Motor Recovery: Challenges and Opportunities. *PM R* **2018**, *10*, S157–S164. [CrossRef] [PubMed]
93. Rossi, C.; Sallustio, F.; Di Legge, S.; Stanzione, P.; Koch, G. Transcranial direct current stimulation of the affected hemisphere does not accelerate recovery of acute stroke patients. *Eur. J. Neurol.* **2013**, *20*, 202–204. [CrossRef] [PubMed]
94. Au-Yeung, S.S.; Wang, J.; Chen, Y.; Chua, E. Transcranial direct current stimulation to primary motor area improves hand dexterity and selective attention in chronic stroke. *Am. J. Phys. Med. Rehabil.* **2014**, *93*, 1057–1064. [CrossRef] [PubMed]
95. Hamoudi, M.; Schambra, H.M.; Fritsch, B.; Schoechlin-Marx, A.; Weiller, C.; Cohen, L.G.; Reis, J. Transcranial Direct Current Stimulation Enhances Motor Skill Learning but Not Generalization in Chronic Stroke. *Neurorehabil. Neural Repair.* **2018**, *32*, 295–308. [CrossRef] [PubMed]
96. Straudi, S.; Fregni, F.; Martinuzzi, C.; Pavarelli, C.; Salvioli, S.; Basaglia, N. tDCS and Robotics on Upper Limb Stroke Rehabilitation: Effect Modification by Stroke Duration and Type of Stroke. *BioMed Res. Int.* **2016**, *2016*, 5068127. [CrossRef] [PubMed]
97. Triccas, L.T.; Burridge, J.H.; Hughes, A.; Verheyden, G.; Desikan, M.; Rothwell, J. A double-blinded randomised controlled trial exploring the effect of anodal transcranial direct current stimulation and uni-lateral robot therapy for the impaired upper limb in sub-acute and chronic stroke. *NeuroRehabilitation* **2015**, *37*, 181–191. [CrossRef]
98. Bernal-Jimenez, J.J.; Dileone, M.; Mordillo-Mateos, L.; Martin-Conty, J.L.; Durantez-Fernandez, C.; Vinuela, A.; Martin-Rodriguez, F.; Lerin-Calvo, A.; Alcantara-Porcuna, V.; Polonio-Lopez, B. Combining transcranial direct current stimulation with hand robotic rehabilitation in chronic stroke patients: A double blind randomized clinical trial. *Am. J. Phys. Med. Rehabil.* **2024**. [CrossRef] [PubMed]
99. Marotta, N.; Demeco, A.; Moggio, L.; Ammendolia, A. The adjunct of transcranial direct current stimulation to Robot-assisted therapy in upper limb post-stroke treatment. *J. Med. Eng. Technol.* **2021**, *45*, 494–501. [CrossRef]
100. van Asseldonk, E.H.; Boonstra, T.A. Transcranial Direct Current Stimulation of the Leg Motor Cortex Enhances Coordinated Motor Output During Walking With a Large Inter-Individual Variability. *Brain Stimul.* **2016**, *9*, 182–190. [CrossRef]

101. Leon, D.; Cortes, M.; Elder, J.; Kumru, H.; Laxe, S.; Edwards, D.J.; Tormos, J.M.; Bernabeu, M.; Pascual-Leone, A. tDCS does not enhance the effects of robot-assisted gait training in patients with subacute stroke. *Restor. Neurol. Neurosci.* **2017**, *35*, 377–384. [CrossRef] [PubMed]
102. Kindred, J.H.; Kautz, S.A.; Wonsetler, E.C.; Bowden, M.G. Single Sessions of High-Definition Transcranial Direct Current Stimulation Do Not Alter Lower Extremity Biomechanical or Corticomotor Response Variables Post-stroke. *Front. Neurosci.* **2019**, *13*, 286. [CrossRef] [PubMed]
103. Klomjai, W.; Aneksan, B.; Pheungphrarattanatrai, A.; Chantanachai, T.; Choowong, N.; Bunleukhet, S.; Auvichayapat, P.; Nilanon, Y.; Hiengkaew, V. Effect of single-session dual-tDCS before physical therapy on lower-limb performance in sub-acute stroke patients: A randomized sham-controlled crossover study. *Ann. Phys. Rehabil. Med.* **2018**, *61*, 286–291. [CrossRef] [PubMed]
104. Klomjai, W.; Aneksan, B.; Chotik-Anuchit, S.; Jitkaew, P.; Chaichanudomsuk, K.; Piriyaprasarth, P.; Vachalathiti, R.; Nilanon, Y.; Hiengkaew, V. Effects of Different Montages of Transcranial Direct Current Stimulation on Haemodynamic Responses and Motor Performance in Acute Stroke: A Randomized Controlled Trial. *J. Rehabil. Med.* **2022**, *54*, jrm00331. [CrossRef]
105. Aneksan, B.; Sawatdipan, M.; Bovonsunthonchai, S.; Tretriluxana, J.; Vachalathiti, R.; Auvichayapat, P.; Pheungphrarattanatrai, A.; Piriyaprasarth, P.; Klomjai, W. Five-Session Dual-Transcranial Direct Current Stimulation with Task-Specific Training Does Not Improve Gait and Lower Limb Performance over Training Alone in Subacute Stroke: A Pilot Randomized Controlled Trial. *Neuromodulation* **2022**, *25*, 558–568. [CrossRef] [PubMed]
106. Klomjai, W.; Aneksan, B. A randomized sham-controlled trial on the effects of dual-tDCS "during" physical therapy on lower limb performance in sub-acute stroke and a comparison to the previous study using a "before" stimulation protocol. *BMC Sports Sci. Med. Rehabil.* **2022**, *14*, 68. [CrossRef] [PubMed]
107. Lima, E.; de Souza Neto, J.M.R.; Andrade, S.M. Effects of transcranial direct current stimulation on lower limb function, balance and quality of life after stroke: A systematic review and meta-analysis. *Neurol. Res.* **2023**, *45*, 843–853. [CrossRef] [PubMed]
108. Li, Y.; Fan, J.; Yang, J.; He, C.; Li, S. Effects of transcranial direct current stimulation on walking ability after stroke: A systematic review and meta-analysis. *Restor. Neurol. Neurosci.* **2018**, *36*, 59–71. [CrossRef] [PubMed]
109. Navarro-Lopez, V.; Molina-Rueda, F.; Jimenez-Jimenez, S.; Alguacil-Diego, I.M.; Carratala-Tejada, M. Effects of Transcranial Direct Current Stimulation Combined with Physiotherapy on Gait Pattern, Balance, and Functionality in Stroke Patients. A Systematic Review. *Diagnostics* **2021**, *11*, 656. [CrossRef]
110. Chew, T.; Ho, K.A.; Loo, C.K. Inter- and Intra-individual Variability in Response to Transcranial Direct Current Stimulation (tDCS) at Varying Current Intensities. *Brain Stimul.* **2015**, *8*, 1130–1137. [CrossRef]
111. Vignaud, P.; Mondino, M.; Poulet, E.; Palm, U.; Brunelin, J. Duration but not intensity influences transcranial direct current stimulation (tDCS) after-effects on cortical excitability. *Neurophysiol. Clin.* **2018**, *48*, 89–92. [CrossRef] [PubMed]
112. Esmaeilpour, Z.; Marangolo, P.; Hampstead, B.M.; Bestmann, S.; Galletta, E.; Knotkova, H.; Bikson, M. Incomplete evidence that increasing current intensity of tDCS boosts outcomes. *Brain Stimul.* **2018**, *11*, 310–321. [CrossRef] [PubMed]
113. Evans, C.; Bachmann, C.; Lee, J.S.A.; Gregoriou, E.; Ward, N.; Bestmann, S. Dose-controlled tDCS reduces electric field intensity variability at a cortical target site. *Brain Stimul.* **2020**, *13*, 125–136. [CrossRef]
114. Elsner, B.; Kugler, J.; Mehrholz, J. Transcranial direct current stimulation (tDCS) for improving aphasia after stroke: A systematic review with network meta-analysis of randomized controlled trials. *J. Neuroeng. Rehabil.* **2020**, *17*, 88. [CrossRef] [PubMed]
115. Inukai, Y.; Saito, K.; Sasaki, R.; Tsuiki, S.; Miyaguchi, S.; Kojima, S.; Masaki, M.; Otsuru, N.; Onishi, H. Comparison of Three Non-Invasive Transcranial Electrical Stimulation Methods for Increasing Cortical Excitability. *Front. Hum. Neurosci.* **2016**, *10*, 668. [CrossRef]
116. Krause, V.; Meier, A.; Dinkelbach, L.; Pollok, B. Beta Band Transcranial Alternating (tACS) and Direct Current Stimulation (tDCS) Applied After Initial Learning Facilitate Retrieval of a Motor Sequence. *Front. Behav. Neurosci.* **2016**, *10*, 4. [CrossRef]
117. Rohner, F.; Breitling, C.; Rufener, K.S.; Heinze, H.J.; Hinrichs, H.; Krauel, K.; Sweeney-Reed, C.M. Modulation of Working Memory Using Transcranial Electrical Stimulation: A Direct Comparison between TACS and TDCS. *Front. Neurosci.* **2018**, *12*, 761. [CrossRef]
118. Kim, J.; Kim, H.; Jeong, H.; Roh, D.; Kim, D.H. tACS as a promising therapeutic option for improving cognitive function in mild cognitive impairment: A direct comparison between tACS and tDCS. *J. Psychiatr. Res.* **2021**, *141*, 248–256. [CrossRef]
119. Senkowski, D.; Sobirey, R.; Haslacher, D.; Soekadar, S.R. Boosting working memory: Uncovering the differential effects of tDCS and tACS. *Cereb. Cortex Commun.* **2022**, *3*, tgac018. [CrossRef]
120. Leonardi, G.; Ciurleo, R.; Cucinotta, F.; Fonti, B.; Borzelli, D.; Costa, L.; Tisano, A.; Portaro, S.; Alito, A. The role of brain oscillations in post-stroke motor recovery: An overview. *Front. Syst. Neurosci.* **2022**, *16*, 947421. [CrossRef]
121. Ray, A.M.; Figueiredo, T.D.C.; Lopez-Larraz, E.; Birbaumer, N.; Ramos-Murguialday, A. Brain oscillatory activity as a biomarker of motor recovery in chronic stroke. *Hum. Brain Mapp.* **2020**, *41*, 1296–1308. [CrossRef] [PubMed]
122. Nicolo, P.; Magnin, C.; Pedrazzini, E.; Plomp, G.; Mottaz, A.; Schnider, A.; Guggisberg, A.G. Comparison of Neuroplastic Responses to Cathodal Transcranial Direct Current Stimulation and Continuous Theta Burst Stimulation in Subacute Stroke. *Arch. Phys. Med. Rehabil.* **2018**, *99*, 862–872.e861. [CrossRef] [PubMed]
123. Espenhahn, S.; Rossiter, H.E.; van Wijk, B.C.M.; Redman, N.; Rondina, J.M.; Diedrichsen, J.; Ward, N.S. Sensorimotor cortex beta oscillations reflect motor skill learning ability after stroke. *Brain Commun.* **2020**, *2*, fcaa161. [CrossRef] [PubMed]
124. Wischnewski, M.; Schutter, D.; Nitsche, M.A. Effects of beta-tACS on corticospinal excitability: A meta-analysis. *Brain Stimul.* **2019**, *12*, 1381–1389. [CrossRef] [PubMed]

125. Storch, S.; Samantzis, M.; Balbi, M. Driving Oscillatory Dynamics: Neuromodulation for Recovery After Stroke. *Front. Syst. Neurosci.* **2021**, *15*, 712664. [CrossRef] [PubMed]
126. Schilberg, L.; Engelen, T.; Ten Oever, S.; Schuhmann, T.; de Gelder, B.; de Graaf, T.A.; Sack, A.T. Phase of beta-frequency tACS over primary motor cortex modulates corticospinal excitability. *Cortex* **2018**, *103*, 142–152. [CrossRef]
127. Alagapan, S.; Schmidt, S.L.; Lefebvre, J.; Hadar, E.; Shin, H.W.; Fröhlich, F. Modulation of Cortical Oscillations by Low-Frequency Direct Cortical Stimulation Is State-Dependent. *PLoS Biol.* **2016**, *14*, e1002424. [CrossRef]

Disclaimer/Publisher's Note: The statements, opinions and data contained in all publications are solely those of the individual author(s) and contributor(s) and not of MDPI and/or the editor(s). MDPI and/or the editor(s) disclaim responsibility for any injury to people or property resulting from any ideas, methods, instructions or products referred to in the content.

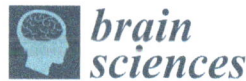

Review

Outcome Measures Utilized to Assess the Efficacy of Telerehabilitation for Post-Stroke Rehabilitation: A Scoping Review

Ardalan Shariat [1], Mahboubeh Ghayour Najafabadi [2,*], Noureddin Nakhostin Ansari [3,4], Albert T. Anastasio [5], Kian Bagheri [6], Gholamreza Hassanzadeh [1,7,8] and Mahsa Farghadan [9]

1. Department of Digital Health, School of Medicine, Tehran University of Medical Sciences, Tehran 1417613151, Iran; a-shariat@sina.tums.ac.ir (A.S.); hassanzadeh@tums.ac.ir (G.H.)
2. Department of Motor Behavior, Faculty of Sport Sciences and Health, University of Tehran, Tehran 1439957131, Iran
3. Department of Physiotherapy, School of Rehabilitation, Tehran University of Medical Sciences, Tehran 141556559, Iran; nakhostin@tums.ac.ir
4. Research Center for War-Affected People, Tehran University of Medical Sciences, Tehran 1417613151, Iran
5. Department of Orthopaedic Surgery, Duke University, Durham, NC 27710, USA; albert.anastasio@duke.edu
6. School of Osteopathic Medicine, Campbell University, Lillington, NC 27546, USA; kian.bagheri@duke.edu
7. Department of Anatomy, School of Medicine, Tehran University of Medical Sciences, Tehran 1417613151, Iran
8. Department of Neuroscience and Addiction Studies, School of Advanced Technologies in Medicine, Tehran University of Medical Sciences, Tehran 1417613151, Iran
9. Department of Artificial Intelligence, Faculty of Computer Engineering, Islamic Azad University of South Tehran Branch, Tehran 4147654919, Iran; farghadanmahsa@gmail.com
* Correspondence: m.ghayournaj@ut.ac.ir

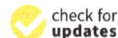

Citation: Shariat, A.; Najafabadi, M.G.; Nakhostin Ansari, N.; Anastasio, A.T.; Bagheri, K.; Hassanzadeh, G.; Farghadan, M. Outcome Measures Utilized to Assess the Efficacy of Telerehabilitation for Post-Stroke Rehabilitation: A Scoping Review. Brain Sci. 2023, 13, 1725. https://doi.org/10.3390/brainsci13121725

Academic Editor: Teng Jiang

Received: 7 November 2023
Revised: 11 December 2023
Accepted: 11 December 2023
Published: 17 December 2023

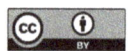

Copyright: © 2023 by the authors. Licensee MDPI, Basel, Switzerland. This article is an open access article distributed under the terms and conditions of the Creative Commons Attribution (CC BY) license (https://creativecommons.org/licenses/by/4.0/).

Abstract: Introduction: Outcome measures using telerehabilitation (TR) in the context of post-stroke rehabilitation are an area of emerging research. The current review assesses the literature related to TR for patients requiring post-stroke rehabilitation. The purpose of this study is to survey the outcome measures used in TR studies and to define which parts of the International Organization of Functioning are measured in trials. Methods: TR studies were searched in Cochrane Central Register of Controlled Trials, PubMed, Embase, Scopus, Google Scholar, and Web of Science, The Cochrane Central Register of Controlled Trials (Cochrane Library), the Cumulative Index to Nursing and Allied Health Literature (CINAHL), and the Physiotherapy Evidence Database (PEDro) from 2016 to June 2023. Two reviewers individually assessed the full text. Discrepancies regarding inclusion or exclusion were resolved by an additional reviewer. Results: A total of 24 studies were included in the current review. The findings were synthesized and presented taking into account their implications within clinical practice, areas of investigation, and strategic implementation. Conclusions: The scoping review has recognized a broad range of outcome measures utilized in TR studies, shedding light on gaps in the current literature. Furthermore, this review serves as a valuable resource for researchers and end users (such as clinicians and policymakers), providing insights into the most appropriate outcome measures for TR. There is a lack of studies examining the required follow-up after TR, emphasizing the need for future research in this area.

Keywords: post-stroke; dependence variable; telerehabilitation; rehabilitation assessment; telecare

1. Introduction

The use of innovative technology for the treatment of cognitive and motor impairments in stroke during the critical golden hour is of paramount importance [1]. Recently, the use of telerehabilitation (TR), which we define as the ability to provide assessment and intervention to people who require rehabilitative services via telecommunication, has emerged as a substitute for in-person therapy [2]. Recent studies have shown that TR can positively affect motor functions such as balance, mobility, and postural control [1,3].

TR offers a potential solution to some of the accessibility challenges faced by individuals living with stroke [2,4]. A study found that TR interventions for stroke found no change between telehealth and face-to-face interventions for activities of daily living, balance, and upper extremity involvement [5]. Within TR, communication between patients and qualified rehabilitation professionals is facilitated via technologies like telephones and internet-based videoconferencing. Analyzing the efficacy of these interventions is pivotal for advancing the field of TR [1]. Numerous tools have been developed to assess both the outcomes and the effectiveness of post-stroke interventions [6].

There is a growing need for improvements in stroke care [7]. The latter study provides strong evidence supporting the effectiveness of both virtual reality (VR) and TR in enhancing stroke care, offering valuable guidance on selecting appropriate outcome measures for assessing the effect of these interventions on survivors of stroke and their families [7]. A recent literature review recognized numerous assessment tools utilized in stroke therapy [8]. Another review of outcome measures utilized in randomized controlled trials (RCTs) identified 30 distinct measures documented in RCTs, which gauged the efficacy of interventions in stroke therapy [9]. The adequacy of TR relative to the status quo is confirmed when outcome measures demonstrate no significant decline in performance compared to traditional treatment [5]. Thus, choice of an appropriate outcome metric to utilize in research and in clinical practice is imperative.

It is important to note that when selecting outcome measures for clinical observation for patient improvement, the consideration should assess not just impairments in motor function, but also encompass various factors such as the patient's lifestyle and daily preferences [9]. There are numerous advantages to employing standardized outcome measures, which include the ability to identify patients at risk of experiencing adverse or unfavorable outcomes, identifying the most effective interventions tailored to specific contexts, and analyzing organizational metrics [2]. Clinicians have supported the utilization of standardized tools in therapy for several years. A study by Diana et al. in 2017 emphasized the importance of clear outcome measurements with a focus on TR and VR [10]. However, there remains a lack of consensus regarding the utilization of outcome measures to enable meaningful appraisals across interventions and studies [4]. This gap in consensus has persisted from January 2015 until the present day, especially within the realm of TR. Considering the COVID-19 pandemic, during which the healthcare industry relied heavily on telerehabilitation interventions, there is a pressing need for establishing a consistent approach in this regard [11]. In addition, using telerehabilitation is beneficial for patients who cannot commute to clinical settings, particularly in rural and isolated areas [12]. Telerehabilitation also has the potential to reduce the costs of hospitalization for some patients [13]. Peretee et al. in 2017 found that telerehabilitation is effective in caring for patients with severe pathologies, such as serious cognitive deficits, enabling them to undergo physiotherapy at home without the need for exhausting transportation [13]. TR is also well-suited for patients residing in rural areas, distant from urban clinical centers, who need rehabilitation during the critical golden hour [13]. Virtual reality serves as a technology for home-based rehabilitation, providing a safe environment for patients to engage in conventional exercises, even though some studies explore the application of TR in virtual environments [14].

The current review is the first to our knowledge that attempts to elucidate the outcome measures employed in the rapidly evolving field of TR. The most recent telerehabilitation technologies include exergames (e.g., the XR-MoBI technology), digital applications, digital health technologies, telecommunication methods, and mobile applications used as treatments for patients [15].

With the aim of establishing comprehensive guidelines for the utilization of outcome measures in TR, particularly within the realm of stroke rehabilitation, we have conducted a scoping review that systematically synthesizes the prevalent outcome measurement practices. Thus, the present study aims to delineate the findings from this scoping review.

2. Methods

The Arksey and O'Malley framework from the University of York was used as guidance for a methodologically rigorous approach to systematically review the outcome metrics utilized to evaluate the efficacy of TR [16]. The York framework has been used broadly in knowledge synthesis trials and consists of the following five stages: (1) classifying the research question; (2) recognizing pertinent studies based on the research question; (3) trial selection; (4) charting the information within the selected trials; and (5) organizing, summarizing, and reporting the findings of the scoping review. The research questions for the current review were as follows: which outcome measures are used in TR stroke therapy trials and at what time points are they controlled (admission, discharge, and follow-up of the patient) subsequent to a stroke? Which functions from the International Classification of Functioning (ICF) are assessed in the outcome measures? This study was carried out in accordance with the Preferred Reporting Items for Systematic Reviews and Meta-Analyses (PRISMA) guidelines [17].

2.1. Eligibility Criteria

The inclusion criteria for this scoping review consisted of trials: (1) including patients that had sustained a stroke, (2) recounting a rehabilitation protocol utilizing TR, (3) written in English, and (4) published after January 2015. The exclusion criteria included: (1) non-English manuscripts, (2) papers omitting outcome measures, (3) papers only reporting laboratory measures, (4) discussion and protocol papers or commentary and qualitative studies, (5) poster presentations, abstracts, or papers lacking information about the treatment, and (6) papers only reporting the change and development of the technology. The search was completed using study design or publication date.

2.2. Search Strategy

The literature search was done by a librarian in the field of therapy. The search included PubMed, Embase, Scopus, Google Scholar, Web of Science, The Cochrane Central Register of Controlled Trials (Cochrane Library), the Cumulative Index to Nursing and Allied Health Literature (CINAHL), and the Physiotherapy Evidence Database (PEDro) (until July 2023) to classify potentially related studies.

2.3. Data Collection Process

Two of the reviewers (MGN and MF) independently investigated the titles and abstracts extracted from the database searches to determine if they fit the inclusion criteria. Disagreements regarding the inclusion or exclusion of a particular manuscript based on the appraisal of its abstract were determined by reaching an agreement or consulting an additional reviewer (AS). Data extraction arrangements were established based on the current literature in the field and on the questions of the research. Extraction of the data was based on essential information according to questions of the current review such as (a) the study's authors, (b) the publication date, (c) the objective(s) of the trial, (d) the design of the trial, (e) country, (f) outcome measures reported, (g) patient characteristics (e.g., age, sex, socioeconomic status, level of education, motor functional level, the phase of the stroke, type of the stroke), (h) related ICF domains, (i) period of time at which the assessment was taken (e.g., admission, discharge, follow-up), (j) technology used for TR, and (k) details on the TR intervention. The outcome measures were categorized based on the ICF domains [16].

2.4. Critical Appraisal of the Included Articles

The modified Critical Appraisal Skills Programme (CASP) tool [18,19] was used for assessing the quality of each of the included studies by the three reviewers (MGN, MF, and AS). The CASP tool is an instrument used for evaluating the strengths and limitations of any qualitative research approach [19]. The tool has 10 questions that each emphasizes different methodological domains of a qualitative study: the identification of the research questions, the relevance of the methodology (including study design), description of the population and sample size, outcomes, suitability of analysis methodologies, relevance, and clarification of results. Information was obtained from studies achieving scores greater than 50% based on the CASP scoring system.

2.5. Quality Assessment

We used the CASP tools for assessing the quality of studies, primarily case-control studies and clinical trials. The CASP RCT checklist evaluates 11 critical criteria:

(1) Did the study address a clearly focused research question?
(2) Was the assignment of participants to interventions randomized?
(3) Were all participants who entered the study accounted for at its conclusion?
(4) Was blinding appropriately addressed for participants, assessors, and therapists?
(5) Were the study groups similar at the start of the randomized controlled trial?
(6) Apart from the experimental intervention, did each study group receive the same level of care (i.e., were they treated equally)?
(7) Were the effects of intervention reported comprehensively?
(8) Was the precision of the estimate of the intervention or treatment effect reported?
(9) Did the benefits of the experimental intervention outweigh the harms and costs?
(10) Could the results be applied to your local population/in your context?
(11) Would the experimental intervention provide greater value to the people in your care than any of the existing interventions?

The CASP case-control study checklist also consists of 11 questions:

(1) Did the study address a clearly focused issue?
(2) Did the authors use an appropriate method to answer their question?
(3) Were the cases recruited appropriately?
(4) Were the controls selected appropriately?
(5) Was the exposure accurately measured to minimize bias?
(6) Aside from the experimental intervention, were the groups treated equally, and did the authors account for the potential confounding factors in the design and/or in their analysis?
(7) How large was the treatment effect?
(8) How precise was the estimate of the treatment effect?
(9) Are the results credible?
(10) Can the results be applied to the local population?
(11) Do the results of this study fit with other available evidence?

Responses to these questions were recorded as "Yes", "No", or "Can't tell". In the current review, seven studies were evaluated using the CASP RCT checklist [20–26] (Table 1).

Table 1. The characteristics of the included studies.

First Author, Year—Country	Design; Participant's Age Group; Sex	Type of Stroke; Phase of Stroke Rehabilitation	Type of VR or TR Brief Description of The System	CASP
Cramer; 2023 [20]—USA	Randomized clinical trial; 124 adults; M = 90, F = 34, age of 61	Stroke with arm motor deficits	TR:	8/11
Toh; 2023 [27]—Hong Kong	Mixed-method study; 11 adults; M = 4, F = 7, age ≥ 18 years	Limb telerehabilitation in persons with stroke	TR: used wearable device, telerehabilitation application	9/9

Table 1. Cont.

First Author, Year—Country	Design; Participant's Age Group; Sex	Type of Stroke; Phase of Stroke Rehabilitation	Type of VR or TR Brief Description of The System	CASP
Contrada, 2022 [28]—Italy	Clinical trial study; 19 patients M=13 F = 6; age: 61.1 ± 8.3 years	Post-stroke patients with a diagnosis of first-ever ischemic (n = 14) or hemorrhagic stroke (n = 5)	TR: The entire TR intervention was performed (online and offline) using the Virtual Reality Rehabilitation System (VRRS) (Khymeia, Italy).	9/9
Allegue; 2022 [29]—Canada	Mixed-method case study; 5 adults M = 3, F = 2; age: 41–89	Stroke survivors	TR+VR: (VirTele): virtual reality combined with telerehabilitation	9/9
Salgueiro; 2022 [30]—Spain	Prospective controlled trial; 49 adults M = 31, F = 18; age: 55–82	Subjects with a worsening of their stroke symptoms or any of the comorbidities (e.g., another neurological disease or orthopedic problem of the lower limbs)	TR: using AppG	9/9
Salgueiro; 2022 [31]—Spain	Prospective, single-blinded, randomized controlled trial; 30 adults M = 20, F = 10; over 18 years of age	Chronic stroke survivors	TR: The practice of specific lumbopelvic stability exercises, known as core-stability exercises	9/11
Anderson; 2022 [32]—USA	Case study design and experimental study;, one participant F = 1; 37 years old	Stroke with the etiology was a subarachnoid hemorrhage caused by a ruptured aneurysm at the left middle cerebral artery bifurcation	TR: framework for telerehabilitation and the effects of team-based remote service delivery	9/9
So Jung Lee; 2022 [26]—Republic of Korea	Randomized control trial (RCT); 17 adults eligible; 14 participants finished M = 10, F = 4; age: experimental group = 9 control group = 8	Patients with subacute or chronic stroke	TR: videoconferencing using Zoom	8/11
Dawson; 2022 [33]—Canada	Pilot, single-blind (assessor), randomized controlled trial (RCT); 17 adults; M = 9, F = 8; age: 42–75	Stroke survivors fluent in written and spoken English and with no severe aphasia	TR: a strategy training rehabilitation approach (tele-CO-OP)	8/11
Uswatte; 2021 [21]—Birmingham	Randomized clinical trial; 24 adults ≥1-year post; age: 48–72 M = 13, F = 11	Upper-extremity hemiparesis after stroke	TR using a computer-generated random numbers table, in-lab or telehealth delivery of CIMT	8/11

Table 1. Cont.

First Author, Year—Country	Design; Participant's Age Group; Sex	Type of Stroke; Phase of Stroke Rehabilitation	Type of VR or TR Brief Description of The System	CASP
Rozevink, 2021 [23]	Randomized controlled; M = 8 F = 3; age = 66.0 ± 8.4	Upper limb function after stroke	TR: home-care arm rehabilitation (MERLIN), a combination of an unactuated training device using serious games and a telerehabilitation platform in the patient's home situation	9/9
Rozevink, 2021 [24]	Randomized controlled; M = 8 F = 4; age = 64.8 ± 8.5	Upper limb function in chronic stroke	TR: home-care arm rehabilitation (MERLIN); telerehabilitation using an unactuated device based on serious games improving the upper limb function in chronic stroke	8/9
Shih-Ching, 2021 [34]	Prospective case-controlled pilot study; 30 patients F = 6 M = 9; age: 51–68	Chronic stroke	TR: three commercially available video games	9/9
Chingyi, 2021 [35]	A single-group trial; 11 participants F = 6 M = 5; age: 44–66	chronic stroke (hemorrhagic/ischemic)	TR: home-based self-help telerehabilitation program assisted by the aforementioned EMG-driven WH-ENMS	7/9
Marin-Pard, 2021 [36]	Case study and clinical trial study; one participant M = 1; age = 67 years old	Chronic stroke with upper extremity hemiparesis	TR: tele-REINVENT system consisting of a laptop computer with all necessary programs preloaded, configured, and displayed in an easy-to-use manner, a pair of EMG sensors with the enclosed acquisition board, and a package of disposable electrodes	7/9

Table 1. Cont.

First Author, Year—Country	Design; Participant's Age Group; Sex	Type of Stroke; Phase of Stroke Rehabilitation	Type of VR or TR Brief Description of The System	CASP
Cramer; 2021 [21]—USA	Prospective, single-group, therapeutic feasibility trial; 13 adults M = 9, F = 4; median age 61	Home-based telerehabilitation after stroke	TR: patients received 12 weeks of TR therapy, 6 days/week, with a live clinic assessment at the end of week 6 and week 12. Patients were free to call the lab with questions	9/9
Kessler; 2021 [37]—Canada	Multiple baseline single-case experimental design; 8 adults M = 6, F = 2; age: 50–83	Stroke survivors	TR: telerehabilitation occupational performance coaching	9/9
Saywell, 2020 [25]	Randomized controlled trial; ACTIV: n = 47; control: n = 48 N = 95 participants M = 49 F = 46	Participants had experienced a first-ever hemispheric stroke of hemorrhagic or ischemic origin and were discharged from inpatient, outpatient, or community physiotherapy services to live in their own home	TR: augmented community telerehabilitation intervention	9/11
Burgos; 2020 [38], Chile	Clinical study; 6 participants M = 3 F = 3	Chronic stage: in early subacute stroke (seven weeks of progress)	TR: low-cost telemedicine (therapist monitoring was carried out by connecting to the web platform and watching games scores daily at the scheduled session time or afterwards based on therapist availability)	9/9
Ora; 2020 [22]—Norway	Pilot randomized controlled trial; 30 adults; M = 19, F = 11; age > 18	Post-stroke with aphasia	TR: using a portable Fujitsu PC (laptop) with necessary software and material	9/11
Huzmeli; 2017 [12]—Turkey	Clinical trial study; 10 adults M = 6, F = 4; age: 45–60	Patients with stroke who were hemiplegic and had sufficient equipment	TR: video communication(TR was applied by contacting the patients via laptops with a camera and microphone and an internet connection)	9/9

Table 1. Cont.

First Author, Year—Country	Design; Participant's Age Group; Sex	Type of Stroke; Phase of Stroke Rehabilitation	Type of VR or TR Brief Description of The System	CASP
Ivanova; 2017 [39]—Germany	Clinical trial study; 6 participants M = 4 F = 1; age: 51–89 years	Motor relearning after stroke (five patients were in the subacute phase; one patient was considered chronic. All participants showed deficits in the motor activity of the shoulder, arm, and hand function)	TR: haptic devices for stroke rehabilitation and robot-based telerehabilitation system	9/9
Dodakian; 2017 [40]—USA	Clinical trial study; 12 adults M = 6, F = 6; age: 26–75	Patients with chronic hemiparetic stroke	TR: individualized exercises and games, stroke education	9/9
Özgün; 2017 [41]—Turkey	Pilot study; 10 adults M = 6, F = 4; age = 44–61	Patients with stroke	TR: giving rehabilitation services with computer-based technologies and communication tool	8/9

Table Legend. VR, virtual reality; TR, telerehabilitation; CASP, cognitive assessment scale for stroke patients; AppG, access to telerehabilitation to perform core stability exercises at home; CIMT, constrained-induced movement therapy; EMG, electromyography; WH-ENMS, wrist/hand exoneuromusculoskeleton.

In addition, when appraising other studies using the CASP case-control study checklist, questions 4 (Were the controls selected appropriately?) and 6 (Aside from the experimental intervention, were the groups treated equally, and did the authors account for the potential confounding factors in the design and/or in their analysis?) were deemed not applicable since the reported trials were uncontrolled trials. Thus, the total number of questions for the latter studies was nine rather than 11. Sixteen out of the 23 trials had scores between 7 and 9 out of 9, with only two studies scoring 7. Six of the included trials had a score between 8 and 9 out of 11, whereas only four studies scored 7.

3. Results

The exploration of the electronic databases recognized 550 manuscripts after duplicate studies were removed. After screening of the titles and abstracts, 136 studies remained. After a full-text review process, 110 articles were excluded, leaving a total of 24 included studies. Reasons for exclusion of studies are depicted in Figure 1.

3.1. Included Studies

The current scoping review encompassed a comprehensive analysis of 24 studies. This review is organized into three key sections: (a) essential characteristics of the trials, which include details about the authors, location, publication year, study design, subject characteristics, type of stroke, TR explanation, and the numerical score of the quality of the studies above 7 from 9 related to pooled studies, (b) TR outcome measures used in assessing post-stroke patients, and (c) areas of the ICF covered by these outcome measures. The included trials were published between 2015 and 2023, and most of the trials were conducted in the USA and Canada. The most common study designs were quantitative approaches such as RCTs, CTs, case studies with one group and two groups with pre- and post-test intervention (Table 1).

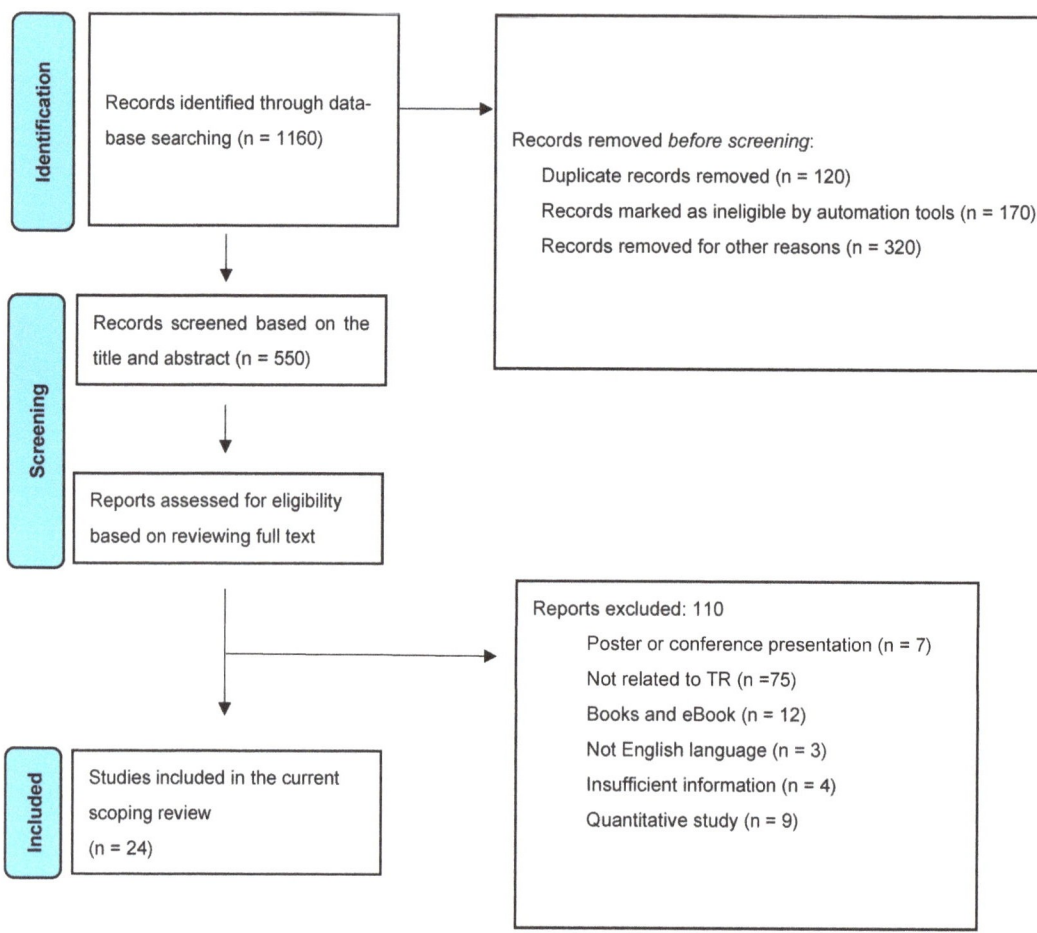

Figure 1. PRISMA 2023 flow diagram for the scoping review about TR and stroke as rehabilitation.

3.2. Participant Characteristics

The study participants primarily consisted of males (335) who had experienced various stroke conditions, including ischemic, subacute, and chronic stroke with symptoms such as hemiparesis, aphasia, and other neurological disorders. These individuals were willing and consenting to begin a rehabilitation protocol. All studies provided detailed information on age, gender distribution, and the total number of participants. Two of the studies included a single case study involving post-stroke patients (Table 1). All the studies used TR intervention and two studies used TR with VR. The TR interventions were provided via various modalities, including video games, an internet-connected computer and laptop, TR application, serious games, and robot-based TR (Table 1)

3.3. Frequently Used Outcome Measures

A total of 20 outcomes were used in the scoping review (15 outcomes in TR studies and 5 outcomes in TR studies with VR). The most used outcomes were the Fugel–Meyer assessment of the recovery of patients with stroke (FMA) [20,24,35,42], balance, and motor function in the upper limb function. All outcome measures were used pre- and post-protocol based on TR (Table 2).

Table 2. Frequency of used outcome measures in TR intervention studies.

Study (First Author, Year)	Standardized Outcome	Instrument	Reported Findings	ICF Domain	Focus of the Outcome
Cramer; 2023 [20]—USA	Upper and lower limb function	Fugel–Meyer motor assessment	Telerehabilitation has the potential to substantially increase access to rehabilitation therapy on a large scale	b730	Suboptimal rehabilitation therapy doses
Toh; 2023 [27]—Hong Kong	Usability of the wristwatch	System usability scale (SUS) questionnaire	Usability of the proposed wristwatch and telerehabilitation system was rated highly by the participants	S730	Upper limb
Contrada, 2022 [28]—Italy	Motor recovery	Barthel Index (BI); Fugel–Meyer motor score (FM) and Motricity Index (MI)	TR tool promotes motor and functional recovery in post-stroke patients	b730	Upper limb
Allegue; 2022 [29]—Canada	Improvement of UE motor function	Berg balance assessment functional gait assessment: activity-specific balance confidence scale independently applied	Most stroke survivors found the technology easy to use and useful	b730	Arm feasibility
Salgueiro; 2022 [30]—Spain	Balance in sitting position	The Spanish-version of the Trunk Impairment Scale 2.0 (S-TIS 2.0), Function in sitting test (S-FIST), Berg Balance Scale (BBS), Spanish-version of postural assessment for Stroke patients (S-PASS), Brunel Balance Assessment (BBA) gait assessment	Greater improvement in balance in both sitting and standing position	b730	Feasibility of core stability exercises
Salgueiro; 2022 [31]—Spain	Balance and gait	Spanish-Trunk Impairment Scale (S-TIS 2.0), sitting test, Spanish postural assessment scale	Improvement in trunk function and sitting balance	b730	Trunk control, balance, and gait
Anderson; 2022 [32]—USA	Feasibility and acceptability, satisfaction	The Canadian Occupational Performance Measure (COPM), a standardized semi-structured interview	Tele-CO-OP was found to be feasible and acceptable	b730	Feasibility and acceptability based exercise

Table 2. Cont.

Study (First Author, Year)	Standardized Outcome	Instrument	Reported Findings	ICF Domain	Focus of the Outcome
So Jung Lee; 2022 [26]—Republic Of Korea	Trunk control and balance function, the functional movement and locomotion necessary for sitting, standing, and walking, dependent walker, ADLs, health-related QoL	Trunk Impairment Scale (TIS) scores, the Berg Balance Scale (BBS), timed up and go (TUG) test, functional ambulation categories (FAC), Korean Modified Barthel Index (K-MBI) scores EuroQoL 5 Dimension (EQ-5D) tool	Significant improvement in the TIS scores	b730	Subacute or chronic stroke
Dawson; 2022 [33]—Canada	Self-identified in everyday life activities and mood	Canadian Occupational Performance Measure (COPM), the PHQ-9	High satisfaction and engagement	b730	Improvements in social participation
Uswatte; 2021 [21]—Birmingham	The outcome is the motor capacity	Built-in sensors and video cameras, participant opinion survey Participant opinion survey, motor activity log (MAL), The Wolf motor function test	Large improvements in everyday use of the more-affected arm	S730	The focus was on upper-extremity hemiparesis
Rozevink, 2021 [23]	Improvement of the upper limb motor ability quality of life, user satisfaction and motivation	Wolf Motor Function test (WMFT), arm function tests, the EuroQoL-5D-5L (EQ-5D), the intrinsic motivation inventory (IMI), system usability scale (SUS) and Dutch–Quebec User	The WMFT, ARAT, and EQ-5D did not show significant differences 6 months after the training period when compared to directly after training. However, the FMA-UE results were significantly better at 6 months than at baseline	S730	Upper limb
Rozevink, 2021 [24]	Limb motor ability, quality of life	Wolf Motor Function Test (WMFT), action research arm test (ARAT), assessment upper extremity (FMA-UE), EuroQoL-5D (EQ-5D)	Progress in monitored game settings, user satisfaction and motivation	S730	Upper limb
Shih-Ching, 2021 [34]	Functional mobility, balance, and fall risk, the degree of perceived efficacy, classifying the strength in each of three lower extremity muscle actions (hip, gait)	Berg Balance Scale (BBS) scores, timed up and go (TUG) test, modified falls efficacy scale, Motricity Index, functional ambulation category	Improvement in balance	b730	Balance

Table 2. Cont.

Study (First Author, Year)	Standardized Outcome	Instrument	Reported Findings	ICF Domain	Focus of the Outcome
Chingyi, 2021 [35]	Upper limb assessment, upper limb voluntary function, functional ability and motion speed of the upper limb, basic quality of participant's ADLs, spasticity	The Fugel–Meyer assessment (FMA), action research arm test (ARAT), Wolf motor function test (WMFT), motor functional independence measure (FIM), modified Ashworth scale (MAS	Improvements in the entire upper limb	S730	Upper limb
Marin-Pard, 2021 [36]	EMG signal processing	Biofeedback, modular electromyography (EMG)	Development of a muscle-computer interface	S730	Upper limb function
Cramer; 2021 [21]—USA	Upper and lower lime function	Fugel–Meyer motor assessment	Assessments spanning numerous dimensions of stroke outcomes were successfully implemented	b730	Limb weakness
Kessler; 2021 [37]—Canada	Satisfaction of using telerehabilitation on the Client Satisfaction Scale (CSS)	Client Satisfaction Scale (CSS), Canadian Occupational Performance Measure (COPM)	High satisfaction and a strong therapeutic relationship	b730	Occupational performance coaching
Saywell, 2020 [25]	Physical function, hand grip strength and balance, self-efficacy, health outcomes	The physical subcomponent of the Stroke Impact Scale), A JAMAR hand-held dynamometer, the stroke self-efficacy questionnaire (SSEQ), overall stroke recovery rating of the SIS3.0	Rehabilitation augmented using readily accessible technology	b730	Physical function
Burgos; 2020 [38], Chile	Balance and functional independence user experience	BBS and Mini-BESTest (MBT), Barthel Index (BI), system usability scale (SUS)	Complementary low-cost telemedicine approach is feasible, and that it can significantly improve the balance of stroke patients	b730	Dosage and overall treatment
Ora; 2020 [22]—Norway	Feasibility and acceptability of speech and language therapy	Videoconference software called Cisco Jabber/Acano	Tolerable technical fault rates with high satisfaction among patients	b730	Post-stroke aphasia

Table 2. Cont.

Study (First Author, Year)	Standardized Outcome	Instrument	Reported Findings	ICF Domain	Focus of the Outcome
Huzmeli; 2017 [12]—Turkey	Balance, Physical function, social role function, Emotional role function, mental health	The Berg Balance scale, short form-36 quality of life scale, The mini mental state	The balance levels significantly improved after the TR program, There was no difference in terms of quality of life and mental status before and after TR	b730	Post-stroke with hemiplegic
Ivanova; 2017 [39]—Germany	Motor relearning collection of instant feedback visualizations, incorporating telerehabilitation, arm motor gains, depression, pain, speed	Collection of instant feedback visualizations	Telehealth system for stroke rehabilitation using haptic therapeutic devices is currently being implemented into full functionality	b730	Stroke patients in recovering voluntary motor movement capability
Dodakian; 2017 [40]—USA	Incorporating telerehabilitation, arm motor gains, depression, pain, speed	Vital signs, magnetic resonance imaging, FM Scale, box and blocks (B&B), NIHSS, Barthel Index, geriatric depression scale (GDS) question form, mini-status exam (MMSE), optimization in primary and secondary control scale [20], Medical Outcomes Study Social Support Survey, Mental Adjustment to Stroke Scale (Fighting Spirit subscore), stroke-specific quality of life scale, modified functional reach forward displacement (cm), shoulder pain gait velocity stroke self-efficacy questionnaire	The results support the feasibility and utility of a home-based system to effectively deliver telerehabilitation	b730	Hemiparetic stroke
Özgün; 2017 [41]—Turkey	Cognitive levels, balance, quality of life	Mini Mental State Examination, Berg Balance Scale, short form-36 (SF-36) quality of life scale	Improvement of using TR programs	b730	TR in patients with hemiplegia

3.4. ICF, Disability, and Health Domain

The ICF serves as a framework comprising domains or categories, offering valuable guidelines for reporting functioning, performance, and health in clinical assessments. In the current study, none of the trials employed the ICF guidelines for outcome measurement encompassing aspects of both upper and lower limb function, structural aspects, and physical activity. The majority of the pooled studies focused on upper limb function (trunk mobility and functional recovery) [21,23,28,32,35,42] and some studies focused on lower limb function (balance and gait) [25,26,30,32,34,38].

4. Discussion

In recent years, TR has emerged as a new technology for treating and rehabilitating stroke patients [34]. In the current review, we identified more than 20 outcome measures (Table 2) that illustrate a broad range of assessments utilized in trials focused on stroke rehabilitation with interventions provided through TR. Among these measures, the most used was the FMA. FMA is a performance-based deficiency index and is designed to measure motor function, balance, awareness, and joint functioning in stroke patients. It serves multiple purposes, including measuring motor recovery, assessing disease severity, and aiding in treatment planning and evaluation.

In contrast, other studies have employed various other tools to assess a common outcome such as balance [7]. These tools encompass diverse measurements, including gait speed, Barthel Index (BI), Berg Balance Scale (BBS), Stroke Impact Scale (SIS), and quality of life (QOL) metrics. Importantly, the FMA has demonstrated outstanding reliability in both inter-rater and intra-rater assessments, exhibits strong construct validity, and is highly responsive to detecting changes in patient's conditions. The intraclass correlation coefficient (ICC) for both the intra- and inter-rater reliability of the FMA both had values above 0.90, consistent with the reliability of this tool for stroke in the chronic and subacute phases. For validation of measuring the strength of association, the ICC and other correlation methods are necessary.

The BBS is another reliable tool, but it is not sensitive enough to detect subtle yet clinically significant changes in balance in individual subjects, particularly those recovering from stroke [15]. It is a relatively inexpensive test and can be used with a wide range of populations, including healthy individuals and patients. It evaluates balance through a comprehensive assessment that encompasses two distinct dimensions, static and dynamic, via a structured questionnaire [43,44].

Gait analysis is another valuable measurement that was utilized in five of the included studies to meticulously assess details of step and gait speed in stroke patients [34]. In addition, the Stroke Impact Scale (SIS) is a widely used measure due to its reliability, validity, and sensitivity to change [45]. The SIS contains a question to evaluate the patient's global perception of their percentage of recovery [46]. Another frequently utilized measure that was used in studies is the Barthel Index (BI). However, there is a strong need for greater consistency in methods, content, and scoring across studies, given that the "BI" acronym is associated with various assessment methodologies. For example, some studies have adopted a 10-item scale, scoring on a range of 0 to 100 with 5-point increments [47]. This approach has been used in several multicenter stroke trials, and we call for more uniform application of this tool for stroke trials. Consistency in result reporting will allow for more appropriate pooling of data for literature review and meta-analysis.

In general, all the aforementioned outcome measures aim to capture important changes in patients who are undergoing stroke rehabilitation, whether by TR or more traditional means. Importantly, most studies have highlighted that patient satisfaction plays a pivotal role in their recovery and motivation to continue with rehabilitation to regain function. Surprisingly, only two studies incorporated a thorough assessment of patient satisfaction and motivation, using tools including the Client Satisfaction Scale (CSS) and the Canadian Occupational Performance Measure (COPM). Upon examining the satisfaction levels of patients who underwent TR following a stroke, the results unequivocally indicate that TR can be a highly effective intervention in the realm of rehabilitation. A study even mentioned maintenance of long exercises in telerehabilitation as feasible; ultimately telerehabilitation can prevent deterioration, improve physical performance, health status, and quality of life [41].

Our scoping review identified various evaluation questions that pertained to changes in health service utilization, intervention costs, and the utilization of comprehensive assessment tools to gauge aspects of patient safety, comfort, ease of use, and the efficiency-related consequences resulting from interactions with the technology [48]. This scoping review focused on motor functions such as upper-extremity function, balance, and postural control, yielding outcomes similar to those observed in previous research, such as the study conducted in 2017 [7]. Notably, the trial of Tate et al. found a limited number of studies (8.8%) that assessed specific motor, sensory, and other bodily functions [47]. It is worth mentioning that most of the studies reviewed in this study predominantly evaluated domains related to mental function [47]. In contrast, our scoping review identified only two studies that used the Mini Mental State Examination (MMSE). Future studies should prioritize outcome measures that support ICF domains using TR. Adhering to the Canadian Best Practice Recommendations for Stroke Care can comprehensively cover the various aspects of the ICF framework during both the short- and long-term recovery in stroke patients.

5. Conclusions

Our review included quantitative studies such as RCTs, CTs, case studies that provided essential information regarding participant demographics, including age and sex, as well as details about the interventions and the specific type of TR employed for rehabilitation. Most of these studies assessed outcomes related to motor function, consistently reporting improvements in this domain. However, it is important to note that most studies did not include information about the cost implications of the interventions, which could provide valuable insights for healthcare providers, clinicians, patients, and their families when making decisions based on using new technology with TR. Future studies should emphasize measuring the utilization and feasibility of these outcomes within the context of TR while also providing detailed cost-related information. Furthermore, future studies should investigate the standards that guide the selection of outcomes by clinicians and investigators. Furthermore, incorporating standard exercises can facilitate the learning and correction of general motor patterns, leading to noticeable improvements. It is crucial to explore the reasons behind the exclusion of certain outcomes, such as the need to establish new protocols for professionals, ensuring the availability of assessment tools in the same language as the patients, managing the time required for assessments, and addressing equipment-related prerequisites for the utilization of specific tools. Understanding and addressing these factors will contribute to the improvement of outcome selection processes in TR and related research. Exploring comprehensive methods to assess intervention costs and investigating potential variation in TR acceptance among different demographic groups could be impactful. The development of an application for assessment based on standardized measurements is essential for telerehabilitation, as physiotherapists can monitor activation and compare movement patterns. On the other hand, future studies must further assess follow-up outcomes for TR and characterize the effect size over the long term.

Funding: This study received no external funding.

Institutional Review Board Statement: Not applicable.

Informed Consent Statement: Not applicable.

Data Availability Statement: Not applicable.

Conflicts of Interest: The authors declare no conflict of interest.

References

1. Vellata, C.; Belli, S.; Balsamo, F.; Giordano, A.; Colombo, R.; Maggioni, G. Effectiveness of telerehabilitation on motor impairments, non-motor symptoms and compliance in patients with Parkinson's disease: A systematic review. *Front. Neurol.* **2021**, *12*, 627999. [CrossRef] [PubMed]
2. Li, F.; Zhang, D.; Chen, J.; Tang, K.; Li, X.; Hou, Z. Research hotspots and trends of brain-computer interface technology in stroke: A bibliometric study and visualization analysis. *Front. Neurol.* **2023**, *17*, 1243151. [CrossRef] [PubMed]
3. Shen, J.; Zhang, X.; Lian, Z. Impact of wooden versus nonwooden interior designs on office workers' cognitive performance. *Percept. Mot. Ski.* **2020**, *127*, 36–51. [CrossRef] [PubMed]
4. Nakhostin Ansari, N.; Bahramnezhad, F.; Anastasio, A.T.; Hassanzadeh, G.; Shariat, A. Telestroke: A Novel Approach for Post-Stroke Rehabilitation. *Brain Sci.* **2023**, *13*, 1186. [CrossRef]
5. Laver, K.E.; Adey-Wakeling, Z.; Crotty, M.; Lannin, N.A.; George, S.; Sherrington, C. Telerehabilitation services for stroke. *Cochrane Database Syst. Rev.* **2020**. [CrossRef] [PubMed]
6. Scuteri, D.; Mantovani, E.; Tamburin, S.; Sandrini, G.; Corasaniti, M.T.; Bagetta, G. Opioids in post-stroke pain: A systematic review and meta-analysis. *Front. Pharmacol.* **2020**, *11*, 587050. [CrossRef]
7. Veras, M.; Kairy, D.; Rogante, M.; Giacomozzi, C.; Saraiva, S. Scoping review of outcome measures used in telerehabilitation and virtual reality for post-stroke rehabilitation. *J. Telemed. Telecare* **2017**, *23*, 567–587. [CrossRef]
8. Zeng, X.; Zhang, Y.; Kwong, J.S.; Zhang, C.; Li, S.; Sun, F. The methodological quality assessment tools for preclinical and clinical studies, systematic review and meta-analysis, and clinical practice guideline: A systematic review. *J. Evid. Based Med.* **2015**, *8*, 2–10. [CrossRef]
9. Gold, D.A. An examination of instrumental activities of daily living assessment in older adults and mild cognitive impairment. *J. Clin. Exp. Neuropsychol.* **2012**, *34*, 11–34. [CrossRef]
10. Diana, C.; Mirela, I.; Sorin, M. Approaches on the relationship between competitive strategies and organizational performance through the Total Quality Management (TQM). *Qual. Access Success* **2017**, *18*, 328–333.
11. Edwards, D.; Kumar, S.; Brinkman, L.; Ferreira, I.C.; Esquenazi, A.; Nguyen, T. Telerehabilitation Initiated Early in Post-Stroke Recovery: A Feasibility Study. *Neurorehabil. Neural Repair.* **2023**, *37*, 131–141. [CrossRef] [PubMed]
12. Huzmeli, E.D.; Duman, T.; Yildirim, H. Efficacy of Telerehabilitation in patients with stroke in turkey: A pilot Study/Turkiye'de Inmeli Hastalarda Telerehabilitasyonun Etkinligi: Pilot Calisma. *Turk. J. Neurol.* **2017**, *23*, 21–26. [CrossRef]
13. Peretti, A.; Amenta, F.; Tayebati, S.K.; Nittari, G.; Mahdi, S.S. Telerehabilitation: Review of the state-of-the-art and areas of application. *JMIR Rehabil. Assist. Technol.* **2017**, *4*, e7511. [CrossRef] [PubMed]
14. Rutkowski, S.; Kiper, P.; Cacciante, L.; Mazurek, J.; Turolla, A. Use of virtual reality-based training in different fields of rehabilitation: A systematic review and meta-analysis. *J. Phys. Med. Rehabil.* **2020**, *52*, 1–16. [CrossRef] [PubMed]
15. Arntz, A.; Weber, F.; Handgraaf, M.; Lällä, K.; Korniloff, K.; Murtonen, K.-P. Technologies in Home-Based Digital Rehabilitation: Scoping Review. *JMIR Rehabil. Assist. Technol.* **2023**, *10*, e43615. [CrossRef] [PubMed]
16. Arksey, H.; O'Malley, L. Scoping studies: Towards a methodological framework. *Int. J. Soc. Res. Methodol.* **2005**, *8*, 19–32. [CrossRef]
17. Tam, W.W.; Tang, A.; Woo, B.; Goh, S.Y. Perception of the Preferred Reporting Items for Systematic Reviews and Meta-Analyses (PRISMA) statement of authors publishing reviews in nursing journals: A cross-sectional online survey. *BMJ Open* **2019**, *9*, e026271. [CrossRef]
18. Stucki, G.; Cieza, A.; Ewert, T.; Kostanjsek, N.; Chatterji, T.B. Application of the International Classification of Functioning, Disability and Health (ICF) in clinical practice. *Disabil. Rehabil.* **2002**, *24*, 281–282. [CrossRef]
19. Long, H.A.; French, D.P.; Brooks, J.M. Optimising the value of the critical appraisal skills programme (CASP) tool for quality appraisal in qualitative evidence synthesis. *Res. Methods Med. Health Sci.* **2020**, *1*, 31–42. [CrossRef]
20. Cramer, S.C.; Young, B.M.; Schwarz, A.; Chang, T.Y.; Su, M. Telerehabilitation Following Stroke. *Phys. Med. Rehabil. Clin. N. Am.* **2023**. [CrossRef]
21. Uswatte, G.; Taub, E.; Lum, P.; Brennan, D.; Barman, J.; Bowman, M.H. Tele-rehabilitation of upper-extremity hemiparesis after stroke: Proof-of-concept randomized controlled trial of in-home constraint-induced movement therapy. *Restor. Neurol. Neurosci.* **2021**, *39*, 303–318. [CrossRef] [PubMed]
22. Øra, H.P.; Kirmess, M.; Brady, M.C.; Sørli, H.; Becker, F. Technical features, feasibility, and acceptability of augmented telerehabilitation in post-stroke aphasia—Experiences from a randomized controlled trial. *Front. Neurol.* **2020**, *11*, 671. [CrossRef] [PubMed]
23. Rozevink, S.G.; van der Sluis, C.K.; Hijmans, J.M. HoMEcare aRm rehabiLItatioN (MERLIN): Preliminary evidence of long term effects of telerehabilitation using an unactuated training device on upper limb function after stroke. *J. Neuroeng. Rehabil.* **2021**, *18*, 141. [CrossRef] [PubMed]
24. Rozevink, S.G.; Van der Sluis, C.K.; Garzo, A.; Keller, T.; Hijmans, J.M. HoMEcare aRm rehabiLItatioN (MERLIN): Telerehabilitation using an unactuated device based on serious games improves the upper limb function in chronic stroke. *J. Neuroeng. Rehabil.* **2021**, *18*, 48. [CrossRef]
25. Saywell, N.L.; Mudge, S.; Kayes, N.M.; Stavric, V.; Taylor, D. A six-month telerehabilitation programme delivered via readily accessible technology is acceptable to people following stroke: A qualitative study. *Physiotherapy* **2023**, *120*, 1–9. [CrossRef]

26. Lee, S.J.; Lee, E.C.; Kim, M.; Ko, S.-H.; Huh, S.; Choi, W. Feasibility of dance therapy using telerehabilitation on trunk control and balance training in patients with stroke: A pilot study. *Medicine* **2022**, *101*, e30286. [CrossRef]
27. Toh, S.F.M.; Gonzalez, P.C.; Fong, K.N. Usability of a wearable device for home-based upper limb telerehabilitation in persons with stroke: A mixed-methods study. *Digit. Health* **2023**, *9*, 20552076231153737. [CrossRef]
28. Marianna, C.; Francesco, A.; Paolo, T.; Loris, P.; Tiziana, M.; Giuseppe, N. Stroke Telerehabilitation in Calabria: A Health Technology Assessment. *Front. Neurol.* **2022**, *12*, 777608.
29. Allegue, D.R.; Higgins, J.; Sweet, S.N.; Archambault, P.S.; Michaud, F.; Miller, W. Rehabilitation of upper extremity by telerehabilitation combined with exergames in survivors of chronic stroke: Preliminary findings from a feasibility clinical trial. *JMIR Rehabil. Assist. Technol.* **2022**, *9*, e33745. [CrossRef]
30. Salgueiro, C.; Urrútia, G.; Cabanas-Valdés, R. Telerehabilitation for balance rehabilitation in the subacute stage of stroke: A pilot controlled trial. *Neurorehabilitation* **2022**, *51*, 91–99. [CrossRef]
31. Salgueiro, C.; Urrútia, G.; Cabanas-Valdés, R. Influence of core-stability exercises guided by a telerehabilitation app on trunk performance, balance and gait performance in chronic stroke survivors: A preliminary randomized controlled trial. *Int. J. Environ. Res. Public Health* **2022**, *19*, 5689. [CrossRef] [PubMed]
32. Anderson, M.; Dexter, B.; Hancock, A.; Hoffman, N.; Kerschke, S.; Hux, K. Implementing Team-Based Post-Stroke Telerehabilitation: A Case Example. *Int. J. Telerehabili.* **2022**, *14*, e6438. [CrossRef]
33. Dawson, D.R.; Anderson, N.D.; Binns, M.; Bar, Y.; Chui, A.; Gill, N. Strategy-training post-stroke via tele-rehabilitation: A pilot randomized controlled trial. *Disabil. Rehabil.* **2022**, *5*, 1–10. [CrossRef] [PubMed]
34. Chen, S.-C.; Lin, C.-H.; Su, S.-W.; Chang, Y.-T.; Lai, C.-H. Feasibility and effect of interactive telerehabilitation on balance in individuals with chronic stroke: A pilot study. *J. Neuroeng. Rehabil.* **2021**, *18*, 1–11. [CrossRef] [PubMed]
35. Nam, C.; Zhang, B.; Chow, T.; Ye, F.; Huang, Y.; Guo, Z. Home-based self-help telerehabilitation of the upper limb assisted by an electromyography-driven wrist/hand exoneuromusculoskeleton after stroke. *J. Neuroeng. Rehabil.* **2021**, *18*, 1–18. [CrossRef] [PubMed]
36. Marin-Pardo, O.; Donnelly, M.R.; Phanord, C.S.; Wong, K.; Pan, J.; Liew, S.-L. Functional and neuromuscular changes induced via a low-cost, muscle-computer interface for telerehabilitation: A feasibility study in chronic stroke. *Front. Neuroergono* **2022**, *3*, 33. [CrossRef]
37. Kessler, D.; Anderson, N.D.; Dawson, D.R. Occupational performance coaching for stroke survivors delivered via telerehabilitation using a single-case experimental design. *Br. Assoc. Occup. Ther.* **2021**, *84*, 488–496. [CrossRef]
38. Burgos, P.I.; Lara, O.; Lavado, A.; Rojas-Sepúlveda, I.; Delgado, C.; Bravo, E. Exergames and telerehabilitation on smartphones to improve balance in stroke patients. *Brain Sci.* **2020**, *10*, 773. [CrossRef]
39. Ivanova, E.; Lorenz, K.; Schrader, M.; Minge, M. Developing motivational visual feedback for a new telerehabilitation system for motor relearning after stroke. In Proceedings of the 31st International BCS Human Computer Interaction Conference (HCI 2017), Sunderland, UK, 3–6 July 2017; Volume 31. [CrossRef]
40. Dodakian, L.; McKenzie, A.L.; Le, V.; See, J.; Pearson-Fuhrhop, K.; Burke Quinlan, E. A home-based telerehabilitation program for patients with stroke. *Neurorehabil. Neural Repair.* **2017**, *31*, 923–933. [CrossRef]
41. Zanaboni, P.; Hoaas, H.; Aarøen Lien, L.; Hjalmarsen, A.; Wootton, R. Long-term exercise maintenance in COPD via telerehabilitation: A two-year pilot study. *J. Telemed. Telecare* **2017**, *23*, 74–82. [CrossRef]
42. Cramer, S.C.; Dodakian, L.; Le, V.; McKenzie, A.; See, J.; Augsburger, R. A feasibility study of expanded home-based telerehabilitation after stroke. *Front. Neurol.* **2021**, *11*, 611453. [CrossRef] [PubMed]
43. Anwer, S.; Waris, A.; Gilani, S.O.; Iqbal, J.; Shaikh, N.; Pujari, A.N. Rehabilitation of upper limb motor impairment in stroke: A narrative review on the prevalence, risk factors, and economic statistics of stroke and state of the art therapies. *Healthcare* **2022**, *10*, 190. [CrossRef] [PubMed]
44. Rossetti, G.; Cazabet, R. Community discovery in dynamic networks: A survey. *ACM Comput. Surv. (CSUR)* **2018**, *51*, 1–37. [CrossRef]
45. Chen, S.; Lach, J.; Lo, B.; Yang, G.-Z. Toward pervasive gait analysis with wearable sensors: A systematic review. *J. Biomed. Inform. X* **2016**, *20*, 1521–1537. [CrossRef]
46. Hauer, K.A.; Kempen, G.I.; Schwenk, M.; Yardley, L.; Beyer, N.; Todd, C. Validity and sensitivity to change of the falls efficacy scales international to assess fear of falling in older adults with and without cognitive impairment. *Gerontology* **2011**, *57*, 462–472. [CrossRef]
47. Quinn, T.J.; Langhorne, P.; Stott, D.J. Barthel index for stroke trials: Development, properties, and application. *Stroke* **2011**, *42*, 1146–1151. [CrossRef]
48. Tate, R.L.; Godbee, K.; Sigmundsdottir, L. A systematic review of assessment tools for adults used in traumatic brain injury research and their relationship to the ICF. *Neurorehabilitation* **2013**, *32*, 729–750. [CrossRef]

Disclaimer/Publisher's Note: The statements, opinions and data contained in all publications are solely those of the individual author(s) and contributor(s) and not of MDPI and/or the editor(s). MDPI and/or the editor(s) disclaim responsibility for any injury to people or property resulting from any ideas, methods, instructions or products referred to in the content.

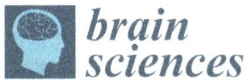

Review

The Application of Soft Robotic Gloves in Stroke Patients: A Systematic Review and Meta-Analysis of Randomized Controlled Trials

Ming-Jian Ko [1], Ya-Chi Chuang [2], Liang-Jun Ou-Yang [3], Yuan-Yang Cheng [2,4], Yu-Lin Tsai [2,*] and Yu-Chun Lee [2,5,6,*]

1. Department of Education, Taichung Veterans General Hospital, Taichung 407219, Taiwan; albert870205@gmail.com
2. Department of Physical Medicine and Rehabilitation, Taichung Veterans General Hospital, Taichung 407219, Taiwan; y065e225@vghtc.gov.tw (Y.-C.C.); s851075@ym.edu.tw (Y.-Y.C.)
3. Department of Physical Medicine and Rehabilitation, Chang Gung Memorial Hospital, Linkou, Taoyuan 333203, Taiwan; ohyoung18287@gmail.com
4. Department of Post-Baccalaureate Medicine, College of Medicine, National Chung Hsing University, Taichung 402202, Taiwan
5. Department of Exercise Health Science, National Taiwan University of Sport, Taichung 404401, Taiwan
6. Department of Industrial Engineering and Enterprise Information, Tunghai University, Taichung 407224, Taiwan
* Correspondence: xok124@vghtc.gov.tw (Y.-L.T.); lyczoj@vghtc.gov.tw (Y.-C.L.)

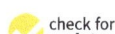

Citation: Ko, M.-J.; Chuang, Y.-C.; Ou-Yang, L.-J.; Cheng, Y.-Y.; Tsai, Y.-L.; Lee, Y.-C. The Application of Soft Robotic Gloves in Stroke Patients: A Systematic Review and Meta-Analysis of Randomized Controlled Trials. *Brain Sci.* **2023**, *13*, 900. https://doi.org/10.3390/brainsci13060900

Academic Editors: Noureddin Nakhostin Ansari, Gholamreza Hassanzadeh and Ardalan Shariat

Received: 13 May 2023
Revised: 30 May 2023
Accepted: 31 May 2023
Published: 2 June 2023

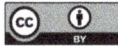

Copyright: © 2023 by the authors. Licensee MDPI, Basel, Switzerland. This article is an open access article distributed under the terms and conditions of the Creative Commons Attribution (CC BY) license (https://creativecommons.org/licenses/by/4.0/).

Abstract: Wearable robotic devices have been strongly put into use in both the clinical and research fields of stroke rehabilitation over the past decades. This study aimed to explore the effectiveness of soft robotic gloves (SRGs) towards improving the motor recovery and functional abilities in patients with post-stroke hemiparesis. Five major bibliographic databases, PubMed, Embase, Cochrane Library, Web of Science, and the Physiotherapy Evidence Database, were all reviewed for enrollment regarding comparative trials prior to 7 March 2023. We included adults with stroke and compared their rehabilitation using SRGs to conventional rehabilitation (CR) on hand function in terms of the Fugl-Meyer Upper Extremity Motor Assessment (FMA-UE), Fugl-Meyer Distal Upper Extremity Motor Assessment (FMA-distal UE), box and blocks test score, grip strength test, and the Jebsen–Taylor hand function test (JTT). A total of 8 studies, comprising 309 participants, were included in the analysis. Compared to CR, rehabilitation involving SRGs achieved better FMA-UE (MD 6.52, 95% CI: 3.65~9.39), FMA-distal UE (MD 3.27, 95% CI: 1.50~5.04), and JTT (MD 13.34, CI: 5.16~21.53) results. Subgroup analysis showed that stroke latency of more than 6 months and training for more than 30 min offered a better effect as well. In conclusion, for patients with stroke, rehabilitation using SRGs is recommended to promote the functional abilities of the upper extremities.

Keywords: soft robotic glove; stroke; rehabilitation; hemiparesis; meta-analysis

1. Introduction

According to the World Stroke Organization, stroke remains the second-leading cause of death and the third-leading cause of death and disability combined in the world [1]. Chronic dysfunction affects 60% of the affected individuals, and of those, 60–80% experience functional dyskinesia in their upper extremities [2].

Developments in the use of robotic devices have shown promise in aiding hand functional recovery [3]. However, previous exoskeleton devices have always presented significant drawbacks due to their heavy and bulky structures, limited range of motion in human joints, and their unaesthetic appearance. Robotic gloves have since emerged as a more compact and intuitive alternative to exoskeletons. These glove-like devices envelop the paretic hand, providing a more comfortable and convenient solution [4] for overcoming a patient's condition. Other advantages of soft robotic wearable devices as compared to exoskeleton devices include maintaining the wearer's mobility and flexibility without over-constraining the joints, less time wearing the device due to there being no need for precise joint alignment, being more comfortable to don and doff (meaning easier to put on and remove) and improving portability due to their reduced overall weight [5].

There are several methods regarding clinical evaluation for those experiencing post-stroke motor function disability. The Fugl-Meyer Assessment (FMA) is a well-designed, feasible, and efficient clinical examination method that has been tested widely in the stroke population. Its primary value is the 100-point motor domain, which has received the most extensive evaluation. Additionally, the method is also responsive to changes in motor impairment following stroke [6]. Another tool that has been widely used in clinical and research settings is the Jebsen-Taylor hand function test (JTT). This test involves seven subsets within the test whom represent a spectrum of hand function, with the patient's performance in each subset timed and compared with the established norms [7]. The box and block test (BBT) is also reliable and valid for patients with stroke as it is used to measure gross manual dexterity. This test measures the number of 1-inch blocks a patient can transport from one box to its adjacent box within 60 s. The greater the number of blocks per minute, the better the performance of gross manual dexterity [8]. Additionally, maximal grip strength measurement is also a great tool which can easily quantify one's weaknesses and recovery following a stroke, and has proven to be reliable in both asymptomatic and symptomatic subjects [9]. All of these measurement tools are capable of providing objective methods to help assess patients and improve their clinical outcomes when diagnosed with hemiparesis.

Over the years, several studies have evaluated the effectiveness of robotic devices on stroke patients, but few of them have confined themselves to only the use of the soft robotic glove (SRG). In recent years, Fardipour et al. and Hernández Echarren et al. have each published systematic reviews regarding the therapeutic effects of wearable robotic gloves on hand function in stroke patients [4,10]. Nevertheless, neither of them involved trials that were all randomized controlled trials and completely focused on SRGs. Therefore, the purpose of this study was to conduct a comprehensive meta-analysis in order to obtain objective outcomes, as well as thoroughly discuss the clinical application of SRGs in stroke patients.

2. Materials and Methods

2.1. Search Strategy and Selection Criteria

The protocol for this review was registered in the International Prospective Register of Systematic Reviews (PROSPERO CRD42023387935). This study was performed in accordance with the Preferred Reporting Items for Systematic Reviews and Meta-analyses (PRISMA) 2020 statement [11] shown in Table S1. Two investigators (K-MJ and T-YL) performed the initial literature screening by reviewing titles and abstracts in five electronic databases (PubMed, Embase, Cochrane Library, Web of Science, and the Physiotherapy Evidence Database (PEDro)) prior to March 7, 2023, without applying any filters. A manual literature search of bibliographies from the retrieved articles and published reviews for eligible publications was also performed. The following keywords and their synonyms were applied to identify relevant publications: "soft robotic glove", "soft wearable robot", and "stroke". A detailed description of the search strategy is provided in Table S2.

We included randomized control trials (RCTs) if they met the following criteria: (1) Population: patients with post-stroke hemiparesis (PSH) who had received or were scheduled to receive rehabilitation; (2) Intervention: rehabilitation programs involving SRGs or other similar devices; (3) Control: conventional rehabilitation (CR) programs, such as physical therapy and occupational therapy; (4) Outcomes: including Fugl-Meyer Upper Extremity Motor Assessment (FMA-UE), Fugl-Meyer Distal Upper Extremity Motor Assessment (FMA-distal UE), grip strength, BBT, and JTT score. Studies were excluded if their data were inaccessible. SRGs were defined as compact and wearable devices but not rigid exoskeleton devices. Participants in the control group received rehabilitation without the use of SRGs or any similar device. Any discrepancies were discussed with a third investigator (C-YC) in order to reach a consensus.

2.2. Outcome Measures

Primary outcomes were determined by FMA-UE and FMA-distal UE scores, while secondary outcomes were based on grip strength, BBT, and JTT scores. The patient's grip strength was recorded in pounds (lbs).

2.3. Data Extraction and Quality Assessment

Two investigators (K-MJ and T-YL) independently screened potential titles and abstracts for eligibility. Subsequently, the full text of each potentially eligible article was assessed. All discrepancies were discussed and resolved in consultation with a third investigator (C-YC). The following variables were extracted: participant characteristics, outcome measurements, follow-up period, and intervention protocol (type of device, training content, frequency, training length, and total training duration). We also contacted the authors for details when data were missing and excluded studies from data analysis when their data were inaccessible or the authors did not respond.

Two investigators (C-YC and K-MJ) independently evaluated the risk of bias for all studies and assessed the quality of the articles included in the analysis using Version 2 of the Cochrane tool to assess the risk of bias in randomized trials (RoB 2.0 tool) [12]. Conflicting opinions were discussed until a consensus was reached, with a third investigator (T-YL) being consulted when necessary.

2.4. Data Synthesis and Statistical Analysis

The results were analyzed using Review Manager V.5.4 software (Cochrane Collaboration, London, UK). Continuous data were expressed as mean ± standard deviation (SD) and summarized as a standardized mean difference (MD) with 95% confidence intervals (CIs). A random effects model was used to assess the pooled estimated effect of the intervention. Subgroup analyses were conducted based on stroke latency, type of device, training length, and total training duration in order to explore the immediate therapeutic effects of SRGs. The heterogeneity of the outcome measures was examined using the Cochrane I^2 statistic and Cochran's Q test. In cases of statistically significant heterogeneity—defined as $I^2 > 75\%$ and Cochran's Q test $p < 0.05$—a sensitivity analysis was performed to explore the possible cause of the heterogeneity. A funnel plot and the Egger regression test were conducted to assess publications bias, and a two-tailed p-value lower than 0.1 was regarded as statistically significant. Egger regression test results were analyzed using comprehensive meta-analysis (CMA 3.0). The Grading of Recommendations Assessment, Development and Evaluation (GRADE) framework was adopted in order to evaluate the certainty of evidence from the included trials [13].

3. Results

3.1. Study Selection and Characteristics

Our electronic search initially yielded a total of 912 studies. After primary screening we identified 156 articles for use in our full-text assessment. Ultimately, eight studies were incorporated into our analysis involving a total of 309 participants after assessment for eligibility [14–21]. The flowchart of the selection procedure is shown in Figure 1. The reasons for exclusion are shown in Table S3.

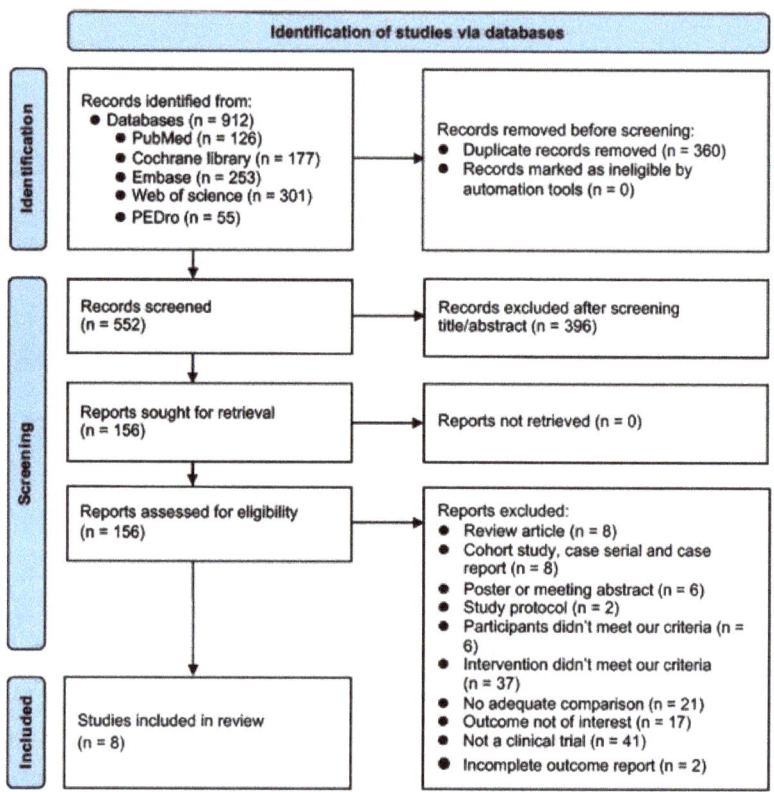

Figure 1. PRISMA2020 flow chart showing the literature search and selection process.

A total of eight randomized controlled studies were included in this meta-analysis. Three studies introduced a rehabilitation program consisting of wearing the RAPAEL Smart Glove [15,17,19]. There were a total of 142 patients who received therapy with SRGs and 134 patients who received CR. The characteristics of these studies are summarized in Table 1, with each study's SRG protocols summarized in Table 2. Six trials measured FMA-UE [14,15,17,19–21], three calculated FMA-distal UE [17,19,20], four recorded JTT scores [15,17–19], three examined grip strength [16,18,19], while two studies examined BBT scores [19,21]. The total training duration ranged from two to four weeks.

Table 1. Characteristics of the included studies.

Study	Design	Location	Participants	Intervention	Outcome Measures	Follow-Up Period
Carmeli et al. (2011) [21]	RCT	Israel	Mean age = 60 years Mean stroke latency = 10 days Stroke type: IS (87%), HS Affected arm, right: 52%	Exp = SRG + PT + OT Con = PT + OT	FMA-UE, BBT	1, 3, 4 weeks
Shin et al. (2016) [17]	RCT	Korea	Mean age = 58 years Mean stroke latency = 14 months Type of stroke: IS (63%), HS Affected arm, right: 44%	Exp = SRG + OT Con = OT	FMA-UE, FMA-distal UE, JTT	2, 4, 8 weeks [a]
Vanoglio et al. (2016) [16]	RCT	Italy	Mean age = 73 years Mean stroke latency = 17 days Stroke type: IS(63%), HS Affected arm, right: 30%	Exp = SRG Con = PT	Grip strength	6 weeks
Kang el al. (2020) [19]	RCT	Korea	Mean age = 57 years Mean stroke latency = 25 days Stroke type: IS (35%), HS Affected arm, right: 52%	Exp = SRG + OT Con = OT + Self-training	FMA-UE, FMA-distal UE, BBT, JTT, Grip strength	2, 6 weeks [b]
Park et al. (2021) [18]	RCT	Korea	Mean age = 61 years Mean stroke latency = ≤1 month Stroke type: N/S Affected arm, right: 61%	Exp = SRG + PT Con = PT	JTT, Grip strength	4 weeks
Guo et al. (2022) [20]	RCT	China	Mean age = 57 years Mean stroke latency = 12 months Stroke type: IS (57%), HS Affected arm, right: 53%	Exp1 = SSVEP-BCI SRG + PT + OT Exp2 = SRG + PT + OT Con = PT + OT	FMA-UE, FMA-distal UE	2, 12 weeks
Shin et al. (2022) [15]	RCT	Korea	Mean age = 60 years Mean stroke latency = 29 days Stroke type: IS (67%), HS Affected arm, right: 39%	Exp = SRG + OT Con = OT	FMA-UE, JTT	4, 8 weeks
Wang et al. (2023) [14]	RCT	China	Mean age = 62 years Mean stroke latency = 95 days Stroke type: IS (42%), HS Affected arm, right: 49%	Exp1 = SRG + PT + OT + Acupuncture Exp2 = rTMS + PT + OT + Acupuncture Con = PT + OT + Acupuncture	FMA-UE	2 weeks

RCT randomised controlled trial, N number, IS ischemic stroke, % percentage, HS haemorrhagic stroke, Exp experimental group, SRG soft robotic glove, PT physical therapy, OT occupational therapy, Con control group, FMA Fugl-Meyer Assessment scores, UE upper extremity, BBT box and blocks test score, JTT Jebsen-Taylor hand function test, N/S not stated, SSVEP-BCI steady-state visually evoked potentials-based brain computer interfaces, rTMS repetitive transcranial magnetic stimulation. [a] Forty-six participants met the inclusion criteria and underwent allocation, but only twenty-three participants completed the follow-up assessment. Intention-to-treat analysis was performed. [b] Twenty-three participants met the inclusion criteria and underwent allocation, but only twenty participants completed the follow-up assessment. Intention-to-treat analysis was performed.

Table 2. Soft robotic gloves training protocol of included studies.

Study	Type of Device	Content	Frequency (per Week)	Training Length (per Session)	Total Training Duration
Carmeli et al. (2011) [21]	HandTutor™ System	Augmented wrist and fingers motion feedback Wrist flexion/extension, fingers flexion/extension Functional task training Visual biofeedback	5	20 to 30 min	3 weeks
Shin et al. (2016) [17]	RAPAEL Smart Glove	Forearm pronation/supination, wrist flexion/extension, wrist radial/ulnar deviation, finger flexion/extension Game-based functional training	5	30 min	4 weeks
Vanoglio et al. (2016) [16]	Gloreha Professional	Finger flexion/extension, thumb-finger opposition movement, wave-like finger movement Visual biofeedback	5	40 min	2 weeks
Kang et al. (2020) [19]	RAPAEL Smart Glove	Forearm pronation/supination, wrist flexion/extension, wrist radial/ulnar deviation, finger flexion/extension Visual biofeedback	5	30 min	2 weeks
Park et al. (2021) [18]	RAPAEL Smart Glove	Game-based functional training and activities of daily living	5	30 min	4 weeks
Guo et al. (2022) [20]	Soft Robotic Gloves with SSVEP-BCI or computer control	Visual biofeedback Finger flexion/extension	5	60 min [a]	2 weeks
Shin et al. (2022) [15]	RAPAEL Smart Glove	Visual biofeedback Game-based functional training	5	30 min	4 weeks
Wang et al. (2023) [14]	Soft Robotic Glove	Wrist flexion/extension and fingers flexion/extension passively or with assistance	7	20 min	2 weeks

SSVEP-BCI steady-state visually evoked potentials-based brain computer interfaces. [a] One hour included 2 lots of 20-min trainings, a 10-min preparation at the beginning, and a 10-min rest.

3.2. Methodological Quality of Included Trials

According to the RoB 2.0, two RCTs [15,17] were considered to have a low risk of bias, while the other six [14,16,18–21] were rated as having some concerns. A summary of the risk of bias is shown in Figure 2. The GRADE framework was introduced for intergroup outcome measure comparison and is presented in Table S4.

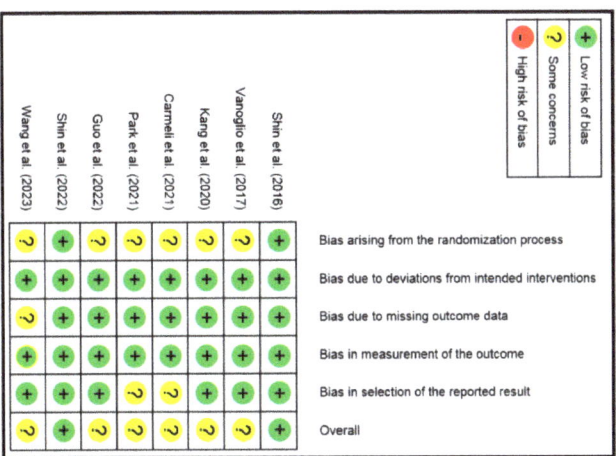

Figure 2. Risk of bias summary for the included trials based on RoB 2.0. Shin et al., 2016 [17]; Vangolio et al., 2017 [16]; Kang et al., 2020 [19]; Carmeli et al., 2021 [21]; Park et al., 2021 [18]; Guo et al., 2022 [20]; Shin et al., 2022 [15]; and Wang et al., 2023 [14].

3.3. Effects of Intervention

3.3.1. Primary Outcome: FMA-UE Scores

A total of 7 trials [14,15,17,19–21] involving 222 patients were included in the quantitative analysis (Figure 3). A significant improvement in FMA-UE scores was demonstrated in those patients receiving therapy with SRGs through the assessment which was made immediately after the intervention (MD 6.52, 95% CI: 3.65~9.39, I^2 = 8%). A total of 6 trials [15,17,19–21] involving 176 patients demonstrated the follow-up assessment, which also revealed a significant improvement in FMA-UE scores (MD 7.79, 95% CI: 5.03~10.55, I^2 = 0%) (Figure 3), with the funnel plot shown in Figure S1. In subgroup analyses, patients who had reached chronic stroke status (latency >6 months) showed significant improvement in their FMA-UE score (MD 4.93, 95% CI: 0.93~8.93, I^2 = 19%), with those whose stroke latency was less than six months also showing significant improvement (MD 8.84, 95% CI: 4.47~13.22, I^2 = 0%). The three trials [15,17,19] which used the RAPAEL Smart Glove revealed significant improvement in FMA-UE scores (MD 8.43, 95% CI: 4.27~12.59, I^2 = 0%), as did the other four studies which involved other devices (MD 5.29, 95% CI: 0.90~9.67, I^2 = 27%). In the subgroup involving a training length of less than 30 min, significant improvement in FMA-UE scores was found (MD 5.85, 95% CI: 2.49~9.21, I^2 = 15%), with those trials whose training length was more than 30 min also showing significant improvement (MD 9.01, 95% CI: 2.77~15.26, I^2 = 3%). Additionally, whether those trials received a total training duration of more than two weeks (MD 7.12, 95% CI: 3.67~10.57, I^2 = 4%) or not (MD 5.51, 95% CI: 0.04~10.98, I^2 = 27%), significant improvements were achieved in both. Further sensitivity analysis was not needed due to a low heterogeneity (I^2 < 50%) being found in all subgroups. The detailed subgroup analysis results are presented in Table 3. The certainty of the evidence ranged from low to moderate according to the GRADE appraisal.

Table 3. Subgroup analyses of the included studies.

Outcome	Categories	Studies	Participants	MD (95% CI)	Heterogeneity I^2	Heterogeneity p-Value	p-Value	Egger's Test	Quality of Evidence
FMA-UE scores									
	All studies	7	222	6.52 (3.65, 9.39)	8%	0.37	**<0.00001**	0.98222	⊕⊕⊕○
	Stroke latency:								
	≤six months	4	136	4.93 (0.93, 8.93)	19%	0.29	**0.02**	0.59725	⊕⊕⊕○
	>six months	3	86	8.84 (4.47, 13.22)	0%	0.60	**<0.0001**	0.51979	⊕⊕⊕○
	Type of device:								
	RAPAEL Smart Glove	3	105	8.43 (4.27, 12.59)	0%	0.61	**<0.0001**	0.13327	⊕⊕○○
	Other device	4	117	5.29 (0.90, 9.67)	27%	0.25	**0.02**	0.73410	⊕⊕⊕○
	Training length:								
	≤30 min	5	182	5.85 (2.49, 9.21)	15%	0.32	**0.0007**	0.80650	⊕⊕⊕○
	>30 min	2	40	9.01 (2.77, 15.26)	3%	0.31	**0.005**	N/A	⊕⊕⊕○
	Total training duration:								
	≤two weeks	4	109	5.51 (0.04, 10.98)	27%	0.25	**0.05**	0.82989	⊕⊕⊕○
	>two weeks	3	113	7.12 (3.67, 10.57)	4%	0.28	**<0.0001**	0.11801	⊕⊕○○
FMA-distal UE scores									
	All studies	4	109	3.27 (1.50, 5.04)	0%	0.46	**0.0003**	0.56538	⊕⊕⊕○
	Stroke latency:								
	≤six months	1	23	−0.40 (−6.15, 5.35)	N/A	N/A	0.89	N/A	N/A
	>six months	3	86	3.66 (1.80, 5.52)	0%	0.66	**0.0001**	0.80182	⊕⊕○○
	Type of device:								
	RAPAEL Smart Glove	2	69	2.52 (−1.27, 6.31)	42%	0.19	0.19	N/A	⊕⊕○○
	Other device	2	40	3.50 (0.80, 6.20)	0%	0.37	**0.01**	N/A	⊕⊕⊕○
	Training length:								
	≤30 min	2	69	2.52 (−1.27, 6.31)	42%	0.19	0.19	N/A	⊕⊕○○
	>30 min	2	40	3.50 (0.80, 6.20)	0%	0.37	**0.01**	N/A	⊕⊕⊕○
	Total training duration:								
	≤two weeks	3	63	2.78 (0.15, 5.40)	11%	0.32	**0.04**	0.81777	⊕⊕○○
	>two weeks	1	46	3.80 (1.24, 6.36)	N/A	N/A	**0.004**	N/A	N/A
JTT scores									
	All studies	4	149	13.34 (5.16, 21.53)	8%	0.35	**0.001**	0.11011	⊕⊕⊕○
Grip strength									
	All studies	3	94	3.11 (−6.25, 12.47)	0%	0.60	0.51	0.66567	⊕⊕○○
BBT scores									
	All studies	2	54	−0.75 (−9.03, 7.54)	0%	0.63	0.86	N/A	⊕⊕○○

FMA Fugl-Meyer Assessment scores, UE upper extremity, JTT Jebsen–Taylor hand function test, BBT box and blocks test score, N/A not assess. Bold values are significant at p-value < 0.05.

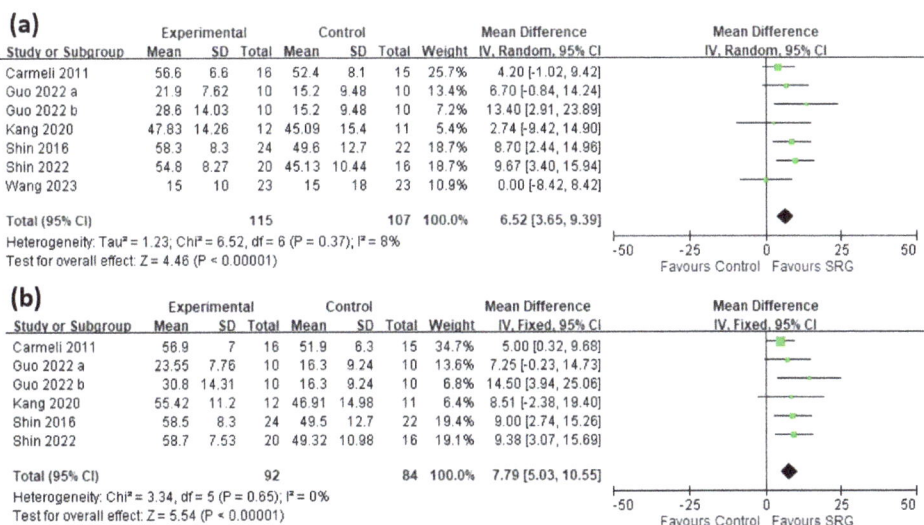

Figure 3. Mean difference (95% CI) of the immediate (**a**) and long-term (**b**) effect of SRGs on FMA-UE compared with CR [14,15,17,19–21]. Guo 2022 a used a steady-state visually evoked potentials-based brain computer interface soft robotic glove [20]. Guo 2022 b used a computer-controlled soft robotic glove [20]. (SRG: soft robotic glove, FMA: Fugl-Meyer Assessment scores, UE: upper extremity, CR: conventional rehabilitation.)

3.3.2. Primary Outcome: FMA-Distal UE Score

A total of 4 trials [17,19,20] involving 109 patients were included in the quantitative analysis (Figure 4). A significant improvement in FMA-distal UE scores was demonstrated in patients receiving therapy with SRGs no matter whether the assessment was performed immediately after the intervention (MD 3.27, 95% CI: 1.50~5.04, $I^2 = 0\%$) or during the follow-up assessment (MD 3.70, 95% CI: 1.92~5.48, $I^2 = 0\%$) (Figure 4), with the funnel plot shown in Figure S2. In subgroup analyses, the three trials whose patients were designated as chronic stroke status (latency >6 months) showed significant improvement in FMA-distal UE scores (MD 3.66, 95% CI: 1.80~5.52, $I^2 = 0\%$). Two trials [17,19] involving the RAPAEL Smart Glove revealed no significant improvement in FMA-distal UE scores (MD 2.52, 95% CI: −1.27~6.31, $I^2 = 42\%$), while the remaining two trials using other devices did see improvement (MD 3.50, 95% CI: 0.80~6.20, $I^2 = 0\%$). In the subgroup involving those undergoing a training length of more than 30 min, significant improvement in FMA-distal UE scores was found (MD 3.50, 95% CI: 0.80~6.20, $I^2 = 0\%$), while those trials where the training length was less than 30 min showed no significant improvement (MD 2.52, 95% CI: −1.27~6.31, $I^2 = 42\%$). As for subgroup analysis regarding total training duration, significant improvement was found no matter whether the duration was for either more or less than two weeks. Further sensitivity analysis was not required due to low heterogeneity ($I^2 < 50\%$) being found in all subgroups. The detailed subgroup analysis results are presented in Table 3. The certainty of the evidence ranged from low to moderate according to the GRADE appraisal.

3.3.3. Secondary Outcome: JTT Scores, Grip Strength, and BBT Scores

Four studies [15,17–19] reported on the effect of therapy involving SRGs when compared to CR on JTT scores, with the results demonstrating both immediate and long-term improvement in a significant manner: (MD 13.34, 95% CI: 5.16–21.53, $I^2 = 8\%$) and (MD 19.38, 95% CI: 9.94–28.82, $I^2 = 0\%$), respectively. The certainty of the evidence was moderate, according to the GRADE appraisal. However, no significant improvement was revealed upon analysis of grip strength (MD 3.11, 95% CI: −6.25~12.47, $I^2 = 0\%$) or BBT scores (MD −0.75, 95% CI: −9.03~7.54, $I^2 = 0\%$) (Figures S3–S5). The certainty of the evidence in each was low, according to the GRADE appraisal.

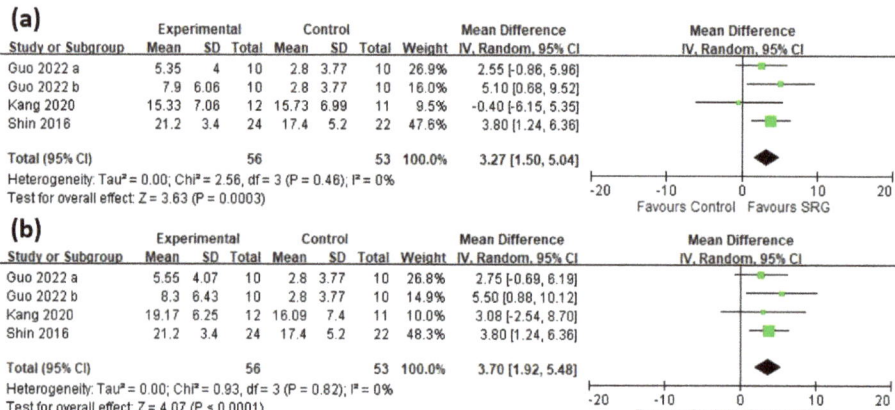

Figure 4. Mean difference (95% CI) of the immediate (**a**) and long-term (**b**) effect of SRGs on FMA-distal UE, compared with CR [17,19,20]. Guo 2022 a used a steady-state visually evoked potentials-based brain computer interface SRG [20]. Guo 2022 b used a computer-controlled soft robotic glove [20]. (SRG: soft robotic glove, FMA: Fugl-Meyer Assessment scores, UE: upper extremity, CR: conventional rehabilitation).

4. Discussion

4.1. Summary and Contributions

In this study, we conducted a meta-analysis to investigate the effectiveness of rehabilitation involving SRGs on hand function in stroke patients. Our results show that rehabilitation with SRGs significantly improved FMA-UE scores, FMA-distal UE scores, and JJT scores when compared to only CR, with these improvements being observed not only immediately after the intervention but also in subsequent follow-up assessments. Regarding distal hand function, our findings suggest that chronic stroke patients who received rehabilitation combined with the use of SRGs may experience a better immediate effect, particularly during training sessions lasting more than 30 min. To the best of our knowledge, this study is the first meta-analysis focusing solely on the effect that SRGs have on hand function in stroke patients.

4.2. Comparison with Previous Studies

Up until now, few systematic reviews or meta-analyses of randomized controlled trials have discussed the effect that SRGs have on hand function in stroke patients. Fardipour et al. published a systematic review in 2022 investigating the therapeutic effects of wearable robotic gloves on improving hand function in stroke patients. However, use of the device was not confined to SRGs, and the included trials were not all randomized controlled trials. Additionally, no meta-analysis was performed. In another study, Luo et al. published a systemic review and meta-analysis evaluating the synergistic effect of combined mirror therapy on the upper extremities in patients with stroke, with one of the experimental groups going through intervention involving mirror therapy with a mesh glove [22]. Fernández-Vázquez et al. published a systematic review and meta-analysis in 2022, but the study focused on intervention involving Haptic Glove Systems in combination with semi-immersive virtual reality (SVR) for use in upper extremity motor rehabilitation after stroke [23]. The study we have performed was the first systematic review and meta-analysis which has purely discussed the effect of SRGs on stroke patients, with the included studies all being randomized controlled trials.

According to previous meta-analysis, we have found similarities in several outcomes, but there were also differences which remained in some of the results. The meta-analysis published by Fernández-Vázquez et al. evaluates the random effect that gloves and SVR have on FMA, JTT, and BBT scores, revealing that the combined use of rehabilitation gloves with SVR produces significant improvements over the use of only CR treatment in the upper extremity functions of stroke patients in both the short and long term, regardless of whether or not associated CR is also performed. As for our study, we precisely analyzed FMA, JTT, and BBT scores, respectively, and found significant improvements in FMA -UE scores, FMA-distal UE scores, and JJT scores. However, no significant improvement in BBT scores was seen in our study. With regards to grip strength, both Fernández-Vázquez et al. and our study revealed no significant improvement over simply using CR.

4.3. Clinical Effect

Concerning the minimal clinically important difference (MCID), this often varies across patient populations and post-onset periods. Thus, it is necessary to have evidence of MCID at each post-onset period and each level of paresis [24]. The recovery time after a stroke is often divided into phases. The Stroke Roundtable Consortium has proposed designating the first 7 days as the acute phase, the first 6 months as the subacute phase, and from 6 months onwards as the chronic phase [25]. The estimated MCID score for upper extremity motor recovery among patients with subacute stroke is 9 to 10 for FMA-UE scores [26]. Therefore, according to our analysis, four studies included patients in the subacute stroke phase. The mean of the increased amount in FMA-UE scores was 10.321 in the soft robotic group but only 4.653 in the control group, which demonstrates that a rehabilitation program involving intervention with SRGs can achieve meaningful clinical improvements in upper extremity motor recovery among subacute stroke patients (Figures S6–S8). Alternatively, the estimated MCID score for upper extremity motor recovery among patients with chronic stroke is 4.25 to 7.25 for FMA-UE scores [24]. Regarding our analysis, three trials included patients in the chronic stroke phase. The mean of the increased amount in FMA-UE scores was 7.377 in the soft robotic glove group but only 1.114 in the control group, which reveals that a rehabilitation program involving intervention with SRGs can also achieve meaningful clinical improvement in upper extremity motor recovery among chronic stroke patients (Figures S6–S8). Conclusively, when compared with the control group, intervention using SRGs can achieve MCID in both subacute and chronic stroke patients.

Regarding proprioception for the orchestration of muscles to better perform targeted motions, biofeedback plays a critical role. Biofeedback can provide the patient with immediate and accurate feedback on messages regarding one's body function by taking intrinsic physiological signals and making them extrinsic. During biofeedback, patients would be connected to electrical sensors which allow medical personnel to help receive information about a patient's body. This technique gains even further significance for its use in the rehabilitation of neurological disorders such as stroke, requiring compensation of motor and sensory functions which may be augmented by biofeedback devices [27]. Most of the soft robotic devices adopted in the trials that we have included here did contain a biofeedback system which could be used in the form of either electromyography which measures muscle tension or electroencephalography which measures brain wave activity. The influences of biofeedback content on robotic post-stroke gait rehabilitation have been studied extensively. A systematic review published by Stanton et al. in 2017 reveals that biofeedback improves performance in lower limb activities more than simply the use of typical therapy in people following stroke [28]. We believe that the improvements SRGs make on hand function are also strongly associated with a biofeedback system.

4.4. Subgroup Analysis

With regards to subgroup analysis, we were impressed by the more significant improvements made in the distal extremities by patients in the chronic stroke phase than those made in the subacute phase. It has become well known that neuroplasticity plays an important role towards improving one's condition after people experience injuries such as stroke or traumatic brain injury. Neuroplasticity is defined as the ability of the nervous system to change its activity in response to intrinsic or extrinsic stimuli by reorganizing its structure, functions, and connections [29]. A previous study has shown that neuroplasticity was most prominent shortly after stroke, particularly during the first thirty days of the post-stroke period, before diminishing over subsequent sessions [30]. We believe that even CR without the use of SRGs could help achieve improvement to some extent for stoke patients in the subacute phase due to neuroplasticity remaining strong. However, since neuroplasticity diminishes gradually over time after stroke, the superiority of the soft robotic glove group over the control group was more obviously seen among stroke patients in the chronic phase. Furthermore, we found that when compared with total training duration, training length had a more positive influence on hand function. The subgroup analysis of FMA-distal UE scores revealed that significant improvement was made only when the training length lasted for more than 30 min per session. This result is reasonable considering that a longer training length would likely have a greater effect on any improvement regarding fine tuning the motor skills of the distal extremities. However, the most suitable training duration involving SRGs for stroke patients remains uncertain, and thus, further research for evaluation of this variable remains necessary.

4.5. Limitations

However, several limitations still exist. Firstly, only a few related trials which completely fulfill our inclusion criteria currently exist, and most of them have been published in an Asian country. Furthermore, it was not only the design of the rehabilitation program and the soft robotic device which were both adopted by each trial that were different, but it was also the long-term follow-up period which was diverse among the different studies that we had included. Additionally, the training period in the control group was prolonged in order to fill the time taken by the SRG training sessions used in several studies [14–17,19–21], which may have caused heterogeneity between the different studies.

4.6. Future Work

To better demonstrate a more comprehensive result, further studies are required in the future in order to maintain consistency in the design of SRGs, the period of each training session, the total training duration, and the follow-up period. These studies should be performed in order to better help achieve a more complete analysis.

5. Conclusions

Our results support the immediate and long-term effectiveness of conventional rehabilitation combined with SRGs in promoting the functions of extremities in patients with PSH, based on improvements seen in FMA-UE, FMA-distal UE, and JTT scores. The effect on distal hand function was most significant when rehabilitation occurred which consisted of SRG use exceeding 30 min per session and when the latency of the stroke was more than six months. These findings offer a perspective on refined SRG prescriptions for patients experiencing PSH. Future randomized controlled trials involving more varied stroke patients and a uniform prescription are still needed in order to better explore the effects of SRGs.

Supplementary Materials: The following supporting information can be downloaded at: https://www.mdpi.com/article/10.3390/brainsci13060900/s1; Table S1: PRISMA 2020 Checklist; Table S2: Electronic database searching strategy; Table S3: Reasons for exclusion; Table S4: Appraisal of the included studies using the GRADE tool; Figure S1: Funnel plot of studies comparing immediate and long-term FMA-UE between the soft robotic gloves and conventional rehabilitation groups; Figure S2: Funnel plot of studies comparing immediate and long-term FMA-distal UE between the soft robotic gloves and conventional rehabilitation groups; Figure S3: Mean difference (95% CI) of the immediate and long-term effect of soft robotic gloves on the Jebsen–Taylor hand function test when compared with conventional rehabilitation; Figure S4: Mean difference (95% CI) of the effect of soft robotic gloves on grip strength when compared with conventional rehabilitation; Figure S5: Mean difference (95% CI) of the effect of soft robotic gloves on box and blocks test scores when compared with conventional rehabilitation; Figure S6: Mean difference (95% CI) of baseline on FMA-UE of subacute stroke patients between groups; Figure S7: Mean difference (95% CI) of baseline on FMA-UE of chronic stroke patients between groups; and, Figure S8: Mean of the increase amount on FMA-UE of stroke patients in the subacute and chronic phases.

Author Contributions: The conceptualization and data curation were performed by L.-J.O.-Y., Y.-C.L. and Y.-L.T.; M.-J.K., Y.-C.C. and Y.-L.T. contributed to software, methodology, formal analysis, and investigation. The first draft of the manuscript was written by M.-J.K., Y.-C.C. and Y.-L.T.; L.-J.O.-Y., Y.-Y.C. and Y.-C.L. reviewed and edited the final draft of the manuscript. This research was supervised by Y.-Y.C. and Y.-C.L. All authors have read and agreed to the published version of the manuscript.

Funding: This research received no external funding.

Institutional Review Board Statement: Because this research is a systematic review and meta-analysis, ethics approval can be waived.

Informed Consent Statement: Consent from participants is not required in a systematic review and meta-analysis.

Data Availability Statement: All data relevant to this research have been extracted from the included studies. They are all included in the article or uploaded as Supplementary Materials.

Conflicts of Interest: The authors declare no conflict of interest.

Abbreviations

Fugl-Meyer assessment (FMA), Jebsen–Taylor hand function test (JTT), box and block test (BBT), soft robotic gloves (SRGs), Preferred Reporting Items for Systematic Reviews and Meta-analyses (PRISMA), randomized control trials (RCTs), post-stroke hemiparesis (PSH), conventional rehabilitation (CR), Fugl-Meyer Upper Extremity Motor Assessment (FMA-UE), Fugl-Meyer Distal Upper Extremity Motor Assessment (FMA-distal UE), standard deviation (SD), mean difference (MD), confidence intervals (CIs), Grading of Recommendations Assessment, Development and Evaluation (GRADE).

References

1. Feigin, V.L.; Brainin, M.; Norrving, B.; Martins, S.; Sacco, R.L.; Hacke, W.; Fisher, M.; Pandian, J.; Lindsay, P. World Stroke Organization (WSO): Global stroke fact sheet 2022. *Int. J. Stroke* **2022**, *17*, 18–29. [CrossRef] [PubMed]
2. Alsubiheen, A.M.; Choi, W.; Yu, W.; Lee, H. The effect of task-oriented activities training on upper-limb function, daily activities, and quality of life in chronic stroke patients: A randomized controlled trial. *Int. J. Environ. Res. Public Health* **2022**, *19*, 14125. [CrossRef]
3. Bertani, R.; Melegari, C.; De Cola, M.C.; Bramanti, A.; Bramanti, P.; Calabrò, R.S. Effects of robot-assisted upper limb rehabilitation in stroke patients: A systematic review with meta-analysis. *Neurol. Sci.* **2017**, *38*, 1561–1569. [CrossRef] [PubMed]
4. Fardipour, S.; Hadadi, M. Investigation of therapeutic effects of wearable robotic gloves on improving hand function in stroke patients: A systematic review. *Curr. J. Neurol.* **2022**, *21*, 125–132. [CrossRef]
5. Bardi, E.; Gandolla, M.; Braghin, F.; Resta, F.; Pedrocchi, A.L.G.; Ambrosini, E. Upper limb soft robotic wearable devices: A systematic review. *J. Neuroeng. Rehabil.* **2022**, *19*, 87. [CrossRef] [PubMed]
6. Gladstone, D.J.; Danells, C.J.; Black, S.E. The fugl-meyer assessment of motor recovery after stroke: A critical review of its measurement properties. *Neurorehabil. Neural. Repair* **2002**, *16*, 232–240. [CrossRef]
7. Sears, E.D.; Chung, K.C. Validity and responsiveness of the Jebsen-Taylor Hand Function Test. *J. Hand Surg. Am.* **2010**, *35*, 30–37. [CrossRef]
8. Ekstrand, E.; Lexell, J.; Brogårdh, C. Test-retest reliability and convergent validity of three manual dexterity measures in persons with chronic stroke. *PM&R* **2016**, *8*, 935–943. [CrossRef]

9. Bertrand, A.M.; Fournier, K.; Wick Brasey, M.G.; Kaiser, M.L.; Frischknecht, R.; Diserens, K. Reliability of maximal grip strength measurements and grip strength recovery following a stroke. *J. Hand Ther.* **2015**, *28*, 356–362. [CrossRef]
10. Hernández Echarren, A.; Sánchez Cabeza, Á. Hand robotic devices in neurorehabilitation: A systematic review on the feasibility and effectiveness of stroke rehabilitation. *Rehabilitacion* **2023**, *57*, 100758. [CrossRef]
11. Page, M.J.; McKenzie, J.E.; Bossuyt, P.M.; Boutron, I.; Hoffmann, T.C.; Mulrow, C.D.; Shamseer, L.; Tetzlaff, J.M.; Akl, E.A.; Brennan, S.E.; et al. The PRISMA 2020 statement: An updated guideline for reporting systematic reviews. *BMJ* **2021**, *372*, n71. [CrossRef]
12. Sterne, J.A.C.; Savović, J.; Page, M.J.; Elbers, R.G.; Blencowe, N.S.; Boutron, I.; Cates, C.J.; Cheng, H.Y.; Corbett, M.S.; Eldridge, S.M.; et al. RoB 2: A revised tool for assessing risk of bias in randomised trials. *BMJ* **2019**, *366*, l4898. [CrossRef]
13. Guyatt, G.H.; Oxman, A.D.; Kunz, R.; Vist, G.E.; Falck-Ytter, Y.; Schünemann, H.J. What is "quality of evidence" and why is it important to clinicians? *BMJ* **2008**, *336*, 995–998. [CrossRef] [PubMed]
14. Wang, T.; Liu, Z.; Gu, J.; Tan, J.; Hu, T. Effectiveness of soft robotic glove versus repetitive transcranial magnetic stimulation in post-stroke patients with severe upper limb dysfunction: A randomised controlled trial. *Front. Neurol.* **2022**, *13*, 887205. [CrossRef] [PubMed]
15. Shin, S.; Lee, H.J.; Chang, W.H.; Ko, S.H.; Shin, Y.I.; Kim, Y.H. A smart glove digital system promotes restoration of upper limb motor function and enhances cortical hemodynamic changes in subacute stroke patients with mild to moderate weakness: A randomized controlled trial. *J. Clin. Med.* **2022**, *11*, 7343. [CrossRef]
16. Vanoglio, F.; Bernocchi, P.; Mulè, C.; Garofali, F.; Mora, C.; Taveggia, G.; Scalvini, S.; Luisa, A. Feasibility and efficacy of a robotic device for hand rehabilitation in hemiplegic stroke patients: A randomized pilot controlled study. *Clin. Rehabil.* **2017**, *31*, 351–360. [CrossRef]
17. Shin, J.H.; Kim, M.Y.; Lee, J.Y.; Jeon, Y.-J.; Kim, S.; Lee, S.; Seo, B.; Choi, Y. Effects of virtual reality-based rehabilitation on distal upper extremity function and health-related quality of life: A single-blinded, randomized controlled trial. *J. Neuroeng. Rehabil.* **2016**, *13*, 17. [CrossRef]
18. Park, Y.S.; An, C.S.; Lim, C.G. Effects of a rehabilitation program using a wearable device on the upper limb function, performance of activities of daily living, and rehabilitation participation in patients with acute stroke. *Int. J. Environ. Res. Public Health* **2021**, *18*, 5524. [CrossRef]
19. Kang, M.G.; Yun, S.J.; Lee, S.Y.; Oh, B.-M.; Lee, H.H.; Lee, S.-U.; Gil Seo, H. Effects of upper-extremity rehabilitation using smart glove in patients with subacute stroke: Results of a prematurely terminated multicenter randomized controlled trial. *Front. Neurol.* **2020**, *11*, 580393. [CrossRef]
20. Guo, N.; Wang, X.; Duanmu, D.; Huang, X.; Li, X.; Fan, Y.; Li, H.; Liu, Y.; Yeung, E.H.K.; To, M.K.T.; et al. SSVEP-based brain computer interface controlled soft robotic glove for post-stroke hand function rehabilitation. *IEEE Trans. Neural. Syst. Rehabil. Eng.* **2022**, *30*, 1737–1744. [CrossRef]
21. Carmeli, E.; Peleg, S.; Bartur, G.; Elbo, E.; Vatine, J.J. HandTutor™ enhanced hand rehabilitation after stroke—A pilot study. *Physiother. Res. Int.* **2011**, *16*, 191–200. [CrossRef]
22. Luo, Z.; Zhou, Y.; He, H.; Lin, S.; Zhu, R.; Liu, Z.; Liu, J.; Liu, X.; Chen, S.; Zou, J.; et al. Synergistic effect of combined mirror therapy on upper extremity in patients with stroke: A systematic review and meta-analysis. *Front. Neurol.* **2020**, *11*, 155. [CrossRef]
23. Fernández-Vázquez, D.; Cano-de-la-Cuerda, R.; Navarro-López, V. Haptic glove systems in combination with semi-immersive virtual reality for upper extremity motor rehabilitation after stroke: A systematic review and meta-analysis. *Int. J. Environ. Res. Public Health* **2022**, *19*, 10378. [CrossRef] [PubMed]
24. Hiragami, S.; Inoue, Y.; Harada, K. Minimal clinically important difference for the Fugl-Meyer assessment of the upper extremity in convalescent stroke patients with moderate to severe hemiparesis. *J. Phys. Ther. Sci.* **2019**, *31*, 917–921. [CrossRef]
25. Grefkes, C.; Fink, G.R. Recovery from stroke: Current concepts and future perspectives. *Neurol. Res. Pract.* **2020**, *2*, 17. [CrossRef]
26. Arya, K.N.; Verma, R.; Garg, R.K. Estimating the minimal clinically important difference of an upper extremity recovery measure in subacute stroke patients. *Top Stroke Rehabil.* **2011**, *18*, 599–610. [CrossRef] [PubMed]
27. Aydin, M.; Mutlu, R.; Singh, D.; Sariyildiz, E.; Coman, R.; Mayland, E.; Shemmell, J.; Lee, W. Novel soft haptic biofeedback-pilot study on postural balance and proprioception. *Sensors* **2022**, *22*, 3779. [CrossRef] [PubMed]
28. Stanton, R.; Ada, L.; Dean, C.M.; Preston, E. Biofeedback improves performance in lower limb activities more than usual therapy in people following stroke: A systematic review. *J. Physiother.* **2017**, *63*, 11–16. [CrossRef]
29. Mateos-Aparicio, P.; Rodriguez-Moreno, A. The impact of studying brain plasticity. *Front. Cell Neurosci.* **2019**, *13*, 66. [CrossRef]
30. Hordacre, B.; Austin, D.; Brown, K.E.; Graetz, L.; Pareés, I.; De Trane, S.; Vallence, A.-M.; Koblar, S.; Kleinig, T.; McDonnell, M.N.; et al. Evidence for a window of enhanced plasticity in the human motor cortex following ischemic stroke. *Neurorehabil. Neural Repair.* **2021**, *35*, 307–320. [CrossRef] [PubMed]

Disclaimer/Publisher's Note: The statements, opinions and data contained in all publications are solely those of the individual author(s) and contributor(s) and not of MDPI and/or the editor(s). MDPI and/or the editor(s) disclaim responsibility for any injury to people or property resulting from any ideas, methods, instructions or products referred to in the content.

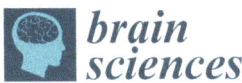

Systematic Review

Effects of Resistance Training on Spasticity in People with Stroke: A Systematic Review

Juan Carlos Chacon-Barba [1], Jose A. Moral-Munoz [1,2,*], Amaranta De Miguel-Rubio [3] and David Lucena-Anton [1,2]

1. Department of Nursing and Physiotherapy, University of Cádiz, 11009 Cadiz, Spain; juancarlos.chaconbarba@alum.uca.es (J.C.C.-B.); david.lucena@uca.es (D.L.-A.)
2. Biomedical Research and Innovation Institute of Cadiz (INiBICA), 11009 Cadiz, Spain
3. Department of Nursing, Pharmacology and Physiotherapy, University of Cordoba, 14004 Cordoba, Spain; z42mirua@uco.es
* Correspondence: joseantonio.moral@uca.es

Abstract: Resistance training induces neuromuscular adaptations and its impact on spasticity remains inadequately researched. This systematic review (PROSPERO: CRD42022322164) aimed to analyze the effects of resistance training, compared with no treatment, conventional therapy, or other therapies, in people with stroke-related spasticity. A comprehensive search was conducted up to October 2023 in PubMed, PEDro, Cochrane, Web of Science, and Scopus databases. Selection criteria were randomized controlled trials involving participants with stroke-related spasticity intervened with resistance training. The PEDro scale was used to evaluate the methodological quality. From a total of 274 articles, 23 full-text articles were assessed for eligibility and nine articles were included in the systematic review, involving 225 participants (155 males, 70 females; mean age: 59.4 years). Benefits were found to spasticity after resistance training. Furthermore, studies measuring spasticity also reported benefits to function, strength, gait, and balance. In conclusion, resistance training was superior to, or at least equal to, conventional therapy, other therapies, or no intervention for improving spasticity, as well as function, strength, gait, and balance. However, the results should be taken with caution because of the heterogeneity of the protocols used. Further research is needed to explore the effects of resistance training programs on people with stroke.

Keywords: stroke; muscle spasticity; resistance training

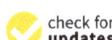

Citation: Chacon-Barba, J.C.; Moral-Munoz, J.A.; De Miguel-Rubio, A.; Lucena-Anton, D. Effects of Resistance Training on Spasticity in People with Stroke: A Systematic Review. *Brain Sci.* **2024**, *14*, 57. https://doi.org/10.3390/brainsci14010057

Academic Editors: Noureddin Nakhostin Ansari, Gholamreza Hassanzadeh and Ardalan Shariat

Received: 18 December 2023
Revised: 2 January 2024
Accepted: 4 January 2024
Published: 6 January 2024

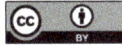

Copyright: © 2024 by the authors. Licensee MDPI, Basel, Switzerland. This article is an open access article distributed under the terms and conditions of the Creative Commons Attribution (CC BY) license (https:// creativecommons.org/licenses/by/ 4.0/).

1. Introduction

Stroke is defined as a sudden loss of neurological function resulting from an infarction or hemorrhage in the brain, spinal cord, or retina and this loss is persistent for over 24 h [1]. It is the second leading cause of death worldwide [2]. In addition, it leads to motor dysfunction and limitations in activities of daily living and quality of life [3]. Spasticity is a motor disorder characterized by an increase in the muscle stretch reflex, accompanied by hypertonia and hyperreflexia, associated with an injury to the upper motor neurons [4]. The neurophysiology of spasticity in stroke involves damage to specific brain areas, such as the superior corona radiata, posterior limb of the internal capsule, thalamus, putamen, premotor cortex, and insula [5]. These brain lesions disrupt the normal inhibitory signals from the brain to the muscles, leading to hyperexcitability of the stretch reflex and increased muscle tone [6]. It is estimated that between 38% and 40% of people with stroke will have some spasticity, with treatment being necessary in 16% of cases. This estimated prevalence varies depending on the time elapsed after the stroke, being 27% in the first month, and 42.6% in periods longer than 3 months [7].

Voluntary muscle contraction and recruitment of muscle fibers in people with stroke may be highly complex because of the exorbitant response it provokes immediately, so it is usually avoided [8]. Traditional stroke treatment programs excluded muscle strengthening because it overexcited the muscle tracts, increasing the spastic process; while muscle weakness was considered as a secondary factor in limiting motor function [9,10]. Nonetheless, it is known that paretic muscle atrophy strongly correlates with reduced fitness levels, so resistance training has the potential to support normal muscle functioning within the affected limb and may counteract the stroke-related decrease of physical fitness as well as the stroke-related sarcopenia [11–13]. Exercise has been shown to create an optimal environment for neuroplasticity in the primary motor cortex and other areas of the brain related to motor control, leading to enhanced motor learning and function [14].

In recent years, it has been shown that there is great evidence of the benefits of resistance training programs in different populations [15–19]. In this sense, resistance training induces a development of power, hypertrophy, and muscle strength, by generating neural and structural adaptations in the medium and long term [20], besides the increase in force production that implies the development of muscle size and cross-section, as well as the modification of the arrangement of muscle fibers [21]. Furthermore, there is an improvement in intermuscular coordination, which is manifested in an intensification in the relaxation capacity of the antagonist muscles during agonist contraction [22], and a greater recruitment of motor units in less time, with an optimization of reflex phenomena. This leads to an increase in the speed and strength of muscle contraction [23]. Nevertheless, it is reasonable to assume that these benefits are present in stroke patients and reduce spasticity, but to date, there is no literature indicating the neurophysiological mechanisms that provoke this phenomenon.

In view of this background, the treatment of spasticity in people with stroke is a main therapeutic goal, but the evidence of using resistance training as an intervention for spasticity is still unclear. This issue was analyzed [15–19] in a systematic review and meta-analysis [11], in which the benefits of resistance training in supporting the recovery of stroke patients were analyzed, and no significant improvements with respect to no intervention or other interventions were found in spasticity. This result was based on only two randomized controlled trials (RCT), highlighting the lack of available evidence on this topic. Therefore, there is no systematic review on the uses of resistance training on spasticity that synthesizes the protocols used and serves as a basis for clinical decision making in stroke rehabilitation.

Therefore, the aim of this systematic review was to analyze the effects of resistance training on spasticity in people with stroke. Furthermore, we aimed to explore the implications on function, strength, gait, and balance in addition to the spasticity. Moreover, the resistance training programs and protocols for the treatment of people with stroke will be analyzed.

2. Methodology

The present study is a systematic review reported according to the guidelines established in the PRISMA 2020 statement (Preferred Reporting Items for Systematic Reviews and Meta-Analyses) [24] (File S1 in Supplementary Material). In addition, this systematic review was registered in the Prospective Register of Systematic Reviews (PROSPERO), register number: CRD42022322164.

2.1. Search Strategy and Selection Process

The literature search for this review was conducted up to October 2023, using the following databases: PubMed, PEDro (Physiotherapy Evidence Database), WoS (Web of Science), Scopus, and CENTRAL (Cochrane Controlled Register of Trials). The search strategy was performed through the combination of different keywords and Boolean operators "AND" and "OR", as shown in Table 1. In the PubMed, CENTRAL, WoS, and Scopus databases, study filters were applied showing only RCT in the case of PubMed, trials in the case of CENTRAL, and articles in the case of WoS and Scopus. For the PEDro database, an advanced search was performed filtering as therapy "strength training", subdiscipline "neurology", and methods "clinical trial". No filters were applied to the date of publication, and no language restriction was established.

Table 1. Search strategy.

Database	Number of Articles	Search Strategy
PubMed	16	("stroke" OR "cerebrovascular accident" OR "hemiparesis" OR "hemiplegia") AND ("Resistance Training" OR "Strength Training" OR "strengthening") AND ("Muscle Spasticity" OR "Muscle Hypertonia" OR "Spastic*" OR "Muscle Tonus") Filter applied: Randomized Controlled Trial
PEDro	39	("Stroke" AND "spasticity) Therapy: strength training Subdiscipline: neurology Methods: clinical trial
Web of Science (All Databases)	30	TS = (("stroke" OR "cerebrovascular accident" OR "hemiparesis" OR "hemiplegia") AND ("Resistance Training" OR "Strength Training" OR "strengthening") AND ("Muscle Spasticity" OR "Muscle Hypertonia" OR "Spastic*" OR "Muscle Tonus")) Document Types: Clinical Trial
Scopus	100	TITLE-ABS-KEY(("stroke" OR "cerebrovascular accident" OR "hemiparesis" OR "hemiplegia") AND ("Resistance Training" OR "Strength Training" OR "strengthening") AND ("Muscle Spasticity" OR "Muscle Hypertonia" OR "Spastic*" OR "Muscle Tonus")
CENTRAL	89	("stroke" OR "cerebrovascular accident" OR "hemiparesis" OR "hemiplegia") AND ("Resistance Training" OR "Strength Training" OR "strengthening") AND ("Muscle Spasticity" OR "Muscle Hypertonia" OR "Spastic*" OR "Muscle Tonus")

The bibliographic information of the retrieved articles was imported into the Mendeley Desktop (version 1.19.4) [25]. An initial manual check was performed to ensure accuracy, followed by grouping and sorting by title to eliminate duplicates. Titles and abstracts were then assessed, and those without human subjects and non-RCTs were discarded. Finally, compliance with inclusion criteria was annotated using the notes tool in Mendeley Desktop [25]. Articles that did not meet the established selection criteria were excluded by evaluating the full-text of the screened articles. The remaining studies were eligible for inclusion in the systematic review.

Two authors (J.C.C.-B. and D.L.-A.) were responsible for the literature search and retrieval of potentially relevant studies. A third reviewer (J.A.M.-M.) took part to reach a consensus when necessary.

2.2. Selection Criteria

The criteria defined for the inclusion of this study were based on the PICOS (Patient, Intervention, Outcomes, and Study type) research model [26]: (P) adults with stroke; (I) resistance training isolated or mixed (such as functional exercise, aerobic training or task-oriented training) programs aiming to develop muscle strength; (C) no treatment, conventional therapy, or other therapies; (O) spasticity; (S) RCT. Studies involving non-active interventions for muscle strength improvement were excluded (e.g., electrostimulation). We also excluded trials that had a mix of people with stroke and other populations and did not report outcomes for people with stroke separately.

2.3. Data Extraction

The extracted data included the characteristics of the study participants, the duration and sessions performed in each intervention, the characteristics of the intervention, the time and tools of measurement, and data on the results. Data extraction was performed by two independent reviewers (J.C.C.-B. and D.L.-A.). A third reviewer (J.A.M.-M.) participated in resolving conflicts during the process.

2.4. Methodological Quality Assessment

The articles included in this review were evaluated using the PEDro scale to assess their methodological quality [27]. The PEDro scale allows users to determine in a simple way the external validity (criterion 1), the internal validity (criteria 2–9), and the statistical information for the interpretation of the results (criteria 10 and 11), being a very useful and specific instrument to evaluate the quality of clinical trials. According to the score obtained on the PEDro Scale, the studies have been classified as low quality (score less than 4), moderate (score of 4–5), good (score of 6–8) or excellent (score of 9–10), with criterion 1 being excluded from the final score [28].

The assessment was performed independently by two authors (J.C.C.-B. and J.A.M.-M.). A third reviewer (A.D.M.-R.) participated to establish a consensus when necessary.

3. Results

A total of 274 articles were found in a first search and a total of 80 duplicate records were removed. The titles and abstracts of the remaining records (194) were screened and 171 were then excluded due to different reasons (not topic and not RCT). The full-texts of the 23 remaining studies were assessed to verify the compliance of the eligibility criteria. Finally, nine articles were included in this review. The PRISMA flowchart in Figure 1 shows the selection of studies for this systematic review.

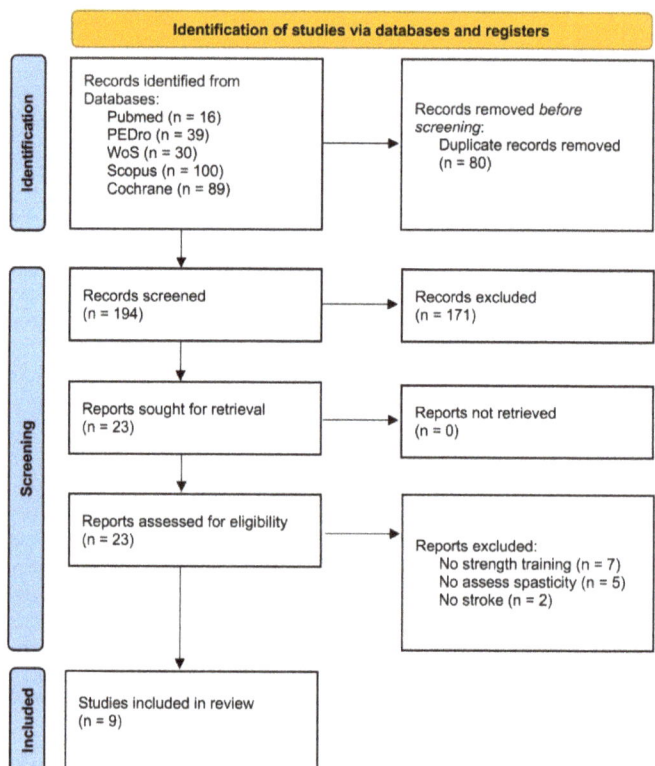

Figure 1. PRISMA flowchart showing the algorithm for the selection of eligible studies.

3.1. Methodological Quality

As shown in Table 2, the mean score of the PEDro scale of the articles included in this review is 5, classified as a moderate mean methodological quality. The studies that score highest on this scale were those of Coroian et al. [29], Dehno et al. [30], and Patten et al. [31], considering them to have a good methodological quality, with a score of 7/10. On the other hand, the study included in this review with the lowest score on the PEDro scale is that of Fernandes et al. [32], with a score of 2/10, therefore having a low methodological quality.

Table 2. PEDro scale score for the studies included in this systematic review.

Study	1	2	3	4	5	6	7	8	9	10	11	Total
Akbari et al. (2006) [33]	-	Yes	No	Yes	No	No	Yes	No	No	Yes	Yes	5
Coroian et al. (2018) [29]	-	Yes	No	Yes	No	No	Yes	Yes	Yes	Yes	Yes	7
Dehno et al. (2021) [30]	-	Yes	Yes	Yes	No	No	Yes	Yes	No	Yes	Yes	7
Fernandes et al. (2015) [32]	-	No	No	No	No	No	No	Yes	No	No	Yes	2
Fernandez et al. (2016) [34]	-	Yes	No	Yes	No	No	Yes	Yes	No	Yes	Yes	6
Flansbjer et al. (2008) [35]	-	Yes	No	Yes	No	No	No	Yes	Yes	Yes	No	5
Mun et al. (2019) [36]	-	Yes	No	Yes	No	No	No	No	No	Yes	Yes	4
Lattouf et al. (2021) [37]	-	Yes	No	Yes	No	No	No	No	No	Yes	Yes	4
Patten et al. (2013) [31]	-	Yes	Yes	Yes	No	No	Yes	Yes	No	Yes	Yes	7

Range: 0–10. Item 1 is not used in the method score. Item 1: Eligibility criteria; Item 2: Random allocation; Item 3: Concealed allocation; Item 4: Baseline similarity; Item 5: Subject blinding; Item 6: Therapist blinding; Item 7: Assessor blinding; Item 8: >85% follow-up; Item 9: Intention-to-treat analysis; Item 10: Between-group statistical comparison; and Item 11: Point and variability measures.

3.2. Participants

The characteristics of the participants included in this study are shown in Table 3. A total of 225 participants were included in this review, with the study by Lattouf et al. [37] reporting the largest number ($n = 37$), while the RCT by Fernandes et al. [32] had the smallest ($n = 16$). The mean age was 59.4 years, with Patten et al. [31] reporting the oldest, 72.9 years, and Akbari et al. [33] reporting the youngest, 48.8 years. The number of women included represented 32% of the total number of participants and only Fernandes et al. is gender-balanced [30]. In contrast, the study by Fernandes et al. [32] only presents male subjects.

The median time elapsed after the cerebrovascular event in the included participants was 21.3 months, with only one study presenting subjects with an acute cerebrovascular event [32]. The study by Fernandez et al. [34] had the participants with the longest time elapsed after stroke.

The proportion of patients with an ischemic-hemorrhagic stroke was reported in all of the studies, with the exception of one study [33]. In this way, ischemic stroke occurred in 73.30% of cases.

Table 3. Main characteristics of the participants included in the systematic review.

Studies	Number of Participants/EG:CG	Age (SD)	Male:Female	Time After Stroke (SD)	Ischemic:Hemorrhagic
Akbari et al. (2006) [33]	N:34 17:17	EG 49.3 (7.1) years	EG 10:7	EG 34.5 (26.37) months	EG ND
		CG 48.8 (3) years	CG 9:8	CG 35.3 (27.5) months	CG ND
Coroian et al. (2018) [29]	N: 20 10:10	EG 63.6 (12.6) years	EG 8:2	EG 32.2 (12.8–629.6) months	EG 9:1
		CG 63.6 (10.6) years	CG 8:2	CG 29.1 (7.6–90.1) months	CG 7:3
Dehno et al. (2021) [30]	N: 26 13:13	EG 53 (9.36) years CG 49.77 (15.48) years	EG 7:6 CG 6:7	EG 95.22 (37.14) days CG 101.62 (32.39) days	EG 11:2 CG 12:1

Table 3. Cont.

Studies	Number of Participants/EG:CG	Age (SD)	Male:Female	Time After Stroke (SD)	Ischemic:Hemorrhagic
Fernandes et al. (2015) [32]	N: 16 9:7	EG 58 (6) years CG 58 (7) years	EG 9:0 CG 7:0	EG 15 (5) days CG 17 (4) days	EG 6:3 CG 5:2
Fernandez et al. (2016) [34]	N: 29 14:15	EG 61.2 (9.8) years CG 65.7 (12.7) years	EG 11:3 CG 11:4	EG 3.5 (3.6) years CG 4.3 (4.9) years	EG 9:5 CG 11:4
Flansbjer et al. (2008) [35]	N: 24 15:9	EG 61 (5) years CG 60 (5) years	EG 9:6 CG 5:4	EG 18.9 (7.9) months CG 20.0 (11.6) months	EG 12:3 CG 6:3
Mun et al. (2019) [36]	N: 20 10:10	EG 53.1 (13.4) years CG 54.0 (9.1) years	EG 8:2 CG 8:2	EG 20.3 (14.4) months CG 15.8 (10.2) months	EG 3:7 CG 7:3
Lattouf et al. (2021) [37]	N: 37 19:18	EG 65.1 (11.7) years CG 68.7 (12.4) years	EG 11:8 CG 11:7	EG 11.61 (4.07) months CG 12.26 (5.41) months	EG 14:5 CG 14:4
Patten et al. (2013) [31]	N: 19 9:10	GA 64.7 (9.7) years GB 72.9 (11.1) years	GA 6:3 GB 9:1	GA 14.7 (2.7) months GB 11.4 (4.3) months	GA 7:2 GB 7:3

CG, Control group; EG, Experimental group; GA, Group A; GB, Group B; ND, Not described.

3.3. Interventions

The characteristics of the interventions included in this review are shown in Table 4. Many of the included studies lasted 4 weeks [30,31,33,37], and two extend up to 12 weeks [32,34]. In terms of the number of sessions, three of the articles covered a total of 12 sessions [30,31,33], while the study by Fernandes et al. [32] stood out for having the highest number of sessions, with a total of 48.

Regarding weekly frequency, it was observed that three of the studies implemented 3 sessions per week [29,30,33], and two had the maximum frequency, with 5 weekly sessions each [36,37]. Two articles showed the lowest frequency, with only two sessions per week [34,35]. It should be noted that Coroian et al. [29] and Lattouf et al. [37] performed two daily sessions with a frequency of three days per week and five days per week, respectively.

In relation to the duration of the sessions, considerable variability was observed among the articles. The average duration of the sessions was 70 min, ranging from the shortest session of 30 min [29,36,37] up to the longest of 3 h [33]. It should be considered that two of the three articles that held 30-min sessions performed two sessions a day [29,37].

In terms of the interventions, four studies focused only on resistance training as an exercise modality [29,34–36]. Two studies combined resistance training with conventional therapy [30,37], while two others did so with task-oriented training [31,32]. Only one intervention complemented resistance training with aerobic and functional exercises [33]. Six workouts were specifically aimed at the lower limbs [32–37], while three focused on the upper limbs [29–31], addressing specific aspects, such as wrist, elbow, and wrist, as well as shoulder and elbow.

Regarding the systems used to perform resistance training, three studies used dynamometers [29–31], and the remaining studies used a leg press [37], sliding stander [36], knee exercise machine [35], and an inertial flywheel [34]. The remaining two studies did not specify the system used. These findings reflect the heterogeneity in the methods and equipment used in the studies reviewed, although there is a consensus that the exercises employ closed kinetic chains.

Table 4. Main characteristics of the interventions included in the systematic review.

Studies	Duration of Intervention; Frequency of Sessions; Session Time	Intervention
Akbari et al. (2006) [33]	4 weeks; 3 weekly sessions; 3 h per session	EG: 3-part program. Part 1: Standing, walking, and aerobic conditioning exercises. Part 2: Functional exercises. Part 3: Strengthening of the lower limbs, with concentric contraction at 70% 1RM, or synergistic contractions for weakened muscles. Ten repetitions of each exercise for each muscle group CG: Same protocol not including the 3rd part
Coroian et al. (2018) [29]	6 weeks; 3 weekly sessions; 2 daily sessions of 30 min	EG: Isokinetic strengthening of the elbow and wrist with dynamometer. A total of 10 min of warm-up (36 reps at 20% 1RM and 15–30° per second) + 30 min of session (six sets of eight reps at 40–70% 1RM, at 15–45° per second) CG: 45 min of passive elbow and wrist mobilization with dynamometer
Dehno et al. (2021) [30]	4 weeks; 3 weekly sessions; 60 min per session for CG and 45 min for EG	EG: CT + Unilateral Resistance Training for Wrist Extensors with Isokinetic Dynamometer. Five sets of six concentric repetitions, at 60°/second, with 2-min breaks between sets CG: CT
Fernandes et al. (2015) [32]	12 weeks; 4 weekly sessions; 70 min per session	EG: Task-oriented training + Lower limb strengthening affect: three sets of 10 reps, increasing resistance in different positions for each muscle group CG: Task-oriented training
Fernandez et al. (2016) [34]	12 weeks; 2 weekly sessions; ND	EG: Unilateral strengthening in the lower limbs with a leg press with an inertial flywheel. Four sets of seven reps maximum, with 3 min of recovery between sets CG: Non-intervention
Flansbjer et al. (2008) [35]	10 weeks; 2 weekly sessions; 90 min per session	EG: Lower limb strengthening on knee exercise machine. Warm-up (5 min. of stationary bike, five reps without resistance and five reps at 25% 1RM) + Session (two sets of six to eight reps at 30–40 s per set, at 80% 1RM). After training, passive stretching of the muscles CG: Usual daily activities
Mun et al. (2019) [36]	6 weeks; 5 weekly sessions; 30 min per session	EG: Strengthening of the lower limbs in a sliding stander. Warm-up and cool-down (reps for 5 min and 25% 1RM) + session (20 min, 3 sets of 15 to 20 reps at 70% 1RM) CG: CT
Lattouf et al. (2021) [37]	4 weeks; 5 weekly sessions; 2 sessions of 30 min	EG: CT + Resistance training in lower limbs in horizontal press (3 phases: concentric, static, and eccentric). Three sets of five repetitions, at 40% 1RM in the first two phases, and at 60% 1RM in the last phase CG: CT
Patten et al. (2013) [31]	4 weeks for each intervention, with 4 weeks off between both interventions; 3 weekly sessions for each intervention; 75 min per session	Functional Physical Therapy Intervention: Functional tasks with progression of six objectives and nine activity categories Hybrid Intervention: Functional Physical Therapy (20–30 min) + shoulder and elbow resistance training with dynamometer (35 min, 3 sets of 10 reps of shoulder abduction/adduction, shoulder flexion/extension, external/internal rotation of the shoulder, and flexion/extension of the elbow; first set in eccentric and the next two in concentric, with gradual increase in speed)

1RM, One-Repetition Maximum CG, Control Group; CT, Conventional Therapy; EG, Experimental Group; ND, Not Described.

The results of the systematic review showed significant variability in exercise intensity, although a considerable number of studies used a load of 70% of repetition maximum, evidencing a common preference for this intensity [29,33,36]. Overall, articles reported a load ranging from 40% to 80% of the maximum repetition. A prominent approach was the inclusion of an inertial exercise, whereby the intensity of the exercise depended on the force applied by the participant himself [34].

Regarding the number of sets and repetitions, the results suggest that, although we did not identify a universally predominant protocol, some notable patterns and trends were evidenced. In terms of the number of repetitions, it was noted that most studies opted for protocols with repetitions ranging from 6 to 15. In particular, the most common protocol consisted of 3 sets of 10 repetitions, this being the standard adopted in several studies [31,34]. Regarding the number of series, a heterogeneous distribution was found. The general preference was to perform between 3 and 5 sets per training session [30–32,34,36,37]. However, some studies presented less conventional approaches, such as that of Flansbjer et al. [35], which proposed 2 sets of 6–8 repetitions. As for the speed of execution, it is only specified in three articles, and there is a discrepancy in this aspect [29,30,35].

It should be noted that there seems to be an interest in the combination of the different forms of contraction, looking for concentric, isometric, and concentric phases during the execution of the repetition [31,32,37]. However, even though many do not specify the type of contraction requested, it can be inferred from the type of exercise to be carried out that the concentric contraction stands out.

3.4. Outcomes Measures

The outcome measures, measuring instruments, and results obtained by the studies are shown in Table 5.

Table 5. Evaluation and results of the articles included in the systematic review.

Studies	Outcome Measures	Results
Akbari et al. (2006) [33]	Two measurement time points (pre and post intervention) - Spasticity: MAS - Strength: Maximum force evaluated with dynamometer.	Spasticity: There was a significant decrease in quadriceps spasticity in EG ($p < 0.0001$), but no change in CG ($p = 0.055$). There was a significant decrease in gastrocnemius spasticity in both EG ($p < 0.0001$) and CG ($p = 0.041$). A significant decrease in spasticity was found in EG compared to CG in both quadriceps ($p = 0.034$) and gastrocnemius ($p = 0.001$). Strength: There was an increase in strength in all muscles in EG on both the affected side ($p < 0.0001$) and the non-affected side ($p < 0.0001$). No differences in strength were found in CG, except in hip and knee extensors ($p < 0.0001$) and ankle flexors ($p = 0.008$) on the non-affected side, and hip extensors ($p = 0.003$) and knee extensors ($p < 0.0001$) on the affected side. A significant increase in muscle strength was found in EG compared to CG ($p < 0.0001$), except in knee extensors ($p = 0.184$).
Coroian et al. (2018) [29]	Four measurement time points (pre and post intervention, 3 months after and 6 months after) - Spasticity: MAS - Function: UL-FMA - Strength: Maximum force evaluated with dynamometer	Spasticity: No significant differences in spasticity were found between the different time points in both groups ($p = 0.4$). No significant differences were found between groups ($p = 0.98$). Function: No significant differences were found pre and post intervention in the total UL-FMA score between the two groups ($p = 2$). No differences were found in the proximal UL-FMA score. In subsequent time points, no significant differences were found in UL-FMA scores between the two groups. There was a significant improvement for EG in the total UL-FMA score pre and post intervention ($p < 0.01$), which was maintained at 3 months ($p < 0.01$) and 6 months ($p < 0.01$) Strength: No significant differences were found in changes in dynamometer scores in different time points for elbow flexors ($p = 0.2$), elbow extensors ($p = 0.3$), wrist flexors ($p = 0.1$) and wrist extensors ($p = 0.1$). No significant differences were found between groups in dynamometer scores for elbow flexors ($p = 0.2$), elbow extensors ($p = 0.8$), wrist flexors ($p = 0.2$) or wrist extensors ($p = 0.3$).
Dehno et al. (2021) [30]	Two intervention measurement time points (pre and post intervention) - Spasticity: MMAS. - Function: UL-FMA. - Strength: On the less affected side, maximum force evaluated with dynamometer. On the most affected side, the Medical Research Council scales.	Spasticity: A significant improvement was found in the MMAS score in EG ($p = 0.002$). There were no differences in the MMAS score in CG ($p = 0.165$). A significant change in spasticity was found in EG compared to CG ($p = 0.014$). Function: Significant improvements were found for both groups between pre and post intervention in the total UL-FMA score (EG $p = 0.001$, CG $p = 0.001$). The improvement in the UL-FMA score in the EG was significantly greater than in the CG ($p = 0.04$). Strength: There was a significant improvement in the strength of the less affected side in EG ($p = 0.001$). There were no significant differences in the strength of the less affected side in CG ($p = 0.106$). There was a significant improvement in the strength of the less affected side between EG and CG ($p = 0.001$). There was a significant improvement in the strength of the most affected side compared to the start of treatment in EG ($p = 0.001$) and CG ($p = 0.001$). There was a significant improvement in EG compared to CG ($p = 0.029$).

Table 5. Cont.

Studies	Outcome Measures	Results
Fernandes et al. (2015) [32]	Two measurement time points (pre and post intervention) - Spasticity: MAS. - Balance: BBS	Spasticity: There were no significant differences between or within the groups ($p \geq 0.05$). Balance: The results in the BBS showed significant differences in both groups (EG $p = 0.002$, CG $p = 0.008$). The comparison between groups after the intervention showed that there was a significant difference, with the EG achieving a greater improvement ($p = 0.008$).
Fernandez et al. (2016) [34]	Two measurement time points (pre and post intervention) - Spasticity: MAS - Strength: Maximum isometric and dynamic force evaluated in leg press - Gait: TUG. - Balance: BBS.	Spasticity: There were no differences between or within the groups. Strength: Differences were found in the isometric strength of the affected leg after the intervention in EG ($p = 0.02$). An improvement in isometric strength was found in EG compared to CG, although it was not significant ($p = 0.06$). There was an improvement in the dynamic strength of both legs after the intervention in EG ($p = 0.03$). A significant improvement in dynamic strength was found in EG compared to CG ($p = 0.03$). Gait: An improvement was found in TUG after the intervention in EG ($p = 0.01$) but not in CG. Significant improvements were found in TUG in EG compared to CG ($p = 0.04$). Balance: An improvement in BBS after the intervention was found in both EG ($p < 0.001$) and CG ($p = 0.01$). Significant improvements were found in EG compared to CG ($p < 0.001$).
Flansbjer et al. (2008) [35]	Three measurement time points (pre and post intervention, and 5 months after the intervention) - Spasticity: MAS. - Strength: Dynamic strength on a knee exercise machine. Maximum isometric force assessed with a dynamometer. - Gait: TUG, Fast Gait Speed, and 6MWT.	Spasticity: A significant improvement in the MAS score was found after the intervention in EG ($p < 0.01$) and CG ($p = 0.02$), which did not continue at follow-up. There were no significant differences between EG and CG after the intervention or at follow-up. Strength: There were significant improvements in dynamic strength both after the intervention and at follow-up in EG ($p < 0.001$), for both paretic and non-paretic limbs. For CG, significant improvements in dynamic strength were found after intervention in the non-paretic limb ($p < 0.05$), but not in the paretic, and at follow-up only non-paretic flexion was significantly higher ($p < 0.05$) than at baseline. There were significant differences between EG and CG after the intervention ($p < 0.001$) and at follow-up ($p < 0.001$). There were significant improvements in isokinetic strength for both limbs both after the intervention and at follow-up in EG ($p < 0.01$). No differences were found for CG in isokinetic strength at intervention or follow-up. There was a significant difference between EG and CG ($p < 0.05$) after the intervention for non-paretic limb extension and flexion, and at follow-up for non-paretic limb extension. Gait: For EG, all gait tests improved significantly ($p < 0.05$) after the intervention, and that change was maintained at follow-up significantly in TUG and 6MWT scores. For CG, only TUG improved significantly ($p < 0.05$) after the intervention. There were no significant differences between EG and CG between pre and post intervention, but there were significant differences at follow-up for TUG score ($p < 0.05$).
Mun et al. (2019) [36]	Two measurement time points (pre and post intervention) - Spasticity: Biodex system assessing the resistance to mobilization within different speed movements. - Gait: TUG - Balance: BBS; Platform for calculating load distribution in standing with eyes open and closed.	Spasticity: There was a decrease in spasticity in EG between pre and post intervention at angular velocities of 60°/sec, 180°/sec, and 240°/sec ($p < 0.05$). There was a decrease in spasticity in CG between pre and post intervention at angular velocities of 180°/sec and 240°/sec ($p < 0.05$). EG decreased spasticity statistically significantly compared to CG at angular velocities of 180°/sec ($p = 0.02$) and 240°/sec ($p = 0.04$). Gait: There was a significant decrease in the TUG score for both groups after the intervention ($p < 0.05$). No statistically significant differences were observed between the two groups ($p = 0.11$). Balance: There was a significant improvement in the BBS score for both groups after the intervention ($p < 0.05$). The BBS score in EG increased significantly compared to the CG ($p < 0.01$). An increase in weight distribution to the paretic side was found in both groups, both with eyes open and closed, after the intervention ($p < 0.05$). EG statistically significantly increased weight distribution with both eyes open ($p = 0.04$) and closed ($p = 0.03$) compared to CG.
Lattouf et al. (2021) [37]	Two measurement time points (pre and post intervention) - Spasticity: MAS - Gait: 10-m Walk Test; 6MWT - Strength: Maximum force calculated from Brzycki's equation	Spasticity: There were no differences between or within the groups. Gait: For both groups, a significant difference was found in the time of the 10-m Walk Test ($p \leq 0.00001$), with a higher walking speed after the intervention. No differences were found in the time of the 10-m Walk Test between the two groups after the intervention. A significant effect was observed in 6MWT between pre and post treatment for CG ($p \leq 0.0003$) and for EG ($p \leq 0.0001$). The results showed a statistically significant difference between the two groups ($p \leq 0.01$). Strength: There was a significant difference between pre and post treatment for both groups (CG $p \leq 0.0001$, EG $p \leq 0.0001$). EG showed a significantly greater increase after treatment than CG ($p \leq 0.014$).

Table 5. *Cont.*

Studies	Outcome Measures	Results
Patten et al. (2013) [31]	Four measurement time points (pre-evaluation, in the rest period, at the end of the interventions, and at 6 months) - Spasticity: Ashworth Scale - Function: WMFT-FAS, UL-FMA, FIM	Spasticity: No significant changes were found in the Ashworth score at the post-intervention assessment or at 6 months ($p > 0.05$). Function: Significant improvements in WMFT-FAS were found after treatment block 1 in both groups ($p < 0.05$). These differences were significantly greater after the Hybrid Group compared to the Functional Physical Therapy group ($p = 0.03$). Tests of a period effect revealed greater improvements in WMFT-FAS after Hybrid versus Functional Physical Therapy ($p = 0.02$), regardless of where they occurred in the order of treatment. Overall, no differences were revealed because of the order of treatment ($p = 0.43$). A significant increase in WMFT-FAS was observed during the 6-month follow-up period ($p = 0.03$). No differences were revealed between Order A and Order B at the 6-month follow-up ($p > 0.05$). A significantly higher proportion of participants (51% vs. 39%) achieved the minimum significant difference of two points or more in the FIM after the Hybrid ($p = 0.05$). These positive changes were observed in 69% of participants at 6 months ($p = 0.05$). Post-intervention improvements were detected in both the total score and the shoulder-elbow portions of the UL-FMA, but these were not statistically significant. Significant differences were found for UL-FMA at 6 months after the intervention, with the minimum significant difference reaching 53% of all participants ($p = 0.04$)

6MWT, 6-Minute Walk Test; BBS, Berg Balance Scale; CG, Control Group; EG, Experimental Group; FIM, Functional Independence Measure; MAS, Modified Ashworth Scale; MMAS, Modified Modified Ashworth Scale; TUG, Timed Up & Go; UL-FMA, Upper Limb Fugl-Meyer Assessment; WMFT-FAS, Wolf Motor Function Test-Functional Abilities Scale.

Concerning the spasticity, four measuring instruments were used, but three of them were versions of the Ashworth scale. Most studies employed the Modified Ashworth Scale [29,32–35,37]. The remaining studies used the Ashworth Scale [31], the Modified Ashworth Scale [30], and the Biodex system [36], which evaluates the resistance to ankle mobilization at different speeds. The section evaluated coincided with the musculature involved in the resistance exercise. Four of the included studies found a significant improvement between pre and post intervention in EG [30,33,35,36]. Three articles found an improvement in EG compared to CG [30,33,36], while the other studies found no differences between groups. The study by Mun et al. [36] found improvements in all angular velocities evaluated. The remaining five articles found no significant differences pre and post intervention in EG.

The function was evaluated in three articles, all of which used the Upper Limb Fugl-Meyer Motor Assessment (UL-FMMA) [29–31]. The study by Patten et al. [31] also assessed the function with the Wolf Motor Function Test-Functional Abilities Scale (WMFT-FAS) and the Functional Independence Measure (FIM). The studies by Dehno et al. [30] and Patten et al. [31] found significant improvements in the EG compared with the CG for improving function, which were also maintained at follow-up time points. Specifically, Dehno et al. [30] found improvements for the UL-FMA score, and Patten et al. [31] for the WMFT-FAS and FIM. The study by Coroian et al. [29] only found pre-post improvements in the EG, but these were not significant in comparison with the CG.

Strength was the most evaluated parameter after spasticity [29,30,33–35,37], studying the maximum strength of the regions worked during the intervention. Dynamic force was studied by two of the studies [34,35]. The study by Dehno et al. [30] studied the strength of the paretic side using the Medical Research Council (MRC) scale. All studies found significant improvements in strength after the EG intervention, as well as significant differences between groups, except the study by Coroian et al. [29]. The study by Fernandez et al. [34] found improvements in dynamic strength, but the improvement in isometric strength did not become significant.

For gait evaluation, the Timed "Up & Go" (TUG) was mostly used [34–36]. The study by Flansbjer et al. [35] also evaluated gait using the Fast Gait Speed (FGS), and the 6-Minute Walk Test (6MWT). Lattouf et al. [37] assessed gait using the 10-m Walk Test and 6-Minute Walk Test (6MWT). The study by Fernandez et al. [34] found significant improvements in EG compared to CG. The study by Lattouf et al. [37] found improvements between groups in the 6MWT but did not find differences in the 10-m Walk Test. Flansbjer et al. [35] did not find changes after the intervention, but it found improvements in EG compared to CG in the follow-up period in TUG. All studies found improvements after the intervention in EG. Moreover, the improvements were maintained in the follow-up evaluation in the study by Flansbjer et al. [35].

Balance was assessed in three of the articles included in this review using the Berg Balance Scale (BBS), the common tool used [32,34,36]. The study by Mun et al. [36] also used a platform that calculates the load distribution when standing, using it both with open and closed eyes. All studies found a significant improvement after the intervention for both groups.

4. Discussion

The purpose of this systematic review was to analyze the current scientific evidence on the use of resistance training programs as a therapeutic option for patients with stroke, and to analyze their effects on spasticity. A total of nine studies studying the application of resistance training programs in stroke populations have been included and reviewed. Benefits to spasticity were reported, as well as to function, strength, gait, and balance, being superior to, or at least equal to, those obtained by the comparison groups. Thus, resistance training programs can bring benefits to people with stroke without causing an increase in spasticity [9,10]. This finding, together with the effectiveness that seems to occur in different parameters related to motor function, makes resistance training an adequate alternative intervention for stroke patients.

Concerning the characteristics of the studies included, samples were relatively small, involving an average of 30 subjects per study. In this sense, it is a common limitation in stroke rehabilitation trials, since it is difficult to obtain large sample sizes because patients are usually treated only in a neurological institution or center, costs are usually high, and inclusion criteria are very narrow [38,39]. Furthermore, profiles of the subjects included had great variability in terms of the time elapsed after stroke, with only one study [32] including patients in an acute stage, and they did not find differences in spasticity, although they did find significant improvements in balance. It is known that most recovery is reached around the third month, with the fastest level of recovery occurring in the first month and a half, because it is the period where the greatest endogenous neuroplasticity occurs [40]. Moreover, the incidence of spasticity in stroke occurs mainly in periods longer than 3 months after stroke, so it may be interesting to know the long-term effects of this intervention in subjects with acute stages of stroke, acting then as a preventive action [7].

Two of the three studies that found improvements in spasticity in EG compared to CG carried out protocols combined with another type of treatment [30,33,36]. Therefore, there was no solid evidence to show that resistance training in isolation improves the degree of spasticity. In this way, Coroian et al. [29] was the only one that performed an isolated resistance training intervention and did not find significant improvements in spasticity. In this regard, isolated resistance training may not be entirely adequate for patient improvement after stroke. According to the current literature [41], combined strength, aerobic, and other physical capacity training would be an appropriate approach for the recovery of stroke patients without increased tone or spasticity.

Regarding the intervention protocol, the superiority of one approach compared to the others is not perceived. However, it seems that there is a consensus to perform between three and five sets, with positive effects in the studies that adopted this number of series in their interventions. Concerning the number of repetitions per set, we found too wide a range to draw conclusions. In this line, the study that opted for the highest number of sets, which in turn contained the highest number of total repetitions, was the one that showed the fewest positive effects [29], which may infer that excessive load on resistance training does not result in beneficial effects in stroke patients. Nevertheless, further studies are needed to confirm this issue.

Despite the variability of the tools used for resistance training, there was agreement on the use of equipment that uses closed kinetic chains. This may be because it offers greater sensory information, which is very favorable in this patient profile [42,43]. There was also some interest in combining different forms of contraction during the execution of the exercise, possibly to take advantage of the different effects they cause [44,45].

In view of the above, the present systematic review provides a comprehensive insight into the effects of resistance training on spasticity among people with stroke. However, several limitations need to be considered. The results should be taken with caution due to the heterogeneity of the participant characteristics and intervention protocols. In this sense, a meta-analysis was not performed because of the high heterogeneity in terms of study interventions and outcome measures, as well as the different body regions assessed, so a meta-analysis is not congruent enough to extract a quantitative synthesis that adds qualitative value to the results of the studies analyzed. Also, the number of articles with long-term follow-up was small, and evidence on the long-term effects of resistance training programs is limited. The inclusion criteria, while well-defined using the PICOS model, might have introduced bias due to the exclusion of certain types of physical interventions for muscle strength improvement. In addition, the lack of information about the specific duration of resistance training in multimodal programs was not reported by some studies and therefore no solid conclusions could be drawn on this issue.

Despite these limitations, the systematic review aims to contribute significantly to understanding the relationship between resistance training and spasticity post-stroke. The comprehensive evidence from this review enables clinicians to make informed decisions when considering the inclusion of resistance training in post-stroke rehabilitation plans. Recognizing its potential benefits in reducing spasticity, as well as improving critical functional areas such as strength, gait, and balance, enables the development of personalized and thorough treatment strategies. Furthermore, by highlighting existing gaps and limitations, this review acts as a catalyst for future research efforts. Finally, this systematic review offers clinicians valuable information for refining rehabilitation strategies, which may result in improved functional performance and quality of life for post-stroke, spastic patients.

5. Conclusions

Resistance training programs were superior to, or at least similar to, no intervention, conventional therapy, or other therapies for managing spasticity. Furthermore, other additional benefits were found to function, strength, gait, and balance in people with stroke. Therefore, the inclusion of this therapy in clinical practice could have a positive impact on people with stroke. However, there was no solid consensus on the optimal training protocol. It seems that the use of closed kinetic chains and the performance of various forms of contraction are those reporting the best results. Despite the results obtained, they should be taken with caution due to the heterogeneity in terms of participants and intervention protocols. We encourage authors to conduct well-designed research protocols including follow-up assessments to explore the long-term effects of resistance training in people with stroke.

Supplementary Materials: The following supporting information can be downloaded at: https://www.mdpi.com/article/10.3390/brainsci14010057/s1, File S1: PRISMA Checklist.

Author Contributions: Conceptualization, J.C.C.-B., D.L.-A. and J.A.M.-M.; methodology and data curation, J.C.C.-B., D.L.-A. and J.A.M.-M.; formal analysis, J.C.C.-B., D.L.-A., A.D.M.-R. and J.A.M.-M.; writing—original draft preparation, J.C.C.-B., D.L.-A., A.D.M.-R. and J.A.M.-M.; writing—review and editing, J.C.C.-B., D.L.-A. and J.A.M.-M. All authors have read and agreed to the published version of the manuscript.

Funding: This research received no external funding.

Institutional Review Board Statement: Not applicable.

Informed Consent Statement: Not applicable.

Conflicts of Interest: The authors declare no conflict of interest.

References

1. Hankey, G.J. Stroke. *Lancet* **2017**, *389*, 641–654. [CrossRef] [PubMed]
2. Feigin, V.L.; Brainin, M.; Norrving, B.; Martins, S.; Sacco, R.L.; Hacke, W.; Fisher, M.; Pandian, J.; Lindsay, P. World Stroke Organization (WSO): Global Stroke Fact Sheet 2022. *Int. J. Stroke* **2022**, *17*, 18–29. [CrossRef] [PubMed]
3. Domínguez-Téllez, P.; Moral-Muñoz, J.A.; Salazar, A.; Casado-Fernández, E.; Lucena-Antón, D. Game-Based Virtual Reality Interventions to Improve Upper Limb Motor Function and Quality of Life after Stroke: Systematic Review and Meta-Analysis. *Games Health J.* **2020**, *9*, 1–10. [CrossRef] [PubMed]
4. Lance, J.W. What Is Spasticity? *Lancet* **1990**, *335*, 606. [CrossRef] [PubMed]
5. Lee, K.B.; Hong, B.Y.; Kim, J.S.; Sul, B.; Yoon, S.C.; Ji, E.-K.; Son, D.B.; Hwang, B.Y.; Lim, S.H. Which Brain Lesions Produce Spasticity? An Observational Study on 45 Stroke Patients. *PLoS ONE* **2019**, *14*, e0210038. [CrossRef] [PubMed]
6. O'Dwyer, N.J.; Ada, L.; Neilson, P.D. Spasticity and Muscle Contracture Following Stroke. *Brain* **1996**, *119*, 1737–1749. [CrossRef]
7. Sainz-Pelayo, M.P.; Albu, S.; Murillo, N.; Benito-Penalva, J. Spasticity in Neurological Pathologies. An Update on the Pathophysiological Mechanisms, Advances in Diagnosis and Treatment. *Rev. Neurol.* **2020**, *70*, 453–460. [CrossRef]
8. Bhakta, B.B.; O'Connor, R.J.; Cozens, J.A. Associated Reactions after Stroke: A Randomized Controlled Trial of the Effect of Botulinum Toxin Type A. *J. Rehabil. Med.* **2008**, *40*, 36–41. [CrossRef]
9. Damiano, D.L.; Vaughan, C.L.; Abel, M.E. Muscle Response to Heavy Resistance Exercise in Children with Spastic Cerebral Palsy. *Dev. Med. Child. Neurol.* **1995**, *37*, 731–739. [CrossRef]
10. Bobath, B. *Adult Hemiplegia: Evaluation and Treatment*, 3rd ed.; Butterworth-Heinemann: Oxford, UK, 1990; 190p.
11. Veldema, J.; Jansen, P. Resistance Training in Stroke Rehabilitation: Systematic Review and Meta-Analysis. *Clin. Rehabil.* **2020**, *34*, 1173–1197. [CrossRef]
12. O'Donovan, G.; Blazevich, A.J.; Boreham, C.; Cooper, A.R.; Crank, H.; Ekelund, U.; Fox, K.R.; Gately, P.; Giles-Corti, B.; Gill, J.M.R.; et al. The ABC of Physical Activity for Health: A Consensus Statement from the British Association of Sport and Exercise Sciences. *J. Sports Sci.* **2010**, *28*, 573–591. [CrossRef] [PubMed]
13. Powell, K.E.; King, A.C.; Buchner, D.M.; Campbell, W.W.; DiPietro, L.; Erickson, K.I.; Hillman, C.H.; Jakicic, J.M.; Janz, K.F.; Katzmarzyk, P.T.; et al. The Scientific Foundation for the Physical Activity Guidelines for Americans, 2nd Edition. *J. Phys. Act. Health* **2018**, *16*, 1–11. [CrossRef] [PubMed]
14. Nicolini, C.; Fahnestock, M.; Gibala, M.J.; Nelson, A.J. Understanding the Neurophysiological and Molecular Mechanisms of Exercise-Induced Neuroplasticity in Cortical and Descending Motor Pathways: Where Do We Stand? *Neuroscience* **2021**, *457*, 259–282. [CrossRef] [PubMed]
15. Mitchell, J.B.; Phillips, M.D.; Yellott, R.C.; Currie, L.M. Resistance and Aerobic Exercise: The Influence of Mode on the Relationship between IL-6 and Glucose Tolerance in Young Men Who Are Obese. *J. Strength Cond. Res.* **2011**, *25*, 1529–1537. [CrossRef] [PubMed]
16. Thent, Z.C.; Das, S.; Henry, L.J. Role of Exercise in the Management of Diabetes Mellitus: The Global Scenario. *PLoS ONE* **2013**, *8*, e80436. [CrossRef] [PubMed]
17. Baigent, C.; Blackwell, L.; Emberson, J.; Holland, L.E.; Reith, C.; Bhala, N.; Peto, R.; Barnes, E.H.; Keech, A.; Simes, J.; et al. Efficacy and Safety of More Intensive Lowering of LDL Cholesterol: A Meta-Analysis of Data from 170,000 Participants in 26 Randomised Trials. *Lancet* **2010**, *376*, 1670–1681. [CrossRef] [PubMed]
18. Figueroa, A.; Park, S.Y.; Seo, D.Y.; Sanchez-Gonzalez, M.A.; Baek, Y.H. Combined Resistance and Endurance Exercise Training Improves Arterial Stiffness, Blood Pressure, and Muscle Strength in Postmenopausal Women. *Menopause* **2011**, *18*, 980–984. [CrossRef]
19. Galvão, D.A.; Nosaka, K.; Taaffe, D.R.; Peake, J.; Spry, N.; Suzuki, K.; Yamaya, K.; McGuigan, M.R.; Kristjanson, L.J.; Newton, R.U. Endocrine and Immune Responses to Resistance Training in Prostate Cancer Patients. *Prostate Cancer Prostatic Dis.* **2008**, *11*, 160–165. [CrossRef]
20. Smith, R.A.; Martin, G.J.; Szivak, T.K.; Comstock, B.A.; Dunn-Lewis, C.; Hooper, D.R.; Flanagan, S.D.; Looney, D.P.; Volek, J.S.; Maresh, C.M.; et al. The Effects of Resistance Training Prioritization in NCAA Division I Football Summer Training. *J. Strength Cond. Res.* **2014**, *28*, 14–22. [CrossRef]
21. Martín-Hernández, J.; Marín, P.; Menéndez, H.; Loenneke, J.; Coelho-e-Silva, M.; García-López, D.; Herrero, A. Changes in Muscle Architecture Induced by Low Load Blood Flow Restricted Training. *Acta Physiol. Hung.* **2013**, *100*, 411–418. [CrossRef]
22. Ross, A.; Leveritt, M.; Riek, S. Neural Influences on Sprint Running: Training Adaptations and Acute Responses. *Sports Med.* **2001**, *31*, 409–425. [CrossRef] [PubMed]
23. Young, W.B.; Rath, D.A. Enhancing Foot Velocity in Football Kicking: The Role of Strength Training. *J. Strength Cond. Res.* **2011**, *25*, 561–566. [CrossRef] [PubMed]
24. Page, M.J.; McKenzie, J.E.; Bossuyt, P.M.; Boutron, I.; Hoffmann, T.C.; Mulrow, C.D.; Shamseer, L.; Tetzlaff, J.M.; Akl, E.A.; Brennan, S.E.; et al. The PRISMA 2020 Statement: An Updated Guideline for Reporting Systematic Reviews. *BMJ* **2021**, *372*, n71. [CrossRef] [PubMed]
25. *Mendeley*, version 1.19.4; Reference Management Software; Available online: https://www.mendeley.com/?interaction_required=true (accessed on 12 September 2023).
26. Costantino, G.; Montano, N.; Casazza, G. When Should We Change Our Clinical Practice Based on the Results of a Clinical Study? Searching for Evidence: PICOS and PubMed. *Intern. Emerg. Med.* **2015**, *10*, 525–527. [CrossRef] [PubMed]

27. Maher, C.G.; Sherrington, C.; Herbert, R.D.; Moseley, A.M.; Elkins, M. Reliability of the PEDro Scale for Rating Quality of Randomized Controlled Trials. *Phys. Ther.* **2003**, *83*, 713–721. [CrossRef] [PubMed]
28. Foley, N.C.; Teasell, R.W.; Bhogal, S.K.; Speechley, M.R. Stroke Rehabilitation Evidence-Based Review: Methodology. *Top. Stroke Rehabil.* **2003**, *10*, 1–7. [CrossRef] [PubMed]
29. Coroian, F.; Jourdan, C.; Bakhti, K.; Palayer, C.; Jaussent, A.; Picot, M.-C.; Mottet, D.; Julia, M.; Bonnin, H.-Y.; Laffont, I. Upper Limb Isokinetic Strengthening Versus, Passive Mobilization in Patients With Chronic Stroke: A Randomized Controlled Trial. *Arch. Phys. Med. Rehabil.* **2018**, *99*, 321–328. [CrossRef] [PubMed]
30. Dehno, N.S.; Kamali, F.; Shariat, A.; Jaberzadeh, S. Unilateral Strength Training of the Less Affected Hand Improves Cortical Excitability and Clinical Outcomes in Patients With Subacute Stroke: A Randomized Controlled Trial. *Arch. Phys. Med. Rehabil.* **2021**, *102*, 914–924. [CrossRef]
31. Patten, C.; Condliffe, E.G.; Dairaghi, C.A.; Lum, P.S. Concurrent Neuromechanical and Functional Gains Following Upper-Extremity Power Training Post-Stroke. *J. Neuroeng. Rehabil.* **2013**, *10*, 1. [CrossRef]
32. Fernandes, B.; Ferreira, M.J.; Batista, F.; Evangelista, I.; Prates, L.; Silveira-Sérgio, J. Task-Oriented Training and Lower Limb Strengthening to Improve Balance and Function after Stroke: A Pilot Study. *Eur. J. Physiother.* **2015**, *17*, 74–80. [CrossRef]
33. Akbari, A.; Karimi, H. The Effect of Strengthening Exercises on Exaggerated Muscle Tonicity in Chronic Hemiparesis Following Stroke. *J. Med. Sci.* **2006**, *6*, 382–388. [CrossRef]
34. Fernandez-Gonzalo, R.; Fernandez-Gonzalo, S.; Turon, M.; Prieto, C.; Tesch, P.A.; García-Carreira, M.D.C. Muscle, Functional and Cognitive Adaptations after Flywheel Resistance Training in Stroke Patients: A Pilot Randomized Controlled Trial. *J. Neuroeng. Rehabil.* **2016**, *13*, 37. [CrossRef] [PubMed]
35. Flansbjer, U.B.; Miller, M.; Downham, D.; Lexell, J. Progressive Resistance Training after Stroke: Effects on Muscle Strength, Muscle Tone, Gait Performance and Perceived Participation. *J. Rehabil. Med.* **2008**, *40*, 42–48. [CrossRef] [PubMed]
36. Mu Mun, B.; Park, J.; Kim, T.H. The Effect of Lower Extremity Strengthening Exercise Using Sliding Stander on Balance and Spasticity in Chronic Stroke: A Randomized Clinical Trial. *J. Korean Phys. Ther.* **2019**, *31*, 311–316. [CrossRef]
37. Lattouf, N.A.; Tomb, R.; Assi, A.; Maynard, L.; Mesure, S. Eccentric Training Effects for Patients with Post-Stroke Hemiparesis on Strength and Speed Gait: A Randomized Controlled Trial. *NeuroRehabilitation* **2021**, *48*, 513–522. [CrossRef] [PubMed]
38. Moreno-Ligero, M.; Lucena-Anton, D.; Salazar, A.; Failde, I.; Moral-Munoz, J.A. MHealth Impact on Gait and Dynamic Balance Outcomes in Neurorehabilitation: Systematic Review and Meta-Analysis. *J. Med. Syst.* **2023**, *47*, 75. [CrossRef] [PubMed]
39. McIntyre, A.; Richardson, M.; Janzen, S.; Hussein, N.; Teasell, R. The Evolution of Stroke Rehabilitation Randomized Controlled Trials. *Int. J. Stroke* **2014**, *9*, 789–792. [CrossRef]
40. Bernhardt, J.; Hayward, K.S.; Kwakkel, G.; Ward, N.S.; Wolf, S.L.; Borschmann, K.; Krakauer, J.W.; Boyd, L.A.; Carmichael, S.T.; Corbett, D.; et al. Agreed Definitions and a Shared Vision for New Standards in Stroke Recovery Research: The Stroke Recovery and Rehabilitation Roundtable Taskforce. *Int. J. Stroke* **2017**, *12*, 444–450. [CrossRef]
41. Ammann, B.C.; Knols, R.H.; Baschung, P.; de Bie, R.A.; de Bruin, E.D. Application of Principles of Exercise Training in Sub-Acute and Chronic Stroke Survivors: A Systematic Review. *BMC Neurol.* **2014**, *14*, 167. [CrossRef]
42. Lee, N.K.; Kwon, J.W.; Son, S.M.; Kang, K.W.; Kim, K.; Hyun-Nam, S. The Effects of Closed and Open Kinetic Chain Exercises on Lower Limb Muscle Activity and Balance in Stroke Survivors. *NeuroRehabilitation* **2013**, *33*, 177–183. [CrossRef]
43. Lee, N.K.; Kwon, J.W.; Son, S.M.; Nam, S.H.; Choi, Y.W.; Kim, C.S. Changes of Plantar Pressure Distributions Following Open and Closed Kinetic Chain Exercise in Patients with Stroke. *NeuroRehabilitation* **2013**, *32*, 385–390. [CrossRef] [PubMed]
44. Oranchuk, D.J.; Storey, A.G.; Nelson, A.R.; Cronin, J.B. Isometric Training and Long-Term Adaptations: Effects of Muscle Length, Intensity, and Intent: A Systematic Review. *Scand. J. Med. Sci. Sports* **2019**, *29*, 484–503. [CrossRef] [PubMed]
45. Franchi, M.V.; Reeves, N.D.; Narici, M.V. Skeletal Muscle Remodeling in Response to Eccentric vs. Concentric Loading: Morphological, Molecular, and Metabolic Adaptations. *Front. Physiol.* **2017**, *8*, 447. [CrossRef] [PubMed]

Disclaimer/Publisher's Note: The statements, opinions and data contained in all publications are solely those of the individual author(s) and contributor(s) and not of MDPI and/or the editor(s). MDPI and/or the editor(s) disclaim responsibility for any injury to people or property resulting from any ideas, methods, instructions or products referred to in the content.

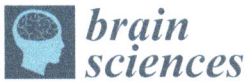

Brief Report

Translation, Adaptation, and Determining the Intra-Rater Reliability of the Balance Evaluation Systems Test (BESTest) for Persian Patients with Chronic Stroke

Mansoureh Sadat Dadbakhsh [1], Afarin Haghparast [2], Noureddin Nakhostin Ansari [3], Amin Nakhostin-Ansari [2] and Soofia Naghdi [1,3,*]

[1] Department of Physiotherapy, School of Rehabilitation, Tehran University of Medical Sciences, Tehran 1417613151, Iran; m-dadbakhsh@razi.tums.ac.ir

[2] Sports Medicine Research Center, Neuroscience Institute, Tehran University of Medical Sciences, Tehran 1417613151, Iran; haghparast.afarin@gmail.com (A.H.); a-nansari@alumnus.tums.ac.ir (A.N.-A.)

[3] Research Center for War-Affected People, Tehran University of Medical Sciences, Tehran 1417613151, Iran; nakhostin@tums.ac.ir

* Correspondence: naghdi@tums.ac.ir; Tel.: +98-912-2979310

Abstract: This study aimed to translate and culturally adapt the BESTest to the Persian language and evaluate its intra-rater reliability in Iranian patients with stroke. A forward-backward translation and expert panel review method was followed. Eighteen patients post-stroke (15 men, 3 female) were included which were assessed by a physiotherapist two times with a one-week interval. The mean total score for the test and retest were 83.66 (SD = 11.98) and 82 (SD = 13.23), respectively. There were no floor and ceiling effects. The intra-rater ICC for the total score was 0.88 (95% CI = 0.73–0.95). The ICC for the BESTest sections ranged from 0.55 (95% CI = 0.12–0.80) to 0.89 (95% CI = 0.55–0.96). The standard error of measurement and the smallest detectable change of the BESTest total score were 8.33 and 22.82, respectively. Our findings confirm the intra-rater reliability of the Persian BESTest for balance assessment of patients with chronic stroke.

Keywords: BESTest; stroke; Persian; reliability

1. Introduction

A stroke is an acute impairment of brain function due to a disruption in blood supply to the brain [1]. In 2017, the incidence of stroke was estimated to be about 11.9 million, and it was the second cause of death in 2019 [2,3]. The trend in the prevalence of stroke in the Middle East and North Africa (MENA) region closely mirrors the global pattern, with a gradual decrease in recent years [4]. Nevertheless, the majority of the stroke burden is concentrated in lower-income and lower-middle-income countries [3]. In Iran, stroke stands out as a significant contributor to disabilities, and its annual incidence varies widely across different regions of the country, spanning from 23 to 103 cases per 100,000 people [5,6]. Hence, stroke stands as a significant contributor to both disability and mortality on a global scale and within Iran.

Stroke could result in life-long persistent physical, psychological, and cognitive impairments [7], with motor disorders affecting approximately 80% to 90% of stroke survivors, making it a significant cause of disability [8]. Among these physical impairments, balance issues are among the most prevalent, affecting an estimated 87.5% of stroke patients [8]. These balance problems are often attributed to weakened muscles, abnormal muscle tone, sensory deficits, cognitive issues, and delayed automatic postural responses [9]. Notably, post-stroke balance problems elevate the risk of falls [10], further impacting the quality of life and increasing healthcare expenses [11,12]. Hence, the assessment of balance in patients with stroke using reliable and valid tools are crucial to monitor changes after using rehabilitation interventions [13–15].

Using a reliable and valid assessment tool for balance is crucial in post-stroke survivors, as balance impairment significantly increases the risk of falls in these individuals [9]. Such assessment tools can help identify the balance issues that would benefit from rehabilitation, determine the specific system contributing to the balance impairment, and monitor progress during treatment [16–19]. Several balance assessment tools have been employed in stroke patients, including the Berg Balance Scale (BBS), Postural Assessment Scale for Stroke Patients (PASS), Community Balance and Mobility Scale (CB & M), Timed Up and Go (TUG), and Dynamic Gait Index (DGI). However, each of these tests has its limitations [20,21]. The BBS is considered the gold standard for balance assessment, but it does not encompass dynamic balance [22,23]. PASS and CB & M exhibit ceiling and floor effects, respectively [23]. TUG serves as a screening test but lacks an in-depth evaluation of the balance system [24]. The complexity of the balance system makes it challenging to determine the specific system responsible for balance impairment. An important drawback of the current balance tests is their inability to evaluate the particular systems contributing to balance impairments [25].

Balance Evaluation Systems Test (BESTest) is a test developed by Horak et al. to identify the disordered systems responsible for poor balance control. The BESTest has 36 items designed to evaluate the performance of six balance systems of biomechanical constraints, stability limits/verticality, transition/anticipatory postural adjustment, reactive postural responses, sensory orientation, and stability during gait [21,25].

Post-stroke survivors experience a range of issues, which can more or less affect all the systems evaluated in the BESTest [26–28]. Previous studies have demonstrated the BESTest has no floor or ceiling effects [29] and is reliable, valid, and responsive to change for assessing balance in patients with stroke [21,25]. BESTest has been translated and culturally adapted into various languages, including German [29], Spanish [30], Norwegian [31], Spanish [32] and Korean [33]. There is no prior research on translating and culturally adapting the BESTest into the Persian language. Therefore, the aim of this study was to translate the BESTest into Persian and assess its intra-rater reliability among patients with stroke.

2. Materials & Methods

2.1. Design

A cross-sectional study was carried out to develop the Persian version of the BESTest and to examine its intra-rater reliability (i.e., between-day reliability) in patients with stroke. The study protocol was approved by the Research Council of the School of Rehabilitation, Tehran University of Medical Sciences (TUMS) (#36621).

2.2. Translation

The guidelines for the previously used forward-backward translation were followed by the expert panel [34–36]. First, two translators independently translated the English BESTest to Persian (forward translation). Then an expert panel (3 physiotherapists, an experienced methodologist, and 2 translators) reviewed the two versions and synthesized one Persian version for back translation. Two different English translators independently back translated the synthesized version to English. The expert panel with all the translators reviewed the documents and approved the pre-final Persian version to be sent to the developer (Prof. Fay B. Horak) for final approval. After approval of the Persian BESTtest by Prof. Horak, the final Persian BESTest emerged (https://www.bestest.us/files/3714/2472/0733/Persian_BESTest.pdf, accessed on 1 November 2023).

2.3. Participants

Participants were stroke patients referred from universities' neurological and physiotherapy clinics. Inclusion criteria were: (1) stroke diagnosis, (2) hemiplegia resulting from stroke with a stable medical condition, (3) aged between 18 and 70 years, (4) ability to follow instructions, and (5) ability to stand and walk 6 m independently. The stroke diagnosis was made by neurologists based on the clinical and radiological findings.

Exclusion criteria were: (1) not willing to participate in the study, (2) inability to complete the tasks, (3) presence of balance disorders due to a medical condition other than stroke (e.g., Parkinson's disease, vestibular disorders, untreated visual or hearing disabilities, pain, or impairments in the musculoskeletal system), (4) history of pathological vertigo, and (5) using medications affecting balance.

2.4. Test Procedure

The study was conducted in the neurological physiotherapy clinic of the school of rehabilitation of TUMS. At the first session, the participants' demographic characteristics, including age, gender, and the time elapsed since the stroke, were collected. The study aims were explained to the participants, and written informed consent was obtained from them. In the next step, an experienced physiotherapist who was trained in the use of the BESTest, and had practiced performing the test items, assessed the participants' balance. Every session included environmental preparation and it took approximately 35 min to complete the test. Both the test and retest were performed in the same environment for every patient. Patients were allowed to rest if they requested. The same physiotherapist assessed the patients again after one week.

2.5. Outcome Measure

The BESTest consists of 27 tasks and 36 items that evaluate six systems contributing to balance. Each item is scored from 0 (worst performance) to 3 (best performance). The sections' scores were the sum of all the related items' scores, and higher scores indicate better performance. The systems of the BESTest include biomechanical constraints (maximum possible score of 15), stability limits/verticality (maximum possible score of 21), transition/anticipatory postural adjustment (maximum possible score of 18), reactive postural responses (maximum possible score of 18), sensory orientation (maximum possible score of 15), and stability in gait (maximum possible score of 21). The total score of 108 is the sum of all the scores of all the sections.

2.6. Statistical Analysis

The mean and standard deviation (SD) was computed for continuous variables. Numbers and percentages were used for categorical variables. Intraclass correlation (ICC), a two-way random effect model, was used to determine the intra-rater reliability. An ICC value of 0.70 was considered as acceptable reliability, and scores were interpreted as excellent (>75), good (0.60–0.75), and fair (0.40–0.59) [37].

The standard error measurement (SEM, $\sigma\sqrt{1-ICC}$) and the smallest detectable change (SDC, $1.96 \times SEM \times \sqrt{2}$) were calculated for the BESTest total score. The percentage of patients that scored the lowest or the highest possible score on the Persian BESTest were calculated for the presence of floor and ceiling effects (cut-off value $\geq 15\%$) [38]. Statistical analyses were performed using the SPSS version 17. $p < 0.05$ was considered statistically significant.

3. Results

A total of 18 participants were included in the study comprising 15 men and 3 women. The mean age was 56.39 (SD = 9.01). The mean time since the stroke was 50.0 months (SD = 35.08). Sixteen patients had ischemic stroke and two patients had hemorrhagic stroke. Ten patients had right hemiplegia. Characteristics of the individuals who participated in the study are presented in Table 1.

There was no issue with translating and adapting the BESTest into Persian, and all items were translated without any difficulties. During pilot testing, the therapist reported the test items that were understandable and easy to apply during the assessment.

The mean of the BESTest total score in the test and retest were 83.66 (SD = 11.98) and 82 (SD = 13.23), respectively. There were no floor and ceiling effects observed for the Persian BESTest total score (no patient scored the minimum or maximum on the Persian

BESTtest). The intra-rater reliability of the BESTest total scores was high (ICC = 0.88, 95% CI = 0.73–0.95), and ICCs for sections ranged from 0.55 (95% CI = 0.12–0.80) for stability limits/verticality to 0.89 (95% CI = 0.55–0.96) for stability in gait (Table 2). The SEM and SDC of the BESTest total score were 8.33 and 22.82, respectively (Table 3).

Table 1. Basic and demographic characteristics of the participants.

Patients Number	Age (Year)	Duration since Stroke (Month)	Gender	Cause	Affected Side
1	65	24	Male	Ischemic	Right
2	56	72	Male	Ischemic	Left
3	66	47	Male	Ischemic	Left
4	55	136	Male	Hemorrhagic	Right
5	60	50	Male	Ischemic	Right
6	75	3	Male	Ischemic	Left
7	63	54	Male	Ischemic	Right
8	62	132	Female	Hemorrhagic	Left
9	46	50	Female	Ischemic	Right
10	61	36	Female	Ischemic	Left
11	43	60	Male	Ischemic	Left
12	46	8	Male	Ischemic	Right
13	45	37	Male	Ischemic	Left
14	57	36	Male	Ischemic	Right
15	45	42	Male	Ischemic	Right
16	63	35	Male	Ischemic	Right
17	49	54	Male	Ischemic	Right
18	58	24	Male	Ischemic	Left

Table 2. Sections and total scores in both sessions and intra-rater reliability for the BESTest.

Subscale	Session 1			Session 2			ICC (95% CI)	p-Value
	Min	Max	Mean (SD)	Min	Max	Mean (SD)		
Biomechanical constraints	6	14	11.61 (2.17)	6	14	10.61 (2.32)	0.72 (0.28–0.89)	<0.001
Stability limits/verticality	12	17	15.11 (1.27)	12	18	15.33 (1.45)	0.55 (0.12–0.80)	0.008
Transition/anticipatory postural adjustment	7	16	12.55 (2.38)	7	16	12.38 (2.50)	0.79 (0.53–0.91)	<0.001
Reactive postural responses	0	18	10.88 (5.01)	0	18	11.72 (5.16)	0.77 (0.49–0.90)	<0.001
Sensory orientation	12	15	14.61 (0.77)	12	15	14.66 (0.76)	0.76 (0.47–0.90)	<0.001
Stability in gait	10	21	18.83 (2.79)	9	21	18 (2.72)	0.89 (0.55–0.96)	<0.001
Total score	47 (43%)	101 (93%)	83.66 (11.98)	46 (42%)	102 (94%)	82 (13.23)	0.88 (0.73–0.95)	<0.001

Table 3. The standard error of measurement (SEM) and smallest detectable change (SDC) for the Persian BESTest.

Systems	SEM	SDC
Biomechanical constraints	2.24	6.06
Stability limits/verticality	1.6	4.38
Anticipatory responses	2.07	5.67
Postural responses	4.46	12.22
Sensory orientation	0.69	1.89
Stability in gait	1.78	4.87
Total score	8.33	22.82

4. Discussion

Balance impairments can significantly impact post-stroke patients' quality of life [39]. Utilizing a reliable and valid instrument for balance evaluation to guide rehabilitation programs is essential. In this study, we translated and culturally adapted the BESTest into the Persian language and investigated its intra-rater reliability for the balance evaluation of Iranian post-stroke patients. The results showed that the Persian BESTest has excellent intra-rater reliability for balance evaluation in stroke patients and therefore can be used as a reliable tool for the assessment of balance in patients with stroke.

In the current study, the Persian version of the BESTest was developed and cross-culturally adapted for Persian patients with stroke. The successful development of the Persian BESTest indicates that the face and content validity of it is consistent with the original English BESTest and translated versions [25,29,31].

All patients in the study participated and completed the test procedure. There were no unexpected events or injuries that occurred during the testing with balance performances. As well, the rater reported no difficulties in conducting the assessment using the Persian BESTest. None of the patients had changes in their balance between the two test sessions. These indicate that the Persian BESTest was acceptable and feasible. The acceptability of the Persian BESTest is in line with those found for the translated versions of the BESTest [29,31,40,41].

Floor or ceiling effects were not present for the Persian BESTest total score. The lack of floor or ceiling effects indicates the content validity and responsiveness of the Persian BESTest. When there are no floor and ceiling effects for an instrument, patients with the lowest or highest possible score can be detected after an intervention. However, the responsiveness of the Persian BESTest was not evaluated in the current study which warrants an investigation designed in the context of a clinical trial. The lack of floor and ceiling effects observed in the present study is consistent with those reported for the translated versions of the BETSTest [31]. The floor and ceiling effects for the BESTest scores are not reported for the original version [25].

The Persian BESTest showed excellent intra-rater reliability. These findings are similar to those of previous studies [25,29,31,42] The original English version of the BESTest has been shown to have high inter- and intra-rater reliability (Horak et al., 2009). The test–retest reliability for the BESTest was high (ICC = 0.88) [42]. A study by Chinsongkram et al. in subacute stroke patients found excellent intra-rater reliability for the BESTest and its sections [40]. Rodrigues et al. (2014) evaluated the intra-rater reliability of the Brazilian BESTest in a sample of 16 chronic stroke patients and found the reliability for the total score (ICC = 0.98) and its sections (ICCs from 0.85 to 0.96) were excellent [40]. The findings indicate that the Persian BESTest in line with the original and other versions [25,31,40,41] can be used as a reliable tool for assessing the balance of patients with stroke.

The ICC for the stability limits/verticality section was the lowest in our study (0.55), in contrast to stability in the gait section, which was the highest (0.89). In the Rodrigues et al. study, ICC was the highest and lowest in the stability in gait and the reactive postural responses sections, respectively [41]. Chinsongkram reported the ICCs for sections ranging from 0.95 and 0.99 [40]. The reasons for discrepancies might be due to the differences in methodology. In the present study, one rater participated in the evaluation of intra-rater reliability and did not score the performances from the video as was done in the previous studies [40]. Future studies using more raters for the evaluation of intra-rater reliability may clarify the intra-rater reliability of the sections, particularly of stability limits/verticality in the Persian BESTest. Nevertheless, we should expect patients to perform differently in the BESTest sections, poor in some sections compared with other ones [25], thus affecting the perception of raters in the level of test performances.

The absolute reliability, presented by SEM and SDC, is an important reliability measure for clinical purposes. The SEM is used to determine the change in test scores which is a real beyond measurement error. The SEM value found in this study was 8.33. A previous study reported the SEM of 3.9/4.3 for two raters [31]. Therefore, the SEM value in our study indicates that the Persian BESTest is a useful tool to identify real changes in patients with stroke. However, the SDC is more important clinically than the SEM as it helps to identify real changes in patients. The SDC was calculated to determine whether an individual patient has achieved a real change after therapy [22]. We found that the SDC value of the Persian BESTest was 22.82. Previous studies reported the SDC as starting from 6.9 [31,43]. Hence, a change of more than 22.82 points in the Persian BESTest score must be observed after an intervention to be interpreted as real and clinically relevant.

There are several limitations of this study worth mentioning. First, in this study, we only evaluated patients with stroke, and our finding might not be applicable to other conditions affecting balance. Therefore, future studies are needed to evaluate the reliability of the Persian BESTest for balance evaluation in other patient groups with balance impairments. Second, we only evaluated intra-rater reliability, SDC, and SEM, and we did not assess other reliability and validity indexes. Future studies are needed to evaluate these indexes, such as construct validity, inter-rater reliability, responsiveness, and discriminative validity. Third, our sample size for reliability evaluation was suboptimal as we only included 18 patients. However, a study conducting power analyses indicated that a minimal sample of 10 participants provides 80% power to detect what would be considered an ICC of 0.70 [44].

5. Conclusions

In this study, we developed the Persian version of the BESTest and found it to be a reliable measure for the balance evaluation of Persian-speaking patients with stroke. This study suggests that the Persian version of the BESTest is a reliable tool which therapists can use for balance evaluation of patients with stroke and determine the system responsible for balance deficits. Further studies on the other psychometric characteristics of the Persian BESTest such as inter-rater reliability in larger sample sizes are warranted.

Author Contributions: Conceptualization, S.N. and N.N.A.; Methodology, S.N., N.N.A. and M.S.D.; Validation, S.N., N.N.A. and M.S.D.; Formal analysis, N.N.A. and M.S.D.; Resources, S.N. and M.S.D.; Data curation, M.S.D.; Writing—Original Draft, A.H., M.S.D. and A.N.-A.; Writing—Review and editing, M.S.D., A.H., N.N.A., A.N.-A. and S.N.; Supervision, S.N. and N.N.A.; Project administration, S.N., N.N.A. and M.S.D. All authors have read and agreed to the published version of the manuscript.

Funding: This research received no external funding.

Institutional Review Board Statement: The study protocol was approved by the Research Council of the School of rehabilitation (#36621, 5 July 2014).

Informed Consent Statement: The study aims were explained to the participants, and written informed consent was obtained from them.

Data Availability Statement: The data that support the findings of this study are available from the corresponding author, S.N., upon reasonable request. The data are not publicly available due to privacy and ethical restrictions.

Conflicts of Interest: The authors declare no conflict of interest.

References

1. Sarkar, S.; Chakraborty, D.; Bhowmik, A.; Ghosh, M.K. Cerebral ischemic stroke: Cellular fate and therapeutic opportunities. *Front. Biosci. -Landmark* **2019**, *24*, 435–450.
2. Avan, A.; Digaleh, H.; Di Napoli, M.; Stranges, S.; Behrouz, R.; Shojaeianbabaei, G.; Amiri, A.; Tabrizi, R.; Mokhber, N.; Spence, J.D.; et al. Socioeconomic status and stroke incidence, prevalence, mortality, and worldwide burden: An ecological analysis from the Global Burden of Disease Study 2017. *BMC Med.* **2019**, *17*, 191. [CrossRef] [PubMed]
3. Feigin, V.L.; Brainin, M.; Norrving, B.; Martins, S.; Sacco, R.L.; Hacke, W.; Fisher, M.; Pandian, J.; Lindsay, P. World Stroke Organization (WSO): Global Stroke Fact Sheet 2022. *Int. J. Stroke* **2022**, *17*, 18–29. [CrossRef] [PubMed]
4. Jaberinezhad, M.; Farhoudi, M.; Nejadghaderi, S.A.; Alizadeh, M.; Sullman, M.J.M.; Carson-Chahhoud, K.; Collins, G.S.; Safiri, S. The burden of stroke and its attributable risk factors in the Middle East and North Africa region, 1990–2019. *Sci. Rep.* **2022**, *12*, 2700. [CrossRef] [PubMed]
5. Sarrafzadegan, N.; Mohammadifard, N. Cardiovascular disease in Iran in the last 40 years: Prevalence, mortality, morbidity, challenges and strategies for cardiovascular prevention. *Arch. Iran. Med.* **2019**, *22*, 204–210. [PubMed]
6. Hosseini, A.A.; Sobhani-Rad, D.; Ghandehari, K.; Benamer, H.T.S. Frequency and clinical patterns of stroke in Iran-Systematic and critical review. *BMC Neurol.* **2010**, *10*, 72. [CrossRef] [PubMed]
7. Mukherjee, D.; Levin, R.L.; Heller, W. The cognitive, emotional, and social sequelae of stroke: Psychological and ethical concerns in post-stroke adaptation. *Top. Stroke Rehabil.* **2006**, *13*, 26–35. [CrossRef] [PubMed]
8. Lendraitienė, E.; Tamošauskaitė, A.; Petruševičienė, D.; Savickas, R. Balance evaluation techniques and physical therapy in post-stroke patients: A literature review. *Neurol. Neurochir. Pol.* **2017**, *51*, 92–100. [CrossRef]
9. Zorowitz, R.D.; Gross, E.; Polinski, D.M. The stroke survivor. *Disabil. Rehabil.* **2002**, *24*, 666–679. [CrossRef]
10. Jalayondeja, C.; Sullivan, P.E.; Pichaiyongwongdee, S. Six-month prospective study of fall risk factors identification in patients post-stroke. *Geriatr. Gerontol. Int.* **2014**, *14*, 778–785. [CrossRef]
11. Hawkins, K.; Musich, S.; Ozminkowski, R.J.; Bai, M.; Migliori, R.J.; Yeh, C.S. The burden of falling on the quality of life of adults with medicare supplement insurance. *J. Gerontol. Nurs.* **2011**, *37*, 36–47. [CrossRef] [PubMed]
12. Novitzke, J.M. The rising cost of falling: Strategies to combat a common post-stroke foe. *J. Vasc. Interv. Neurol.* **2008**, *1*, 61. [PubMed]
13. Iatridou, G.; Pelidou, H.S.; Varvarousis, D.; Stergiou, A.; Beris, A.; Givissis, P.; Ploumis, A. The effectiveness of hydrokinesiotherapy on postural balance of hemiplegic patients after stroke: A systematic review and meta-analysis. *Clin. Rehabil.* **2017**, *32*, 583–593. [CrossRef] [PubMed]
14. Dominguez-Romero, J.G.; Molina-Aroca, A.; Moral-Munoz, J.A.; Luque-Moreno, C.; Lucena-Anton, D. Effectiveness of Mechanical Horse-Riding Simulators on Postural Balance in Neurological Rehabilitation: Systematic Review and Meta-Analysis. *Int. J. Environ. Res. Public Health* **2020**, *17*, 165. [CrossRef] [PubMed]
15. Chen, L.; Lo, W.L.; Mao, Y.R.; Ding, M.H.; Lin, Q.; Li, H.; Zhao, J.L.; Xu, Z.Q.; Bian, R.H.; Huang, D.F. Effect of Virtual Reality on Postural and Balance Control in Patients with Stroke: A Systematic Literature Review. *Biomed. Res. Int.* **2016**, *2016*, 7309272. [CrossRef] [PubMed]
16. Felius, R.A.W.; Geerars, M.; Bruijn, S.M.; Wouda, N.C.; Van Dieën, J.H.; Punt, M. Reliability of IMU-based balance assessment in clinical stroke rehabilitation. *Gait Posture* **2022**, *98*, 62–68. [CrossRef]
17. Pollock, C.L.; Eng, J.J.; Garland, S.J. Clinical measurement of walking balance in people post stroke: A systematic review. *Clin. Rehabil.* **2011**, *25*, 693–708. [CrossRef]
18. Mancini, M.; Horak, F.B. The relevance of clinical balance assessment tools to differentiate balance deficits. *Eur. J. Phys. Rehabil. Med.* **2010**, *46*, 239.
19. Blum, L.; Korner-Bitensky, N. Usefulness of the Berg Balance Scale in Stroke Rehabilitation: A Systematic Review. *Phys. Ther.* **2008**, *88*, 559–566. [CrossRef]
20. Naghdi, S.; Nakhostin Ansari, N.; Forogh, B.; Khalifeloo, M.; Honarpisheh, R.; Nakhostin-Ansari, A. Reliability and Validity of the Persian Version of the Mini-Balance Evaluation Systems Test in Patients with Stroke. *Neurol. Ther.* **2020**, *9*, 567–574. [CrossRef]
21. Chinsongkram, B.; Chaikeeree, N.; Saengsirisuwan, V.; Horak, F.B.; Boonsinsukh, R. Responsiveness of the Balance Evaluation Systems Test (BESTest) in people with subacute stroke. *Phys. Ther.* **2016**, *96*, 1638–1647. [CrossRef] [PubMed]
22. Oyama, C.; Otaka, Y.; Onitsuka, K.; Takagi, H.; Tan, E.; Otaka, E. Reliability and validity of the Japanese version of the mini-balance evaluation systems test in patients with subacute stroke. *Prog. Rehabil. Med.* **2018**, *3*, 20180015. [CrossRef]
23. Whitney, S.; Wrisley, D.; Furman, J. Concurrent validity of the Berg Balance Scale and the Dynamic Gait Index in people with vestibular dysfunction. *Physiother. Res. Int.* **2003**, *8*, 178–186. [CrossRef] [PubMed]
24. Joshua, A.M.; Karnad, S.D.; Nayak, A.; Suresh, B.v.; Mithra, P.; Unnikrishnan, B. Effect of foot placements during sit to stand transition on timed up and go test in stroke subjects: A cross sectional study. *NeuroRehabilitation* **2017**, *40*, 355–362. [CrossRef] [PubMed]
25. Horak, F.B.; Wrisley, D.M.; Frank, J. The balance evaluation systems test (BESTest) to differentiate balance deficits. *Phys. Ther.* **2009**, *89*, 484–498. [CrossRef] [PubMed]

26. Priplata, A.A.; Patritti, B.L.; Niemi, J.B.; Hughes, R.; Gravelle, D.C.; Lipsitz, L.A.; Veves, A.; Stein, J.; Bonato, P.; Collins, J.J. Noise-enhanced balance control in patients with diabetes and patients with stroke. *Ann. Neurol.* **2006**, *59*, 4–12. [CrossRef] [PubMed]
27. Lee, N.G.; You, J.S.; Chung, H.Y.; Jeon, H.S.; Choi, B.S.; Lee, D.R.; Park, J.M.; Lee, T.H.; Ryu, I.T.; Yoon, H.S. Best Core Stabilization for Anticipatory Postural Adjustment and Falls in Hemiparetic Stroke. *Arch. Phys. Med. Rehabil.* **2018**, *99*, 2168–2174. [CrossRef] [PubMed]
28. De Oliveira, C.B.; De Medeiros, Í.R.T.; Frota, N.A.F.; Greters, M.E.; Conforto, A.B. Balance control in hemiparetic stroke patients: Main tools for evaluation. *J. Rehabil. Res. Dev.* **2008**, *45*, 1215–1226. [CrossRef]
29. Haselwander, M.; Henes, Y.; Weisbrod, M.; Diermayr, G. Balance Evaluation Systems Test: German translation, cultural adaptation and preliminary results on psychometric properties. *Z. Gerontol. Geriatr.* **2023**, *56*, 125–131. [CrossRef]
30. Dominguez-Olivan, P.; Gasch-Gallen, A.; Aguas-Garcia, E.; Bengoetxea, A. Validity and reliability testing of the Spanish version of the BESTest and mini-BESTest in healthy community-dwelling elderly. *BMC Geriatr.* **2020**, *20*, 444. [CrossRef]
31. Hamre, C.; Botolfsen, P.; Tangen, G.G.; Helbostad, J.L. Interrater and test-retest reliability and validity of the Norwegian version of the BESTest and mini-BESTest in people with increased risk of falling. *BMC Geriatr.* **2017**, *17*, 92. [CrossRef] [PubMed]
32. Torres-Narvaez, M.R.; Luna-Corrales, G.A.; Rangel-Pineros, M.C.; Pardo-Oviedo, J.M.; Alvarado-Quintero, H. Transcultural adaptation to the Spanish language of the Balance Evaluation Systems Test (BESTest) in older adults. *Rev. Neurol.* **2018**, *67*, 373–381. [PubMed]
33. Jeon, Y.J.; Kim, G.M. A Study of Translation Conformity on Korean Version of a Balance Evaluation Systems Test. *Phys. Ther. Korea* **2018**, *25*, 53–61. [CrossRef]
34. Beaton, D.E.; Bombardier, C.; Guillemin, F.; Ferraz, M.B. Guidelines for the process of cross-cultural adaptation of self-report measures. *Spine* **2000**, *25*, 3186–3191. [CrossRef] [PubMed]
35. Naghdi, S.; Ansari, N.N.; Raji, P.; Shamili, A.; Amini, M.; Hasson, S. Cross-cultural validation of the Persian version of the Functional Independence Measure for patients with stroke. *Disabil. Rehabil.* **2016**, *38*, 289–298. [CrossRef] [PubMed]
36. Nakhostin Ansari, N.; Naghdi, S.; Eskandari, Z.; Salsabili, N.; Kordi, R.; Hasson, S. Reliability and validity of the Persian adaptation of the Core Outcome Measure Index in patients with chronic low back pain. *J. Orthop. Sci.* **2016**, *21*, 723–726. [CrossRef]
37. Fleiss, J.L.; Levin, B.; Cho Paik, M. *Statistical Methods for Rates and Proportions*, 3rd ed.; John Wiley & Sons, Inc.: Hoboken, NJ, USA, 2004; pp. 1–760. Available online: https://onlinelibrary.wiley.com/doi/book/10.1002/0471445428 (accessed on 6 November 2023).
38. Terwee, C.B.; Van Der Windt, D.A.; Dekker, J.; Bot, S.D.M.; De Boer, M.R.; Bouter, L.M.; Knol, D.L.; de Vet, H.C.W. *Quality Criteria Were Proposed for Measurement Properties of Health Status Questionnaires*; Elsevier: Amsterdam, The Netherlands, 2007. Available online: https://www.sciencedirect.com/science/article/pii/S0895435606001740 (accessed on 6 November 2023).
39. Schmid, A.A.; van Puymbroeck, M.; Altenburger, P.A.; Miller, K.K.; Combs, S.A.; Page, S.J. Balance is associated with quality of life in chronic stroke. *Top. Stroke Rehabil.* **2013**, *20*, 340–346. [CrossRef]
40. Chinsongkram, B.; Chaikeeree, N.; Saengsirisuwan, V.; Viriyatharakij, N.; Horak, F.B.; Boonsinsukh, R. Reliability and Validity of the Balance Evaluation Systems Test (BESTest) in People With Subacute Stroke. *Phys. Ther.* **2014**, *94*, 1632–1643. [CrossRef]
41. Rodrigues, L.C.; Marques, A.P.; Barros, P.B.; Michaelsen, S.M. Reliability of the Balance Evaluation Systems Test (BESTest) and BESTest sections for adults with hemiparesis. *Braz. J. Phys. Ther.* **2014**, *18*, 276–281. [CrossRef]
42. Leddy, A.L.; Crowner, B.E.; Earhart, G.M. Functional Gait Assessment and Balance Evaluation System Test: Reliability, Validity, Sensitivity, and Specificity for Identifying Individuals With Parkinson Disease Who Fall. *Phys. Ther.* **2011**, *91*, 102–113. [CrossRef]
43. Huang, M.H.; Miller, K.; Smith, K.; Fredrickson, K.; Shilling, T. Reliability, Validity, and Minimal Detectable Change of Balance Evaluation Systems Test and Its Short Versions in Older Cancer Survivors: A Pilot Study. *J. Geriatr. Phys. Ther.* **2016**, *39*, 58–63. [CrossRef] [PubMed]
44. Bujang, M.A.; Baharum, N. A simplified guide to determination of sample size requirements for estimating the value of intraclass correlation coefficient: A review. *Arch. Orofac. Sci. J. Sch. Dent. Sci. USM Arch Orofac Sci.* **2017**, *12*, 1–11.

Disclaimer/Publisher's Note: The statements, opinions and data contained in all publications are solely those of the individual author(s) and contributor(s) and not of MDPI and/or the editor(s). MDPI and/or the editor(s) disclaim responsibility for any injury to people or property resulting from any ideas, methods, instructions or products referred to in the content.

MDPI AG
Grosspeteranlage 5
4052 Basel
Switzerland
Tel.: +41 61 683 77 34

Brain Sciences Editorial Office
E-mail: brainsci@mdpi.com
www.mdpi.com/journal/brainsci

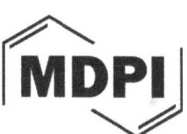

Disclaimer/Publisher's Note: The title and front matter of this reprint are at the discretion of the . The publisher is not responsible for their content or any associated concerns. The statements, opinions and data contained in all individual articles are solely those of the individual Editors and contributors and not of MDPI. MDPI disclaims responsibility for any injury to people or property resulting from any ideas, methods, instructions or products referred to in the content.

www.ingramcontent.com/pod-product-compliance
Lightning Source LLC
LaVergne TN
LVHW070610100526
838202LV00012B/610